Informatik aktuell

Herausgeber: W. Brauer
im Auftrag der Gesellschaft für Informatik (GI)

Ziel der Reihe ist die möglichst schnelle und weite Verbreitung neuer Forschungs- und Entwicklungsergebnisse, zusammenfassender Übersichtsberichte über den Stand eines Gebietes und von Materialien und Texten zur Weiterbildung. In erster Linie werden Tagungsberichte von Fachtagungen der Gesellschaft für Informatik veröffentlicht, die regelmäßig, oft in Zusammenarbeit mit anderen wissenschaftlichen Gesellschaften, von den Fachausschüssen der Gesellschaft für Informatik veranstaltet werden. Die Auswahl der Vorträge erfolgt im allgemeinen durch international zusammengesetzte Programmkomitees.

Thomas M. Deserno · Heinz Handels
Hans-Peter Meinzer · Thomas Tolxdorff
Herausgeber

Bildverarbeitung
für die Medizin 2014

Algorithmen – Systeme – Anwendungen

Proceedings des Workshops
vom 16. bis 18. März 2014 in Aachen

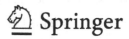

Herausgeber

Thomas Martin Deserno, geb. Lehmann
Uniklinik RWTH Aachen
Institut für Medizinische Informatik
Pauwelsstr. 30, 52074 Aachen

Hans-Peter Meinzer
Deutsches Krebsforschungszentrum
Abteilung für Medizinische
und Biologische Informatik
Im Neuenheimer Feld 280, 69120 Heidelberg

Heinz Handels
Universität zu Lübeck
Institut für Medizinische Informatik
Ratzeburger Allee 160, 23562 Lübeck

Thomas Tolxdorff
Charité – Universitätsmedizin Berlin
Institut für Medizinische Informatik
Hindenburgdamm 30, 12200 Berlin

ISSN 1431-472X
ISBN 978-3-642-54110-0   ISBN 978-3-642-54111-7   (eBook)
DOI 10.1007/978-3-642-54111-7

CR Subject Classification (1998): A.0, H.3, I.4, I.5, J.3, H.3.1, I.2.10, I.3.3, I.3.5, I.3.7, I.3.8, I.6.3

Die Deutsche Nationalbibliothek verzeichnet diese Publikation in der Deutschen Nationalbibliografie; detaillierte bibliografische Daten sind im Internet über http://dnb.d-nb.de abrufbar.

Gedruckt auf säurefreiem und chlorfrei gebleichtem Papier

Springer DE ist Teil der Fachverlagsgruppe Springer Science+Business Media (www.springer.com)

Bildverarbeitung für die Medizin 2014

Veranstalter

IMI	Institut für Medizinische Informatik, Uniklinik RWTH Aachen
i3ac	Interdisciplinary Imaging and Vision Institute Aachen e.V.

Unterstützende Fachgesellschaften

BVMI	Berufsverband Medizinischer Informatiker e.V.
CURAC	Deutsche Gesellschaft für Computer- und Roboterassistierte Chirurgie e.V.
	Fachgruppe Medizinische Informatik der
DGBMT	Deutschen Gesellschaft für Biomedizinische Technik im Verband Deutscher Elektrotechniker (VDE) e.V.
DAGM	Deutsche Arbeitsgemeinschaft für Mustererkennung e.V.
GMDS	Gesellschaft für Medizinische Informatik, Biometrie und Epidemiologie e.V. AG Medizinische Bild- und Signalverarbeitung (AG MBV)
IEEE	Joint Chapter Engineering in Medicine and Biology, German Section
GI	Gesellschaft für Informatik Fachbereich Informatik in den Lebenswissenschaften e.V.

Tagungsvorsitz

Prof. Dr. Thomas M. Deserno
Institut für Medizinische Informatik, Uniklinik RWTH Aachen

Tagungssekretariat

Michaela Huth
Institut für Medizinische Informatik, Uniklinik RWTH Aachen

Postanschrift:	52057 Aachen
Lieferanschrift:	Pauwelsstr. 30, 52074 Aachen
Telefon:	+49 241 80 88790
Telefax:	+49 241 80 3388790
Email:	bvm2014@mi.rwth-aachen.de
Web:	http://bvm-workshop.org

Lokales BVM-Komitee

Prof. Dr. Thomas Deserno, RWTH Aachen, Fakultät 10
Prof. Dr. Torsten Kuhlen, RWTH Aachen, Fakultät 1
Prof. Dr. Dorit Merhof, RWTH Aachen, Fakultät 6
Prof. Dr. Robert Schmitt, RWTH Aachen, Fakultät 4
Prof. Ingrid Scholl, FH Aachen, Fachbereich 5
Prof. Dr. Ulrich Schurr, Forschungszentrum Jülich

Verteilte BVM-Organisation

Prof. Dr. Thomas M. Deserno, Jan Dovermann
Rheinisch-Westfälische Technische Hochschule Aachen (Tagungsband)

Prof. Dr. Heinz Handels, Dr. Jan-Hinrich Wrage
Universität zu Lübeck (Beitragsbegutachtung)

Prof. Dr. Hans-Peter Meinzer, Dr. Alexander Seitel
Deutsches Krebsforschungszentrum Heidelberg (Anmeldung)

Prof. Dr. Thomas Tolxdorff, Dr. Thorsten Schaaf
Charité – Universitätsmedizin Berlin (Internetpräsenz)

Programmkomitee

Prof. Dr. Dr. Johannes Bernarding, Universität Magdeburg
Prof. Dr. Oliver Burgert, Universität Leipzig
Prof. Dr. Thorsten Buzug, Universität zu Lübeck
Prof. Dr. Thomas Deserno, RWTH Aachen
Prof. Dr. Hartmut Dickhaus, Universität Heidelberg
Dr. Jan Ehrhardt, Universität zu Lübeck
Prof. Dr. Heinz Handels, Universität zu Lübeck
Priv.-Doz. Dr. Peter Hastreiter, Universität Erlangen
Dr. Tobias Heimann, Siemens Corporate Technology Erlangen
Prof. Dr. Joachim Hornegger, Universität Erlangen
Prof. Dr. Dr. Klaus Kabino, Uniklinik RWTH Aachen
Prof. Ron Kikinis, MD, Fraunhofer MEVIS Bremen
Prof. Dr. Leif Kobbelt, RWTH Aachen
Prof. Dr. Torsten Kuhlen, RWTH Aachen
Priv.-Doz. Dr. Lena Maier-Hein, DKFZ Heidelberg
Prof. Dr. Dorit Merhof, RWTH Aachen
Prof. Dr. Hans-Peter Meinzer, DKFZ Heidelberg
Prof. Dr. Jan Modersitzki, Fraunhofer MEVIS Lübeck
Prof. Dr. Heinrich Müller, Technische Unversität Dortmund
Prof. Dr. Henning Müller, Université Sierre Schweiz
Prof. Dr. Nassir Navab, Technische Universität München
Prof. Dr. Heinrich Niemann, Universität Erlangen
Prof. Dr. Christoph Palm, OTH Regensburg
Prof. Dr. Regina Pohle-Fröhlich, Hochschule Niederrhein
Prof. Dr. Bernhard Preim, Universität Magdeburg
Priv.-Doz. Dr. Karl Rohr, Universität Heidelberg
Prof. Ingrid Scholl, FH Aachen
Prof. Dr. Robert Schmitt, RWTH Aachen
Prof. Dr. Hauke Schramm, Fachhochschule Kiel
Dr. Hanno Scharr, Forschungszentrum Jülich
Dr. Stefanie Speidel, KIT Karlsruhe
Prof. Dr. Thomas Tolxdorff, Charité-Universitätsmedizin Berlin

Dr. Gudrun Wagenknecht, Forschungszentrum Jülich
Dr. Stefan Wesarg, Fraunhofer IGD Darmstadt
Prof. Dr. Herbert Witte, Universität Jena
Priv.-Doz. Dr. Thomas Wittenberg, Fraunhofer IIS, Erlangen
Dr. Stefan Wörz, Universität Heidelberg
Prof. Dr. Ivo Wolf, HS Mannheim

Sponsoren des Workshops BVM 2014

Die BVM wäre ohne die finanzielle Unterstützung der Industrie in ihrer so erfolgreichen Konzeption nicht durchführbar. Deshalb freuen wir uns sehr über langjährige kontinuierliche Unterstützung mancher Firmen sowie auch über das neue Engagement anderer.

Platin-Sponsor

VISUS Technology Transfer GmbH
Universitätsstraße 136, 44799 Bochum
http://www.visus.com

Sponsoren

Nikon GmbH
Tiefenbroicher Weg 25, 40472 Düsseldorf
http://www.nikon.de

Schneider Digital Josef J. Schneider e.K.
Maxlrainer Straße 10, D-83714 Miesbach
http://www.schneider-digital.com

Siemens AG, Healthcare Sector
Karlheinz Kaske Straße 2, D-91052 Erlangen
http://www.healthcare.siemens.de/

Stiftung von Preisgeldern

CHILI GmbH Digital Radiology
Burgstraße 61, D-69121 Heidelberg, http://www.chili-radiology.com

Springer Science & Business Media Deutschland GmbH
Heidelberger Platz 3, D-14197 Berlin, http://www.springer.com

Preisträger des BVM-Workshops 2013 in Heidelberg

Der mit 1.000 € dotierte BVM-Award wird von der Jury an eine herausragende Diplom-, Bachelor-, Master- oder Doktorarbeit vergeben. Die besten wissenschaftlichen Beiträge werden vom Programmkommittee mit drei Preisen á 300 €, 250 € und 150 € ausgezeichnet. Die Publikumspreise werden unter den Teilnehmern des Workshops abgestimmt und sind mit je 150 € dotiert.

BVM-Award 2013 für eine herausragende Dissertation

René Werner mit *Mirko Marx, Jan Ehrhardt, Heinz-Peter Schlemmer, Heinz Handels* (Institut für Medizinische Informatik, Universität zu Lübeck)
Bewegungsfeldschätzung und Dosisakkumulation anhand von 4D-Bilddaten für die Strahlentherapie atmungsbewegter Tumoren

BVM-Preis 2013 für die beste wissenschaftliche Arbeit

Keno März mit *Alfred Michael Franz, Bram Stieltjes, Alexandra Zahn, Alexander Seitel, Justin Iszatt, Boris Radeleff, Hans-Peter Meinzer, Lena Maier-Hein* (Junior-Gruppe: Computer-assistierte Interventionen, DKFZ Heidelberg)
Navigierte ultraschallgeführte Leberpunktion mit integriertem EM Feldgenerator

Caspar Goch mit *Bram Stieltjes, Romy Henze, Jan Hering, Hans- Peter Meinzer, Klaus H. Fritzsche* (Abteilung Medizinische und Biologische Informatik, DKFZ Heidelberg)
Quantification of Changes in Language-Related Brain Areas in Autism Spectrum Disorders Using Large-Scale Network Analysis

BVM-Preis 2013 für die drittbeste wissenschaftliche Arbeit

Simon Eck mit *Stefan Wörz, Andreas Biesdorf, Katharina Müller-Ott, Karsten Rippe, Karl Rohr* (Dept. of Bioinformatics and Functional Genomics, Biomedical Computer Vision Group, BIOQUANT Center IPMB and DKFZ Heidelberg)
Segmentation of Heterochromatin Foci Using a 3D Spherical Harmonics Intensity Model

BVM-Publikumspreis 2013 für den besten Vortrag

Constantin Heck mit *Lars Ruthotto, Siawoosh Mohammadi, Jan Modersitzki, Nikolaus Weiskopf* (Institute of Mathematics and Image Computing, University of Lübeck)
HySCO: Hyperelastic Susceptibility Artifact Correction of DTI in SPM

BVM-Publikumspreis 2013 für das beste Poster

Alfred Franz mit *Keno März, Alexander Seitel, Michael Müller, Sascha Zelzer, Marco Nodeln, Hans-Peter Meinzer, Lena Maier-Hein* (Junior-Gruppe: Computer-assistierte Interventionen, DKFZ Heidelberg)
MITK-US: Echtzeitverarbeitung von Ultraschallbildern in MITK

Vorwort

Die Analyse und Verarbeitung medizinischer Bilddaten hat sich zu einem festen Baustein moderner Diagnose- und Therapiesysteme entwickelt. In den letzten Jahren haben auch Systeme zur computerbasierten Operationsplanung ihren Weg in die klinische Routine gefunden. Hierbei steht stets das Ziel im Vordergrund, die Behandlung des Patienten sicherer und effizienter zu gestalten, um somit zu dessen bestmöglicher Genesung beizutragen. Neben einer stetigen Verbesserung bestehender Ansätze und der Entwicklung neuer, praxistauglicher Verfahren steht die gründliche Evaluierung als bedeutende Herausforderung im Vordergrund, wobei auch immer die Relevanz im klinischen Alltag kritisch hinterfragt werden muss.

Der Workshop „Bildverarbeitung für die Medizin" bietet in diesen Themenfeldern eine ideale Plattform. Seit nun schon über zwanzig Jahren treffen sich hier Experten aus dem interdisziplinären Umfeld der medizinischen Bildverarbeitung, um neue Ideen zu diskutieren und zukünftige Ziele festzulegen. Auch für junge Nachwuchswissenschaftler stellt der Workshop ein hervorragendes Podium dar, um über ihre Bachelor-, Master-, Promotions- oder Habilitationsprojekte zu berichten.

Der diesjährige Workshop findet zum vierten Mal in Aachen statt und vereint in diesem Jahr insbesondere wissenschaftlich hochaktuelle Themen mit dem klinischen Alltag. Hierfür konnten drei renommierte Gastredner gewonnen werden:

- *Prof. Dr. Horst Hahn*, Fraunhofer-Institut für Bildgestützte Medizin MEVIS, Bremen zeigt in seinem Vortrag „Future Challenges of Medical Image Computing" die herausfordernden Perspektiven der medizinsichen Bildverarbeitung der nächsten Jahre auf.
- *Prof. Dr. Josien Pluim*, Image Sciences Institute, University Medical Center Utrecht, The Netherlands, spricht zum Thema „Image Registration: Evaluation and Error Detection".
- *Dr. Hans Henrik Thodberg*, Visiana ApS, Holte, Denmark, machte sich mit seinem Promotionsthema zur automatischen Knochenaltersbestimmung aus Radiographien selbstständig und wird in seinem Vortrag „Commercialization of Medical Image Analysis" vor allem über den steinigen Weg vom Algorithmus zum erfolgreichen Produkt berichten.

Die Organisation des Workshops wurde wie immer auf Institutionen aus Aachen, Berlin, Heidelberg und Lübeck verteilt. Dies erwies sich ein weiteres Mal als vorteilhaft für die Durchführung der Veranstaltung. Nach Begutachtung aller eingereichten Beiträge durch jeweils drei unabhängige Gutachter – organisiert von den Kollegen aus Lübeck – wurden insgesamt 70 Beiträge angenommen, wobei hiervon 39 als Vorträge, 25 als Poster und 4 als Softwaredemonstrationen auf dem Workshop präsentiert werden. Erstmalig wurden auch 2 Kurzbeiträge von Bachelor-Absolventen zur Präsentation angenommen. Die schriftlichen

Langfassungen aller Beiträge sind von den Aachener Kollegen in diesem Tagungsband zusammengefasst worden und die Proceedings werden wieder vom Springer-Verlag in der bewährten Reihe „Informatik Aktuell" der Gesellschaft für Informatik (GI) elektronisch publiziert. Die Anmeldung zum Workshop wird von den Heidelberger Kollegen abgewickelt. Weitere Informationen zum Workshop sind auf der von den Berliner Kollegen gepflegten Internetpräsenz zu finden:

http://www.bvm-workshop.org

Als zusätzliches Rahmenprogramm werden am Tag vor dem wissenschaftlichen Programm drei Tutorien angeboten:

- *Dr. rer. medic. Dipl.-Inform. Stephan Jonas*, Institut für Medizinische Informatik, Uniklinik RWTH Aachen gibt in dem Tutorium „Das Smartphone als bildgebende Modalität" eine Einführung in die wichtigsten Grundelemente der Bildgebung und -verarbeitung auf dem Smartphone.
- *Dr. rer. nat. Dipl.-Inform. Jakob Valvoda*, Anwaltssozietät Boehmert und Boehmert, München, gibt mit dem Patent-Tutorial „Schutz von Erfindungen in der Informatik und der medizinischen Bildverarbeitung" eine Einführung in den Themenkomplex der Patentierung von Erfindungen und richtet insbesondere den Fokus auf computer-implementierte Erfindungen (Software) im Bereich der medizinischen Bildverarbeitung.
- *Dr. sc. hum. Dipl.-Inform. Med. Marco Nolden, Dr. sc. hum. Mag. rer. nat. Sascha Zelzer, Dipl.-Inform. Med. Andreas Fetzer* und *Dipl.-Inform. Med. Jasmin Metzger*, Medizinische und Biologische Informatik, Deutsches Krebsforschungszentrum (DKFZ), Heidelberg geben im Tutorium „Entwicklung interaktiver Bildverarbeitungssysteme mit MITK und CTK" eine Einführung in die Erstellung interaktiver medizinischer Bildverarbeitungssysteme auf Basis des Medical Imaging Interaction Toolkits (MITK) und der zugrundeliegenden Bibliotheken Insight Toolkit (ITK), Visualization Toolkit (VTK) und Common Toolkit (CTK).

Angrenzend zur BVM findet am 19.3. in Aachen das AG Meeting der GI Fachgruppe „Visual Computing in Biologie und Medizin" statt. Informationen hierzu sind im Internet zu finden (www.fg-medvis.de).

Als wesentliche Neuerung der BVM 2014 wurde erstmals bei der Einreichung die gewünschte Präsentationssprache der Autoren erfasst und bei der inhaltlichen Gruppierung der Vorträge zu Sessions berücksichtigt. Am bewährten Konzept zweier paralleler Vortragssessions festhaltend ist es gelungen, einen vollständig englischsprachigen und einen deutschsprachigen Track gegenüberzustellen. Wir kommen damit der zunehmenden Zahl internationaler Workshopteilnehmer entgegen, die Vorträge und Software-/Posterpräsentationen in englischer Sprache bevorzugen.

An dieser Stelle möchten wir allen, die bei den umfangreichen Vorbereitungen und der Durchführung des Workshops beteiligt waren und sind, unseren herzlichen Dank für ihr Engagement bei der Organisation aussprechen: den Referenten der Gastvorträge, den Autoren der Beiträge, den Referenten der Tutorien, den Industrierepräsentanten, dem Programmkomitee, den Fachgesellschaften, den Mitgliedern des BVM-Organisationsteams und allen Mitarbeitern des Instituts für Medizinische Informatik, Uniklinik RWTH Aachen. Namentlich nennen möchten wir Herrn Tobias Fürtjes, der als Geschäftsführer des Interdisciplinary Imaging & Vision Institute Aachen (i3ac, http://www.i3ac.de) die Industriekontakte aufgebaut und die den Workshop begleitende Industrieausstellung organisiert hat.

Wir wünschen allen Teilnehmerinnen und Teilnehmern des Workshops BVM 2014 lehrreiche Tutorien, viele interessante Vorträge, Gespräche an den Postern, bei den Softwaredemonstrationen und bei der Industrieausstellung sowie spannende neue Kontakte zu Kolleginnen und Kollegen aus dem Bereich der medizinischen Bildverarbeitung.

Januar 2014

Thomas Deserno (Aachen)
Heinz Handels (Lübeck)
Hans-Peter Meinzer (Heidelberg)
Thomas Tolxdorff (Berlin)

Inhaltsverzeichnis

Die fortlaufende Nummer am linken Seitenrand entspricht den Beitragsnummern, wie sie im endgültigen Programm des Workshops zu finden sind. Dabei steht V für Vortrag, P für Poster und S für Softwaredemonstration.

Eingeladene Vorträge

Tutorien

Softwaredemonstrationen

Imaging & Reconstruction
(Oral Session 1, Monday 10:00 am, Lecture Hall 5)

Computerunterstützte Diagnostik
(Vortragssitzung 2, Montag 10:00 Uhr, Hörsaal 6)

Endoscopy
(Oral Session 3, Monday 11:30 am, Lecture Hall 5)

Bilderzeugung
(Vortragssitzung 4, Montag 11:30 Uhr, Hörsaal 6)

Fundus Imaging & Motion Tracking
(Oral Session 5, Monday 1:30 pm, Lecture Hall 5)

3D Segmentierung

(Vortragssitzung 6, Montag 13:30 Uhr, Hörsaal 6)

Medical Informatics

(Poster Session 1, Monday 3:00 pm, Seminar Hall)

Segmentierung & Registrierung
(Posterpräsentationen 2, Montag 15:00 Uhr, Seminarraum)

3D Imaging
(Oral Session 7, Tuesday 9:30 am, Lecture Hall 5)

Bildbasierte Messungen
(Vortragssitzung 8, Dienstag 9:30 Uhr, Hörsaal 6)

Phantoms & Virtual Techniques
(Oral Session 9, Tuesday 10:50 am, Lecture Hall 5)

Simulationstechniken
(Vortragssitzung 10, Dienstag 10:50 Uhr, Hörsaal 6)

Tracking & Navigation
(Poster Session 3, Tuesday 12:00 noon, Seminar Hall)

Medizinische Informatik & Informationstechnik
(Posterpräsentation 4, Dienstag 12:00 Uhr, Seminarraum:)

Segmentation
(Oral Session 11, Tuesday 2:40 pm, Lecture Hall 5)

Mikroskopie
(Vortragssitzung 12, Dienstag 14:40 Uhr, Hörsaal 6)

Kategorisierung der Beiträge

Image Registration
Evaluation and Error Detection

Josien Pluim

Image Sciences Institute, University Medical Center Utrecht, The Netherlands
j.pluim@umcutrecht.nl

Knowing how accurate the results of a registration method are is an important question, yet one that is very hard to answer. This holds especially for deformable registration, for which the quality of alignment can vary across the image volume. The complexity of evaluating image registration is reflected in the imbalance in the list of recent image analysis challenges (www.grand-challenge.org/index.php): the majority is on image segmentation and only the odd one is on image registration.

The presentation will include a brief overview of methods on evaluation of image registration and on error detection. The presentation will further highlight some of the work of the UMC Utrecht in this area, including a method for fast generation of reference standards for evaluation and a method for automatic evaluation of local registration quality in deformable registration. It will then be shown how these approaches and the principle of boosting can be combined to improve registration results.

Commercialization of Medical Image Analysis

Hans Henrik Thodberg

Visiana ApS, Holte, Denmark
thodberg@visiana.com

The motivation for most researchers in medical image analysis is to develop technology that can benefit the patients, but in practice very few methods makes it all the way to widespread clinical use. The talk describes the main obstacles on this road to utility, using concepts from the book Biodesign by Zenios et al. [1].

For illustration is used the BoneXpert product, a CE-marked medical device, www.BoneXpert.com, which is a pure-software image analysis device that automatically determines the bone age of a child from a digital X-ray of the hand. Bone age expresses how far the child has advanced in its maturation (pubertal development), and parents typically request a bone age assessment of their child to predict its adult height. BoneXpert is based on active appearance models which are briefly described and compared to non-rigid registration. The product has been licensed and installed as an integral part of picture archiving and communication systems (PACS) in 30 hospitals across Europe (including six in Germany).

References

1. Zenios S, Makower J, Yock P, et al. Biodesign: The Process of Innovating Medical Technologies. Cambridge University Press; 2010.

Future Challenges of Medical Image Computing

Horst Karl Hahn

Fraunhofer MEVIS, Institute for Medical Image Computing, Bremen, Germany
`horst.hahn@mevis.fraunhofer.de`

The last decade has seen an enormous increase in medical image computing research and development and this trend continues to gain further speed, driven by the vast amount of multimodal medical image data but also by the broad spectrum of computer assisted applications. At the same time, user expectations with respect to diagnostic accuracy, robustness, speed, automation, workflow efficiency, broad availability, as well as ease of use have reached a high level already. It appears that generic solutions will hardly exist and that software development and optimization will continue to be highly application specific. More recently, cloud computing has entered the field of medical imaging, providing means for more flexible workflows including the support of mobile devices and even a medical imaging equivalent of the App Store paradigm. We discuss current and emerging challenges of medical image computing both from a methodological and from a technological perspective.

Das Smartphone als bildgebende Modalität

Stephan Jonas

Institut für Medizinische Informatik, Uniklinik RWTH Aachen
sjonas@mi.rwth-aachen.de

Die rasante Entwicklung und Verbreitung von Smartphones hat weitreichende Implikationen für die medizinische Klinik und Forschung. Dieses Tutorial widmet sich insbesondere der Bildakquisition und -verarbeitung auf Smartphones und Tablets. Hierbei werden die drei verbreiteten Betriebssysteme Android, iOS und Windows Phone 8 mit Vertiefung der Kamera- und Sensorunterstützung betrachtet. Dazu werden verschiedene Beispielapplikationen besprochen, die jeweils unterschiedliche Ansätze der Bildakquisition wie den Image-Picker oder die direkte Anbindung der Kamera durch die API verfolgen. Die Anbindung externer Kameramodule wird ebenso thematisiert wie neue Smart Devices und deren Kapazitäten. Die Bildverarbeitung auf dem Smartphone wird anhand von Beispielanwendungen aus den Bereichen mHealth, eHealth und Ambient Assisted Living demonstriert.

Das Ziel dieses Tutorials ist es, den Teilnehmern wichtige Grundelemente der Bildgebung und -verarbeitung auf dem Smartphone zu vermitteln. Die Entwicklung anhand einfacher Fallbeispiele soll helfen, den Einstieg in die Entwicklung von Smartphone-Applikationen in der medizinischen Bildverarbeitung zu vereinfachen. Das Tutorium richtet sich an Informatiker, Ingenieure und Naturwissenschaftler mit grundlegenden Programmierkenntnissen.

Schutz von Erfindungen in der Informatik und der medizinischen Bildverarbeitung

Jakob Valvoda

Boehmert & Boehmert Anwaltssozietät München
valvoda@boehmert.de

Das Patent-Tutorial gibt eine Einführung in den Themenkomplex der Patentierung von Erfindungen und richtet insbesondere den Fokus auf computerimplementierte Erfindungen (Software) im Bereich der medizinischen Bildverarbeitung. Nach einer Einführung in die grundlegenden Begriffe der Patentierbarkeit und spezielle Anforderungen an die Patentfähigkeit von computer-implementierten Erfindungen wird ein kurzer Exkurs zu weiteren Schutzrechten und insbesondere zu der Open Source-Thematik gegeben. Das Tutorial wird mit konkreten Fallbeispielen abgerundet, wobei mit den Teilnehmern interaktiv Patentansprüche entworfen und analysiert werden sollen.

Das Tutorium richtet sich an alle BVM Teilnehmer jeglicher Disziplin und erfordert keine Vorkenntnisse.

Entwicklung interaktiver Bildverarbeitungssysteme mit MITK und CTK

Marco Nolden, Sascha Zelzer, Andreas Fetzer, Jasmin Metzger

Medizinische und Biologische Informatik Deutsches Krebsforschungszentrum (DKFZ)
Heidelberg
m.nolden@dkfz-heidelberg.de

Das Tutorial gibt eine Einführung in die Erstellung interaktiver medizinischer Bildverarbeitungssysteme auf Basis des Medical Imaging Interaction Toolkits (MITK) und der zugrundeliegenden Bibliotheken Insight Toolkit (ITK), Visualization Toolkit (VTK) und Common Toolkit (CTK). Die vier Bibliotheken beschäftigen sich mit verschiedenen Bereichen der medizinischen Bildverarbeitung und ergänzen sich gegenseitig. ITK ist ein algorithmisches Framework für Segmentierung und Registrierung, VTK bietet mächtige Visualisierungsverfahren und MITK fügt Applikations- und Interaktionskomponenten für die Erstellung klinisch einsetzbarer medizinischer Bildverarbeitungssysteme hinzu. Mittels CTK können auf flexible Weise andere Plattformen und Technologien wie z.B. Matlab angebunden werden. Die Teilnehmer erhalten einen Überblick über die grundlegenden Konzepte, die den Toolkits gemeinsam sind. Anhand der Entwicklung einer Beispielanwendung mit MITK werdenDatenmanagements- und GUI-Komponenten vorgestellt sowie die Nutzung der wichtigsten ITK Komponenten zur Segmentierung und Registrierung und der wichtigsten VTK Komponenten zur Visualisierung gezeigt. Ferner wird die Anbindung weiterer Toolkits und eigener Anwendungen mit den Konzepten und Schnittstellentechnologien des CTK demonstriert. Eine Demonstration der MITK Workbench gibt außerdem einen Überblick über die wichtigsten Funktionen wie DICOM Import, Visualisierung und Segmentierung für anwendungsorientierte Nutzer. Ziel ist die Präsentation aktueller Plattform-Technologien in der medizinischen Bildverarbeitung sowie die Einführung in verschiedene Werkzeuge, um Algorithmen und Verfahren in unterschiedlichen Plattformen zu entwickeln und in klinische Workflows zu integrieren.

Das Tutorium richtet sich an Informatiker, Ingenieure und Naturwissenschaftler mit Kenntnissen in C++ Programmierung.

Automated Assessment of Pleural Thickening
Towards an Early Diagnosis of Pleuramesothelioma

Kraisorn Chaisaowong[1,2], Peter Faltin[1], Thomas Kraus[3]

[1]Institute of Imaging & Computer Vision, RWTH Aachen University
[2]King Mongkut's University of Technology North Bangkok, Thailand
[3]Institute and Out-Patient Clinic of Occupational Medicine, Uniklinik RWTH Aachen
kraisorn.chaisaowong@lfb.rwth-aachen.de

Abstract. Assessment of the growth of pleural thickenings is crucial for an early diagnosis of pleuramesothelioma. The presented automatic system supports the physician in comparing two temporally consecutive CT data-sets to determine this growth. The algorithms perform the determination of the pleural contours. After surface-based smoothing, anisotropic diffusion, a model-oriented probabilistic classification specifies the thickening's tissue. The volume of each detected thickening is determined. While doctors still have the possibility to supervise the detection results, a full automatic registration carries out the matching of the same thickenings in two consecutive datasets to fulfill the change follow-up, where manual control is still possible thereafter. All algorithms were chosen and designed to meet runtime requirements, which allow an application in the daily routine.

1 Introduction

1.1 Objective

Malignant pleuramesothelioma (MPM) is a high-grade malignant tumor of the pleura, of which 70%-90% can be traced back to asbestos exposure [1]. Without any therapy MPM can rapidly lead to death. Thus, an early diagnosis and subsequent therapy are important to extend patients' life expectancy. To detect MPM in its early stage, physicians have to examine and observe significant changes of pleural thickenings out of consecutive CT scans taken at different points in time from those asbestos-exposed workers (Fig. 1). This diagnosis is not only a time-consuming and tedious task, but underlies both inter- as well as intra-reader variability [2]. An integration of a computer-aided diagnosis system may reduce the expenditure of time by providing the physician with a quantitative and repeatable documentation of the thickenings' growth rate [3].

1.2 State of the art

A reported semi-automatic computer-assisted system to estimate the dimension of MPM starts with automatic lung detection in combination with an user estimation of the outer margin of the tumor at a desired measurement site [4].

Fig. 1. Observation of thickening's growth is the key to an early diagnosis of pleuramesothelioma.

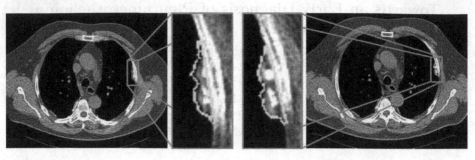

A further development allows the direct visual, but still manual comparison between a baseline and a follow-up study [5]. Another system for automated detection of pleural thickenings differentiates between diffuse pleural thickenings with its smooth appearance and pleural plaques as local and sharply defined bumps [6]. Pleural plaques are initially detected by subtracting the original segmented lung contour from its convex hull. By applying a radial walk, the lung's contour is dilated iteratively pixel by pixel. For every pixel of the dilated contours, various features are extracted. These features encode local information for each thickening and are used for later classification. No follow-up study was carried out with this system.

2   Materials and methods

The implemented system (Fig. 2) consists of the determination of the pleural contours, the detection of the thickening's tissue, and the volumetry of the detected thickenings. A full automatic registration of two consecutive CT data carries out the matching of the same thickenings to fulfill the change follow-up, while doctors still have the possibility to supervise the assessment results.

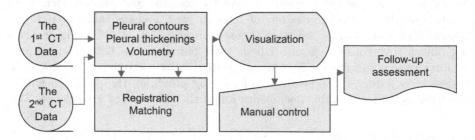

Fig. 2. Schematic workflow of the new implemented automated assessment system for pleural thickenings with consecutive CT data as input and the follow-up assessment report as output.

2.1   Automatic segmentation of pleural contour

1. After an initial segmentation using the 3D histogram by supervised range-constrained Otsu thresholding twice, the 3D histogram of connected pulmonary organs is modeled as a finite mixture of c Gaussian distributions $p(x, \phi)$ to detect and remove trachea and bronchi. Parameters ϕ are estimated using the Expectation-Maximization algorithm with all n voxels: $L(\phi) = \prod_{i=1}^{n} p(x_i, \phi)$. Application of the maximum a posteriori criterion to map all voxels i to discrete labels $L_k = \underset{x_k = \{1,...,c\}}{\mathrm{argmax}}\ p(i | x_k, \phi)$ leads to the classification of that pulmonary region. After removing trachea and bronchi, left and right lungs are separated.

2. A Gibbs-Markov random field describes the prior probability of the Markov random field X that contains the class $x_k \in \{1, \ldots, c\}$ in each CT slice with $P(X) = \frac{1}{Z} \exp\left(-\frac{n_A A + n_B B}{T}\right)$, where Z, T are constant, n_A is the number of horizontal and vertical, and n_B of diagonal inhomogeneous second order cliques. The diagonal potential B is set to $1/\sqrt{2}$, the horizontal and vertical potential A to 1. The maximum a posteriori rule is applied to estimate the optimal final labeling

$$\hat{X} = \underset{x_k = \{1,...,c\}}{\mathrm{argmax}}\ p(X|Y) \propto \underset{x_k = \{1,...,c\}}{\mathrm{argmax}}\ p(Y|X)P(X) \qquad (1)$$

By assuming $p(Y|X)$ takes a Gaussian distribution, the contour relaxation can be done for all pixels lying along the contour of the current lung region according to

$$\frac{\left(N_{0|\hat{x}=0}\ln\hat{\sigma}^2_{0|\hat{x}=0} + N_{1|\hat{x}=0}\ln\hat{\sigma}^1_{0|\hat{x}=0}\right) + n_{A|\hat{x}=0} + \sqrt{2}n_{B|\hat{x}=0}}{\left(N_{0|\hat{x}=1}\ln\hat{\sigma}^2_{0|\hat{x}=1} + N_{1|\hat{x}=1}\ln\hat{\sigma}^1_{0|\hat{x}=1}\right) + n_{A|\hat{x}=1} + \sqrt{2}n_{B|\hat{x}=1}} \overset{\hat{x}_i = 0}{\underset{\hat{x}_i = 1}{\lessgtr}} 1 \qquad (2)$$

where $N_{c|\hat{x}}$ represents the pixel number in either region $c = 1$ for the lung inside, or $c = 0$ for the outside, and $\hat{\sigma}^2_{c|\hat{x}}$ is the estimated variance corresponding to the class of $\hat{x}$, while N is the total number of all pixels.

2.2   Detection and volumetry of pleural thickenings

A topology-oriented and tissue-specific detection algorithm was applied which allows the separation of pleural thickenings from the surrounding thoracic tissue. The 3D detection of pleural thickenings is accomplished by the so-called adaptive surface-based smoothing (ASBS) algorithm [7].

1. Since pleural thickenings can be understood as fine-scale occurrences on the rather large-scale lung surface, the applied algorithm creates a "healthy" volume model of the pleura by smoothing the roughness of the pleural surface by the local adaptation of smoothing degree. Differences between the healthy model and the original data are considered as potential pleural thickenings.

2. For a model-based tissue-specific segmentation, a probabilistic Hounsfield Unit (HU) model for pleural plaques was created. A pre-processing step performs an orientation-based anisotropic diffusion filtering on the region-of-interest around the initially detected thickenings. For the first estimation, a significance test was carried out to initially label each voxel to be either a member of pleural thickenings tissue or of other residual thoracic tissue. The final determination was carried out with the application of posterior probability in combination with Gibbs-Markov random field.

3. In order to determine the volume of a pleural thickening, all voxels of each thickening are counted, its volume can be calculated according to the voxel dimensions.

2.3   Registration and spatiotemporal matching

Several registration techniques were explored regarding their precision and especially their runtime. Comprising the extracted lung mask from sec. 2.1, a Markov-Gibbs random field based approach yields robust results in a short runtime [8]. Due to the following matching process and the typically size and distribution of the findings, registration accuracy does not have a significant influence on the matching. Two features are used to match pleural thickenings of two temporally consecutive CT data-sets, i.e. 3D centroids of the thickenings $c = (x, y, z)^T$ and their mean values over all voxels' Hounsfield units μ. Difference of each feature $\nu \in \{x, y, z, \mu\}$ can be calculated as $\Delta_\nu(i, j) = \nu_j - -\nu_i$, with $i = 1 \ldots I$, $j = 1 \ldots J$, where I is the number of thickenings detected in the first data-set and J the number of thickenings detected in the second temporally successive CT data-set. Every difference component $\Delta_\nu(i, j)$ is separately normalized on its extreme value in order to obtain a finite and unique feature space [9], since the range of z values, representing the number of slices, is different to the range of x and y values representing width and height of the slice image

$$\hat{\Delta}_\nu(i, j) = \frac{\Delta_\nu(i, j) - \min\limits_{\substack{i=1\ldots I \\ j=1\ldots J}} (\Delta_\nu(i, j))}{\max\limits_{\substack{i=1\ldots I \\ j=1\ldots J}} (\Delta_\nu(i, j)) - - \min\limits_{\substack{i=1\ldots I \\ j=1\ldots J}} (\Delta_\nu(i, j))} \in [0, 1] \tag{3}$$

To match two corresponding thickenings, a decision rule $i \mapsto r(i)$ is set up to assign a thickening i to the thickening j by minimizing the cost function

$$r(i) = \operatorname*{argmin}_j \{ \sqrt{ \hat{\Delta}_x^{\,2}(i, j) + \hat{\Delta}_{y(i,j)}^{\,2} + \hat{\Delta}_z^{\,2}(i, j) } + w \, \| \hat{\Delta}_\mu(i, j) \| \} \tag{4}$$

consisting of the normalized Euclidean distance between two centroids c_i, c_j and the weighted absolute value of the normalized HU mean difference $\hat{\Delta}_\mu(i, j)$. Since the HU mean is the feature, which describes the tissue's character of the thickening, and in order to avoid a decision, only based on a topological neighborhood, difference of HU mean value $\hat{\Delta}_\mu(i, j)$ should have more influence on the cost function than the topological feature $\hat{d}(i, j)$. This can be done by assigning a high value to the weight w.

3   Results

In order to realize such a system, different components were implemented, including the handling of DICOM data, the analysis algorithms, and the visualization of the results, based on the software framework MITK [10] (Fig. 3). Physicians' requirements were taken into account during the development. In order to verify the whole automated system, 20 CT data sets have been applied in two steps. For the reliability of the detection of pleural thickenings, three occupational physicians marked and the machine detected, respectively. This primary analysis was carried out on each CT-slice of two CT data sets, containing 397 and 348 slices. All marked results were overlapped to determine the total number of considered areas. Gold standard has been set up as consensus between human and machine results. Altogether, 4537 thickening areas are processed. 30 working hours have been spent on the verification. The evaluation showed that 71.4% of the thickenings found to be correctly detected. The system showed high sensitivity, but low specificity of 35.2% as expected. The sensitivity of the computer-aided detection together with doctors was 89.0% which demonstrated an improvement of the total detection rate in comparison to human reader only of 86.5%. To validate the automatic matching of thickenings from the machine, physicians have evaluated the matching results using further 18 CT data from 9 patients. After the evaluation, the matching revealed to be correct in 95% of all cases, which reflected high sensitivity as well.

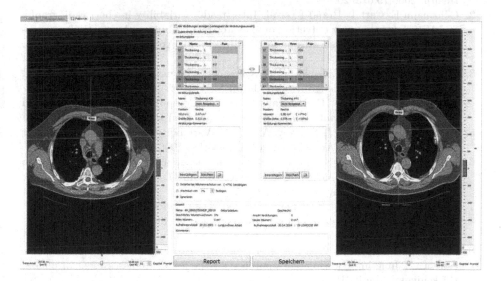

Fig. 3. GUI of the implemented automated assessment system for pleural thickenings displays CT data of the same patient from different point in time. The matching results are displayed in the middle and can be manually supervised. Doctors have the possibility to comment each case individually, while report output as well as documentation are provided.

4   Discussion

With the improvement of the total detection rate in comparison to human reader only, the system demonstrated the ability to increase the reliability of diagnosis. This system, which has never existed elsewhere before, comprises fully automatic algorithms for the detection and assessment. Also the spatiotemporal matching of the detected pleural thickenings from consecutive 3D CT data at different points in time was carried out automatically. A comparison to previous works is difficult since purpose and usage of each system vary. The only similarity among them was the detection of pleural anomalies. All algorithms were implemented to meet runtime requirements (i.e. the processing of all steps for a pair of each 700 slices takes ca. 8 min on an Intel®Core™i7 2600k Quad-Core with 16 GB RAM), therefore promise to reduce physicians' workload, while they still have access to modify the results at every step. However, to improve the specificity of the detection, error due to anatomic condition such as spinal cord indentations might be reduced by enhancement the algorithm with the anatomic information. This will be the future task.

References

1. Hagemeyer O, Otten H, Kraus T. Asbestos consumption, asbestos exposure and asbestos-related occupational diseases in Germany. Int Arch Occup Environ Health. 2006;79:613–20.
2. Ochsmann E, Carl T, Brand P, et al. Inter-reader variability in chest radiography and HRCT for the early detection of asbestos-related lung and pleural abnormalities in a cohort of 636 asbestos-exposed subjects. Int Arch Occup Environ Health. 2010;83:39–46.
3. Lehmann T, Meinzer H, Tolxdorff T. Advances in biomedical image analysis past, present and future challenges. Methods Inf Med. 2004;43(4):308–14.
4. Sensakovic W, Armato III S, Straus C, et al. Computerized segmentation and measurement of malignant pleural mesothelioma. Med Phys. 2011;38(1):238–44.
5. Armato III S, Ogarek J, Starkey A, et al. Variability in mesothelioma tumor response classification. Am J Roentgenol. 2006;186:1000–6.
6. Rudrapatna M, Mai V, Sowmya A, et al. Knowledge-driven automated detection of pleural plaques and thickening in high resolution CT of the lung. Proc Int Conf Inf Process Med Imaging. 2005; p. 270–85.
7. Bürger C, Chaisaowong K, Knepper A, et al. A topology-oriented and tissue-specific approach to detect pleural thickenings from 3D CT data. Proc SPIE. 2009;7259:72593D–1–11.
8. Faltin P, Chaisaowong K, Kraus T, et al. Markov-Gibbs model based registration of CT lung images using subsampling for the follow-up assessment of pleural thickenings. Proc ICIP. 2011;18:2229–32.
9. Ohm JR. Multimedia Communication Technology: Representation, Transmission and Identification of Multimedia Signals. Springer; 2004.
10. Wolf I, Vetter M, Wegner I, et al. The medical imaging interaction toolkit. Med Image Anal. 2005;9:594–604.

Visualization and Navigation Platform for Co-Registered Whole Tissue Slides

Ralf Schönmeyer, Maria Athelogou, Günter Schmidt, Gerd Binnig

Definiens AG, München
rschoenmeyer@definiens.com

Abstract. The routine use of digital pathology by clinicians is just beginning to grow rapidly. This adoption will be accelerated by new software applications that increase pathologists' productivity and quality of work. Increasingly specific stains are available to better diagnose diseases such as cancer. Pathologists are confronted with growing complexity when correlating images from differently stained tissue sections. Here traditional microscopy, which generally allows local viewing of only one image at a time, reaches its limits. Digital pathology can offer tools to facilitate such tasks when assessing complex cases. In this contribution we present a visualization and navigation platform prototype. The basic viewing functions are implemented in a style analogous to Google Maps. The principles of meaningful navigation, however, are based on two sophisticated image analysis types. Firstly, the user interface is designed to intuitively handle panels of automatically co-registered whole-slide images; secondly, heat maps – the result of quantitative image analysis – help the user to quickly navigate to the relevant regions. Under the assumption that the general image analysis challenges can be met robustly, this prototype was used to collect feedback from more than ten pathologists and to analyze how they operated the system. These results are the basis for product development requirements for clinical pathology applications.

1 Introduction

Digital pathology is a lively research topic [1, 2], significantly driven by the increasing availability of whole slide imaging (WSI) from stained tissue slices. In recent years the quality, data handling and costs of WSI – also known as virtual slides – have reached levels competitive with traditional optical microscopy. For routine clinical applications, digital pathology is still in its infancy [3, 4], as institutes are traditionally equipped with high-quality optical microscopes and already have established workflows taught by generations of pathologists. Digital scanners are an additional investment and only make sense when there is a significant need.

One area where digital pathology is already commonly used is remote consulting [5, 6]. Here a computer displays a scanned tissue slide and replaces direct interaction with a microscope, supporting the appraisal of specific cases.

New applications must go beyond these possibilities and add value in a convenient, intuitive and user-friendly way. In contrast to analog microscopy – as we demonstrate in this contribution – digital images can be processed and enriched by automated image analysis, and quantitative measurements can be made.

Histochemistry is continually advancing and pathologists often have to evaluate growing numbers of specific stains – for example when diagnosing or stratifying a type of cancer. They are confronted by increasing complexity when faced with consecutive biopsy slices.

Therefore we developed a prototype of a new visualization platform, which offers extended functionality compared to the standard viewers provided by manufacturers of digital slide scanners. It introduces an easy-to-use interface and some practical tools to approach co-registered virtual slides and related quantitative image analysis data.

2   Materials and methods

An important premise was a Google Maps-style approach for handling and presenting large amounts of image data. The ability to switch from a map to a satellite view has been adapted to allow users to switch from one stain to

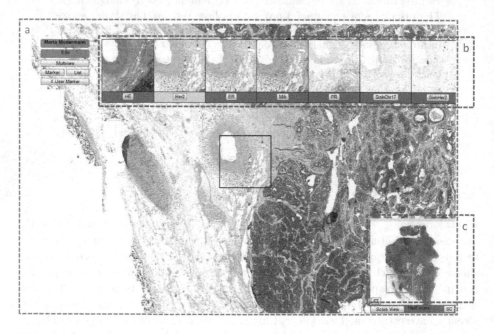

Fig. 1. Screenshot from the graphical user interface of the prototype: (a) main view with full-screen presentation of a virtual tissue slide. (b) Multiview panel with co-registered views of other stains. The box frame in the center of the main view indicates the portion of the image shown for each available stain. (c) Thumbnail overview shows the section on display in the main view (green box frame) and allows for fast navigation.

another, or to an image analysis result. In this sense, an image of a stain corresponds to a satellite image, and an image analysis result corresponds to a map (such as a classification view of nuclei). Consecutive sections of a biopsy, which typically have a thickness of $3\mu m$, enable co-registration, where a location in one section closely relates to a corresponding region in another. Co-registration itself is a widely researched field [7] but for this prototype we decided on an affine transformation provided by three manually selected landmarks on each stain. The Google Maps API, in combination with a JavaScript framework, turned out to be very useful for rapid application development. It is web-based and offers a user experience with fast and smooth transitions of images, which has been proven by millions of users. In addition to its core functionality – the intuitive switching from one stain or classification result view to another, while keeping corresponding regions in the center of the main view (Fig. 1 a) – the user interface was extended with the following views and functions:

- Multiview: views of corresponding regions of multiple serial sections stained with multiple markers, by means of a panel with several (small) viewports (Fig. 1 b).
- Heat map: a visualization of quantitative image analysis results as an overlay (Fig. 2 a).
- Thumbnail overview: provide an overview of a stain or heat map, also displaying the current origin of the contents of the main view (Fig. 1 c).
- Flags: interactively mark points of interest, which are bookmarked in a list for fast retrieval (Fig. 2 b).
   Polygon: interactively mask regions of interest, with live updates of score calculations (Fig. 2 c).
- Smart cursor: provide quantitative data from image analysis to the stain region currently indicated by the mouse cursor.

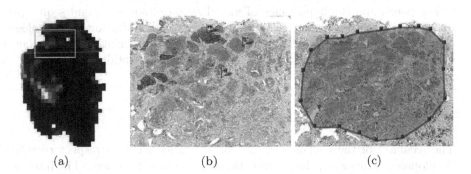

(a)   (b)   (c)

Fig. 2. (a) Heat map representation of a quantitative image analysis result as colored overlay to an overview of the virtual slides. As an example the spatial distribution of the expression of a progesterone receptor staining is shown. (b) Detailed view from a section of this staining where some sample points of interest are marked by flag symbols. Different colors of the flags indicate on which stain they have been set. (c) Detailed view with an example of a polygon annotation of the same region but showing a MIB-1 staining as underlaying.

– Data table: display a sheet with quantitative image analysis data. Columns can be interactively sorted and the locations, where each data row originates from, can be centered directly in the main view.

A high-resolution 40x scan of a tissue slide can typically reach a size of 150 k × 150 k pixels. For the prototype, a sample image set from a breast biopsy – consisting of an H&E stain and IHC stains for Her2, ER, PR, Mib, SishChr17 and SishHer2 – was selected and analyzed with Definiens software [8, 9]. Differently stained regions in each section were classified and a variety of cell types identified. The original images and corresponding images of analysis results were converted to a common coordinate system and stored in a format compatible with the Google Maps API. Again a workflow based on Definiens Developer and Server software was used to transform data. It works on a tile-by-tile basis to process several portions of image data in parallel.

3   Results

At differing stages of development we demonstrated the prototype to 11 pathologists from clinics including the Technical University Munich, the Ludwig Maximilian University Munich and the Charité Berlin. Presentations were conducted informally and experts could operate the prototype themselves on a 17" Windows 7 notebook. As two instructors were present for most sessions, one could concentrate on explaining the system and the other could focus on observing pathologists' reactions and gather feedback. After each session the two instructors noted their impressions independently, then met to form a consensus on the following categories: the usefulness of the graphical user interface (GUI), the importance of co-registered tissue slides, the availability of analysis-based navigation, the importance of analysis result visualization, the usefulness of the Multiview panel, and the importance of visualization of statistics and scores (heat map and data table view). Without beeing given any limitation all pathologists provided positive feedback ranging from moderate appreciation (ok) to enthusiasm (excellent). The diagram in Fig. 3 gives a more detailed overview of the results.

4   Discussion

The feedback of the pathologists has been considered with respect to further developments, including the specifications of potential products. The interviews provided valuable insights into the requirements of applications in the clinical routine.

The presence of a working prototype made a big difference to the quality of the feedback, compared to a feature list and specification outline, in written or oral form. Potential users could experience the prototype hands-on and subtle reactions – such as how comfortable the user felt when operating certain functions – could be observed. This allowed important fine-tuning and improved further development based on real user experience. This seeing-is-believing approach convinced all participating pathologists of the benefits of the system, including those who were previously skeptical about digital pathology in general. Although image analysis visualization had the lowest rating in the evaluation shown in Fig. 3, image analysis is a prerequisite for all software features (including registration and Multiview). We learned that users experienced no benefits when image analysis results were displayed as detailed maps; this feature was subsequently no longer promoted. Pathologists instead favored quantitative data, such as score calculations or heat maps, which guide to regions of interest in a more efficient way. The ability to display classification results, however, may be of increasing interest in the future, when they constitute some kind of artificial stain – in particular when they highlight image properties that are hard to recognize by visual inspection at low magnification. For example, the locations of mitotic cells could be identified by automated image analysis on a small scale and be made visible at low magnification through high contrast or object enlargement.

Further developments will concentrate on fully automated slide co-registration, considered to be the most important feature – in the prototype this was simulated using manually selected landmarks. Automated image analysis combined with quantitative evaluations – such as stain intensity and score calculations – are not available to traditional microscopists and will add further value to digital pathology applications. The prototype gives an example for such an application, which is not only a viewer for whole tissue slides but also a platform for a tissue navigation system. It offers a new user-friendly interface to assess co-registered images and related image analysis results in a uniquely integrated way: additionally to the possibility of a seamless switching from one stain to another stain in the main view – and in contrast to all other known viewers – a pathologist always is able to also overview corresponding locations of many stains simultaneously via the Multiview functionality. Together with other tools and extensions described in this contribution this makes it possible

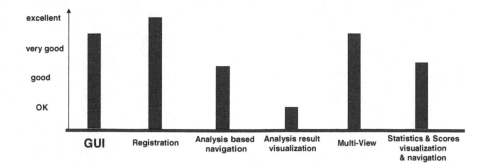

Fig. 3. Summary of feedback with ranked importance or usefulness of presented features: mean values of 11 pathologists.

to better handle the required complexity today's pathologists have to face when investigating slices of differently stained consecutive biopsy slices.

The tissue navigation system helps to translate knowledge from research into clinics faster, providing the pathologist with the latest innovative tissue-based diagnostic applications for optimal therapeutic decisions.

References

1. Al-Janabi S, Huisman A, Van Diest PJ. Digital pathology: current status and future perspectives. Histopathology. 2012;61:1–9.
2. Pantanowitz L, Valenstein PN, Evans AJ, et al. Review of the current state of whole slide imaging in pathology. J Pathol Inform. 2011;2:36.
3. Pantanowitz L. Digital images and the future of digital pathology. J Pathol Inform. 2010;1.
4. Krupinski EA. Optimizing the pathology workstation "cockpit": Challenges and solutions. J Pathol Inform. 2010;1:19.
5. Park S, Parwani AV, Aller RD, et al. The history of pathology informatics: A global perspective. J Pathol Inform. 2013;4:7.
6. Al Habeeb A, Evans A, Ghazarian D. Virtual microscopy using whole-slide imaging as an enabler for teledermatopathology: A paired consultant validation study. J Pathol Inform. 2012;3:2.
7. Wolf JC, Schmidt-Richberg A, Werner R, et al. Optimierung nicht-linearer Registrierung durch automatisch detektierte Landmarken. Proc BVM. 2011; p. 89–93.
8. Schäpe A, et al. Fraktal hierarchische, prozeß- und objektbasierte Bildanalyse. Proc BVM. 2003; p. 206–10.
9. Athelogou M, Schönmeyer R, Schmidt G, et al. Bildanalyse in Medizin und Biologie: Beispiele und Anwendungen. Medizintechnik – Life Science Engineering. 2008; p. 983–1005.

Gestaltung patientenspezifischer Annuloplastieringe

Bastian Graser[1], Sameer Al-Maisary[2], Manuel Grossgasteiger[3],
Sandy Engelhardt[1], Raffaele de Simone[2], Norbert Zimmermann[2],
Matthias Karck[2], Hans-Peter Meinzer[1], Diana Wald[1], Ivo Wolf[4]

[1]Abteilung für Medizinische und Biologische Informatik, Deutsches
Krebsforschungszentrum (DKFZ) Heidelberg
[2]Klinik für Herzchirurgie, Universitätsklinikum Heidelberg
[3]Klinik für Anästhesiologie, Universitätsklinikum Heidelberg
[4]Institut für Medizinische Informatik, Hochschule Mannheim
b.graser@dkfz.de

Kurzfassung. Mitralinsuffizienz ist eine weit verbreitete Krankheit, welche durch die Implantation von Annuloplastieringen behandelt werden kann. Die Wahl eines geeigneten Ringes gestaltet sich aufgrund uneindeutiger Mess- und Selektionskriterien jedoch schwierig. Durch das vorgestellte Verfahren zur patientenspezifischen Gestaltung von Annuloplastieringen wird eine gute Passgenauigkeit gewährleistet. Das individuelle Ringdesign ermöglicht eine geringere maximale Deformation des Mitralannulus über den Herzzyklus gegenüber den untersuchten kommerziellen Ringe, wodurch die Gefahr einer Ringdehinszenz gemindert werden kann. Durch die Herstellung eines entsprechenden implantierfähigen Annuloplastierings mit Hilfe von Rapid-Prototyping Technologien wird zusätzlich gezeigt, dass eine Einbindung in die Klinik zeitlich und preislich vertretbar ist.

1 Einleitung

Mitralinsuffizienz ist eine der häufigsten Herzklappenerkrankungen in Europa [1]. Sie beschreibt eine Undichtigkeit der Mitralklappe in der systolische Herzphase, was einen Blutrückfluss in die Lungen verursacht und die Pumpfunktion des Herzens einschränkt. Zu den Symptomen zählen Erschöpfung, Atemnot und Herzrhythmusstörungen. In schweren Fällen ist ein chirurgischer Eingriff notwendig um die Mitralklappe zu rekonstruieren und ihre Schließfähigkeit wiederherzustellen. Dabei wird im Normalfall eine Annuloplastie durchgeführt. Hierbei wird der die Mitralklappe umschließende Ringmuskel (Mitralannulus) durch die Implantation eines Annuloplastierings stabilisiert.

Die Form und Größe des Annuloplastierings spielt dabei eine wichtige Rolle und sollte entsprechend der individuellen Anatomie und Pathologie gewählt werden [2]. Schlecht angepasste Ringe beeinträchtigen die Qualität und die Altersbeständigkeit der Behandlung [3] und können durch hohe Zugkräfte sogar

zu einer Ablösung des Rings vom Gewebe führen (Ringdehiszenz) mit lebens-
bedrohlichen Folgen [4]. Da oft unterschiedliche Verfahren und Strategien zur
Ringselektion angewandt werden sind die Ergebnisse meist schlecht reproduzierbar, stark geprägt von der persönlichen Erfahrung des Chirurgen und eventuell
nicht optimal an den Patienten angepasst. Manche Experten bezeichnen daher
die gegenwärtige Praxis zur Annuloplastieringselektion als „Voodoo" [5]. Um eine bessere Anpassung an den Patienten zu erlauben, ist es möglich neuartige
Annuloplastieringe mittels Rapid-Prototyping Verfahren zu erstellen [6, 7, 8].
Im Folgenden wird ein Verfahren vorgestellt, das diese Technologie nutzt um
Annuloplastie Ringe patientenspezifisch und nach verständlichen Kriterien herzustellen.

2   Material und Methoden

In der klinischen Routine werden für gewöhnlich 3D transösophageal Echokar-
diogramme (TEE) präoperativ aufgenommen. Basierend auf diesen Bilddaten
wird mit einem bereits publizierten Ansatz [9] ein 4D Modell des Mitralannulus
erstellt. Für jeden aufgenommenen Zeitschritt des Herzzyklus beinhaltet das Modell 16 Punkte, die mit Subdivisionskurven verbunden sind. Die Punktkonstel-
lationen der einzelnen Zeitschritte werden anschließend aufeinander ausgerichtet
mittels einer punktbasierten Registrierung, die lediglich Rotation und Translation zulässt. Die jeweils korrespondierenden Punkte der registrierten Modelle werden daraufhin gemittelt, um ein durchschnittliches 3D Modell des Mitralannulus

Abb. 1. Zwei Konzepte zur Gestaltung   patientenspezifischer
Annuloplastieringe.

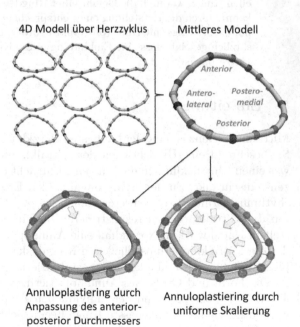

Tabelle 1. Die durchschnittliche und maximale Deformation des Mitralannulus über den gesamten Herzzyklus in Millimeter.

	Durchschnittliche Deformation	Maximale Deformation
Konzept 1	2.68 (± 0.71)	6.84 (± 1.51)
Konzept 2	3.98 (± 0.33)	7.94 (± 1.25)
Edward's Classic	4.97 (± 0.75)	11.81 (± 1.88)
Edward's GeoForm	5.87 (± 0.79)	15.03 (± 2.59)
Edward's IMR Etlogix	4.70 (± 0.78)	11.63 (± 2.14)
Edward's Myxo Etlogix	3.20 (± 0.66)	9.09 (± 2.11)
St. Jude's Rigid Saddle Ring	4.09 (± 0.73)	10.35 (± 2.12)

zu erhalten. Basierend auf diesem Modell werden zwei Konzepte zur Erstellung von Annuloplastie-Ringen vorgestellt (Abb. 1).

Ein Konzept (Konzept 1) beschreibt die Wiederherstellung des natürlichen Verhältnisses des anterior-posterior Durchmessers zum anterolateral-posteromedial Durchmesser von 3:4 [10]. Dazu werden alle Punkte des mittleren Mitralannulusmodells auf der anterior Seite in posteriorer Richtung verschoben und umgekehrt, wobei die anterolaterale und posteromediale Kommissurpunkte statisch bleiben.

Ein zweites Konzept (Konzept 2) beschreibt die isotrope Verkleinerung des Mitralannulus, um dessen pathologisch bedingter Dilatation [2] entgegenzuwirken. Hierfür werden die Abstände aller Punkte des mittleren Modells zum gemeinsamen Mittelpunkt um 20% reduziert.

3 Ergebnisse

Die in [9] vorgestellte Modellierungssoftware wurde verwendet um 4D Modelle des Mitralannulus von 42 Patienten zu erstellen basierend auf klinischen 3D transösophageal Echokardiogrammen. Die Patienten waren zwischen 11 und 78 Jahren alt und wurden mit leichter bis schwerer Mitralinsuffizienz diagnostiziert. Die Aufnahmen wurden im Live-3D Modus des Philips ultrasound system iE33 xMatrix mit einer Philips X7-2t matrix array Sonde erstellt (Philips Healthcare, Andover, MA, USA).

Für jeden Patient wurde nach den beiden vorgestellten Konzepten patientenspezifische Annuloplastieringmodelle gestaltet. Anschließend wurde mit der verwendeten Software [9] die Deformation der Annuloplastieringmodelle auf den jeweiligen Patienten simuliert und verglichen mit der entsprechenden simulierten Deformation von fünf verschiedenen kommerziellen Annulostplastieringformen. Es wurde die durchschnittliche und die maximale Deformation über den gesamten Herzzyklus berechnet und gemittelt für alle Patienten. Die Ergebnisse sind dargestellt in Tabelle 1.

Abb. 2. Mittels Rapid-Prototyping wurde ein patientenspezifischer Annuloplastiering aus bio-kompatiblen Titan hergestellt (links). Zum Vergleich ist rechts ein kommerzieller Annuloplastiering abgebildet (Edwards Lifescience Physio).

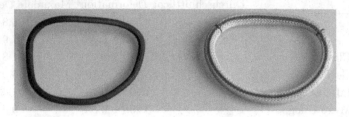

4   Diskussion

Die Ergebnisse in Tab. 1 zeigen, dass beide Gestaltungskonzepte eine geringere maximale Deformation über den Herzzyklus verursachen als die untersuchten kommerziellen Ringformen, wodurch das Risiko einer Ringdehiszenz gemindert werden kann. Auch die durchschnittliche Deformation über den Herzzyklus ist bei beiden Konzepten niedrig. Das Konzept zur Wiederherstellung des natürlichen Durchmesserverhältnisses (Konzept 1) bewirkt dabei etwas geringere durchschnittliche und maximale Deformationen als das Konzept der isotropen Verkleinerung (Konzept 2). Mittels Rapid-Prototyping wurde ein patientenspezifisch gestalteter Annuloplastiering hergestellt aus einer bio-kompatiblen Titanlegierung, wie sie für medizinische Implantate üblich ist (Abb. 2). Die Herstellung dauerte ca. sieben Tage und war mit Kosten von ca. 300 Euro verbunden. Dies zeigt, dass die Produktion patientenspezifischer Annuloplastieringe möglich ist. Durch die Anpassung an die individuelle Anatomie wird eine gute Passform des Annuloplastierings sichergestellt. Basierend auf den vorgestellten Erkenntnissen können weitere Experimente zur Implantation und funktionalen Auswirkung von patientenspezifischen Annuloplastieringen auf die Herzfunktion durchgeführt werden.

Literaturverzeichnis

1. Enriquez-Sarano M, Akins CW, Vahanian A. Mitral regurgitation. Lancet. 2009 Apr;373(9672):1382–94.
2. Carpentier A, Adams DH, Filsoufi F. Carpentier's reconstructive valve surgery. Saunders W.B. Saunders/Elsevier; 2010.
3. Flameng W, Herijgers P, Bogaerts K. Recurrence of mitral valve regurgitation after mitral valve repair in degenerative valve disease. Circulation. 2003;107(12):1609–13.
4. Gillinov AM, Wierup PN, Blackstone EH, et al. Is repair preferable to replacement for ischemic mitral regurgitation? J Thorac Cardiovasc Surg. 2001;122(6):1125–41.
5. Bothe W, Miller DC, Doenst T. Sizing for mitral annuloplasty: where does science stop and voodoo begin? Ann Thorac Surg. 2013;95(4):1475–83.
6. Diaz Lantada A, Valle-Fernandez RD, Morgado PL, et al. Development of personalized annuloplasty rings: combination of CT images and CAD-CAM tools. Ann Biomed Eng. 2010;38:280–90.

7. Suendermann SH, Gessat M, Perrin N, et al. Implantation of personalized, biocompatible mitral annuloplasty rings: feasibility study in an animal model. Interact Cardiovasc Thorac Surg. 2013.

8. Tenenholtz NA, Hammer PE, Fabozzo A, et al. Fast simulation of mitral annuloplasty for surgical planning. Proc FIMH. 2013.

9. Graser B, Seitel M, Al-Maisary S, et al. Computer-assisted analysis of annuloplasty rings. Proc BVM. 2013; p. 75–80.

10. Carpentier AF, Lessana A, Relland JY, et al. The "physio-ring": an advanced concept in mitral valve annuloplasty. Ann Thorac Surg. 1995;60:1177–86.

GPGPU-beschleunigter anisotroper ICP zur Registrierung von Tiefendaten

Eric Heim[1]*, Thomas Kilgus[2]*, Sven Haase[3], Justin Iszatt[1,2],
Alfred M. Franz[2], Alexander Seitel[2], Michael Müller[1], Markus Fangerau[1],
Joachim Hornegger[3], Hans-Peter Meinzer[1], Lena Maier-Hein[2]

[1]Abteilung für Medizinische und Biologische Informatik, DKFZ Heidelberg
[2]Juniorgruppe: Computer-assistierte Interventionen, DKFZ Heidelberg
[3]Lehrstuhl für Mustererkennung, Friedrich-Alexander-Universität Erlangen-Nürnberg
e.heim@dkfz-heidelberg.de

Kurzfassung. Methoden zur Oberflächenregistrierung sind häufig zentraler Bestandteil verschiedener Anwendungen basierend auf Tiefenbildkameras. Der Iterative Closest Point (ICP) Algorithmus wird oft für die rigide Feinregistrierung verwendet, bezieht jedoch a-priori Wissen über die für Tiefenbildkameras typischen anisotropen Messfehler nicht in die Transformationsberechnung mit ein. Eine kürzlich vorgestellte, als anisotroper ICP (A-ICP) bezeichnete Erweiterung des ICP kompensiert diese Probleme, konnte wegen der hohen Laufzeit bislang jedoch nicht für zeitkritische Anwendungen eingesetzt werden. In dieser Arbeit zeigen wir, dass man die Laufzeit des A-ICP mittels General Purpose Computation on Graphics Processing Unit (GPGPU)-Implementierung deutlich verringern kann. Eine in silico Studie auf öffentlich verfügbaren Daten lieferte abhängig von der Oberflächengröße einen Geschwindigkeitsgewinn um den Faktor 22 (1000 Punkte pro Oberfläche) bis 149 (50.000 Punkte pro Oberfläche) im Vergleich zur Central Processing Unit (CPU) Implementierung. Des Weiteren zeigen wir anhand einer Softwaredemonstration auf der BVM 2014, dass die GPU-basierte Variante des A-ICP für die Echtzeitvisualisierung im Kontext der mobilen erweiterten Realität geeignet ist.

1 Einleitung

Oberflächenregistrierung ist in der Regel zentraler Bestandteil von Anwendungen basierend auf Tiefenbildkameras. Dabei ist der Iterative Closest Point (ICP) Algorithmus die meist genutzte Methode zur rigiden Feinregistrierung von 3D Modellen. Gegeben zwei Punktwolken, welche die zu registrierenden Oberflächen repräsentieren, berechnet er iterativ (1) Punktkorrespondenzen zwischen den Eingangsdaten anhand ihrer aktuellen Lage relativ zueinander und (2) eine Transformation zur Registrierung der Punktwolken anhand der aktuellen Korrespondenzen. Hierbei wird jedoch implizit angenommen, dass die Daten mit isotropem Gauss'schem Rauschen behaftet sind. In der Praxis sind statistische Fehler bei der Lokalisierung von Punkten allerdings meist anisotrop [1]. Beispielsweise haben Laser Scanner, sowie Time-of-Flight- und Stereokameras [1] typischerweise eine wesentlich größere Unsicherheit in Blickrichtung der Kamera. In [1] haben wir eine Generalisierung des ICP namens anisotroper ICP (A-ICP) vorgestellt, welche anisotrope Unsicherheiten im Registrierungsprozess berücksichtigt. Der statistische Fehler bei der Lokalisierung eines Punktes wird mit einer Kovarianzmatrix repräsentiert, die vom Nutzer definiert oder direkt aus Daten berechnet werden kann. Obwohl der A-ICP eine signifikante Verbesserung der Genauigkeit für viele Anwendungen zeigte [1], findet er bisher in der Praxis kaum Verwendung, was auf die erhöhte Laufzeit (mehrere Minuten für moderate Punktmengen) im Vergleich zum ICP zurückzuführen ist. Aus diesem Grund stellen wir eine massiv parallele Implementierung des A-ICP auf der Graphics Processing Unit (GPU) vor und zeigen auf öffentlich verfügbaren Daten die Verbesserung der Laufzeit. Des Weiteren zeigen wir in einer Softwaredemonstration auf der BVM 2014 die Anwendung des GPGPU A-ICP auf ein zuvor vorgestelltes Konzept [2] der erweiterten Realität zur intuitiven Visualisierung von medizinischen Daten auf einem mobilen Display.

2 Material und Methoden

In diesem Abschnitt beschreiben wir kurz den Ablauf des A-ICP sowie die Parallelisierung auf der GPU (Abschnitt 2.1), Experimente zur Laufzeitevaluation (Abschnitt 2.2) und die Anwendung des GPGPU A-ICP auf ein Konzept der mobilen erweiterten Realität (Abschnitt 2.3).

2.1 GPGPU-beschleunigter anisotroper ICP-Algorithmus

Der A-ICP ermittelt in einem iterativen Verfahren die Transformation τ zur Registrierung zweier Punktmengen X (Source) und Y (Target), welche den gewichteten Fiducial Registration Error (FRE) FRE_w minimiert. Der detaillierte Ablauf des Algorithmus kann in [1] nachgelesen werden. Die für das Verständnis der Parallelisierung essentiellen Schritte sind im Folgenden aufgeführt:

1. Setze $FRE_\mathrm{w}^0 = \infty$, $k = 0$, $X^0 = X$, $\tau^0 = I$ und erzeuge KD-Baum[1] aus Y.
2. Suche $\forall \ \boldsymbol{x}_\mathrm{i}^k \in X^k$ im KD-Baum eine Korrespondenz $\boldsymbol{z}_\mathrm{i}^k \in Y$ mit dem gewichteten Abstand $d_w(\boldsymbol{x}_\mathrm{i}^k, Y) = min\|W_{\boldsymbol{x}_\mathrm{i}^k \boldsymbol{y}_\mathrm{j}}^k (\boldsymbol{x}_\mathrm{i}^k - \boldsymbol{y}_\mathrm{j})\|$ mit $\boldsymbol{y}_\mathrm{j} \in Y$.
3. Berechne die Transformation τ^k mit dem Verfahren aus [1].
4. Transformiere X^k mit τ^k zu X^{k+1} und propagiere alle Kovarianzmatrizen.
5. Berechne FRE_w^{k+1} und wiederhole Schritt 2.-5. bis $|FRE_\mathrm{w}^k - FRE_\mathrm{w}^{k+1}| < \epsilon$.

In jeder Iteration (Schritt 3) wird anhand der gefundenen Korrespondenzen $(\boldsymbol{x}_\mathrm{i}^k, \boldsymbol{z}_\mathrm{i}^k)$ mit $\boldsymbol{z}_\mathrm{i}^k \in Y$ die Transformation mit der in [1] vorgestellten iterativen Methode berechnet. Z wird eingeführt, um den Umgang mit den Indizes zu vereinfachen. Z enthält dieselbe Anzahl an Punkten wie X und hat die Eigenschaft, dass der Punkt $\boldsymbol{x}_\mathrm{i}$ die Korrespondenz zu $\boldsymbol{z}_\mathrm{i}$ ist. Dann folgt:

---

[1] KD-Baum: GPU Implementierung eines K-dimensionalen Baumes aus [3].

A. Setze $\tilde{X}^0 = X^k$, $n = 0$, $F\tilde{R}E_{\mathrm{w}}^0 = \infty$, $\tilde{\tau}^0 = I$. Bestimme initiale Transformation τ_{isotrop} welche X^k und Z^k nach der Methode von Horn [4] aufeinander registriert. Wende sie auf $\tilde{X}^0$ an und propagiere alle Gewichtsmatrizen.

B. Berechne die Gewichtsmatrix $W^k_{\tilde{x}_i^n z_i^k}$ $\forall$ $(\tilde{x}_i^n, z_i^k)$ durch die Methode aus [1].

C. Berechne die Transformation $\tilde{\tau}^{n+1}$ durch die Methode von Danilchenko und Fitzpatrick [5].

D. Transformiere $\tilde{X}^n$ mit $\tilde{\tau}^{n+1}$ zu $\tilde{X}^{n+1}$

E. Berechne $F\tilde{R}E_{\mathrm{w}}^{n+1}$ und wiederhole Schritt B.-E. bis $|F\tilde{R}E_{\mathrm{w}}^n - F\tilde{R}E_{\mathrm{w}}^{n+1}| < \epsilon$

F. Gebe $\tilde{\tau}^{n+1}$ als Ergebnis zurück, falls $\tilde{\tau}^{n+1}$ einen besseren FRE_{w} liefert als τ_{isotrop} und die Identitätsfunktion.

Abb. 1 zeigt, welche Schritte auf der GPU parallelisiert werden. Der Datenaustausch zwischen GPU und CPU wird minimal gehalten, da er zu den

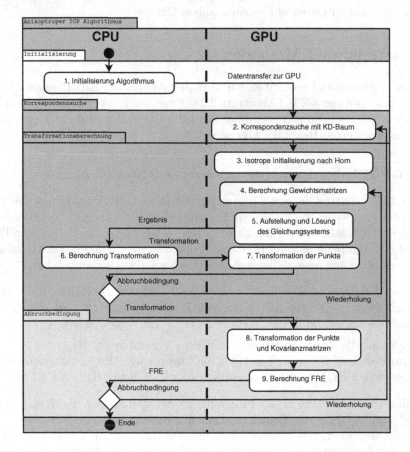

Abb. 1. Schematische Darstellung des GPGPU Anisotropen-ICP. Schritte auf der CPU links; auf der GPU rechts. Der K-dimensionale Baum (KD-Baum) in Schritt 2. basiert auf einer GPU Implementierung aus [3]. Die Berechnung des gewichteten Fiducial Registration Errors (FRE) erfolgt über das bekannte Prinzip der parallelen Reduktion.

zeitintensivsten Operationen im GPGPU-Computing gehört [6]. Lediglich die Berechnung der Transformation und das Überprüfen der Abbruchkriterien erfolgt auf der CPU, weil es sich um wenige, sequentielle Rechnungen handelt. Die Software in diesem Projekt basiert auf dem Medical Imaging Interaction Toolkit[2] (MITK) [7] und dessen open-source Modulen MITK-ToF [8] und MITK-Ocl [9]. Zur GPU Programmierung wurde der OpenCL Standard[3] verwendet, wodurch der Code auf allen gängigen Grafikkarten einsetzbar ist.

2.2 Experimente zur Laufzeit

In dieser Studie wird die Laufzeit des GPGPU-beschleunigten A-ICP mit der Laufzeit der in [1] beschriebenen CPU Variante anhand des öffentlich verfügbaren Stanford Bunny[4] Datensatz verglichen. Alle Experimente wurden durchgeführt wie beschrieben in [1]. Größere Datensätze wurden mittels Catmull-Clark Subdivision generiert. Zur Evaluation der Laufzeit wurde ein Desktop PC mit einer NVIDIA® GTX 580 3GB GPU und Intel® Core i7™ 970 verwendet.

2.3 Anwendung auf mobile erweiterte Realität

Unter Verwendung des GPGPU A-ICP wurde ein Konzept zur mobilen erweiterten Realität, aus einer vorhergehenden Arbeit [2] als Demonstrationsanwendung entwickelt. Um eine hohe Genauigkeit und Bildwiederholfrequenz zu erreichen, führen wir erst den ICP aus und danach reichen wenige (<10) Iterationen des

---

[2] http://www.mitk.org
[3] http://www.khronos.org/opencl/
[4] http://graphics.stanford.edu/data/3Dscanrep/

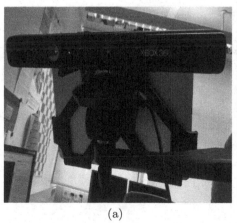
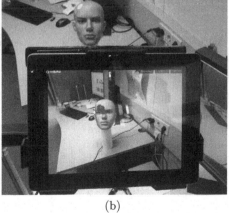

| (a) | (b) |

Abb. 2. Erster Prototyp für die markerlose mobile erweiterten Realität. (a) Apple iPad 4 als Display und Microsoft Kinect als Tiefenbildkamera. (b) Intuitive direkte Visualisierung an einem Puppenkopf mit Tumor (rot).

GPGPU A-ICP aus, um nah an die optimale Lösung zu kommen. Der Hardware-Aufbau besteht aus einer Tiefenbildkamera, die an einem Tablet-PC befestigt wird und einem Server. Die Kamera akquiriert Tiefendaten, welche auf dem Server mittels des GPGPU A-ICP mit medizinischen Daten registriert werden. Das Ergebnis der Registrierung ermöglicht einen Blick ins Innere des Patienten mittels eines mobilen Displays (Abb. 2).

3   Ergebnisse

Tab. 1 zeigt die Laufzeit für die GPGPU-beschleunigte A-ICP Version und den Geschwindigkeitsgewinn ($\frac{T_{CPU}}{T_{GPU}}$) im Vergleich zur CPU Version aus [1]. Es ist bereits bei kleinen Punktmengen (je 1.000) eine Verbesserung um den Faktor 22 zu sehen. Bei je 50.000 Punkten beträgt der Faktor sogar 149. Die Beschleunigung steigt proportional zur Anzahl der Sourcepunkte. Bei einer steigenden Anzahl an Targetpunkten fällt die Beschleunigung geringer aus. Abb. 3 zeigt die Laufzeit im Detail für ausgewählte Daten. Auf der Konferenz erfolgt zusätzlich eine Softwaredemonstration des in Abschnitt 2.3 vorgestellten Konzeptes.

4   Diskussion

Diese Arbeit beschreibt die GPGPU-Implementierung des A-ICP, einer Generalisierung des ICP, die anisotrope Unsicherheiten bei der Registrierung berücksichtigt. Die Ergebnisse zeigen eine Beschleunigung bereits bei relativ kleinen Punktmengen und ermöglichen den Einsatz des A-ICP in zeitkritischen Anwendungen. Außerdem wird der GPGPU A-ICP in einem Konzept zur mobilen erweiterten Realität eingesetzt. In Zukunft muss untersucht werden, ob der GPGPU A-ICP, bei selber Laufzeit mit weniger Punkten, ein besseres Ergebnis erzielen kann als der ICP mit deutlich mehr Punkten.

Abb. 3. Durchschnittliche Laufzeit einer Iteration des CPU bzw. GPGPU Anisotropen-ICP für unterschiedlich große Eingangspunktmengen Source und Target ± Standardabweichung. Zu beachten ist die logarithmische Skala der vertikalen Achse.

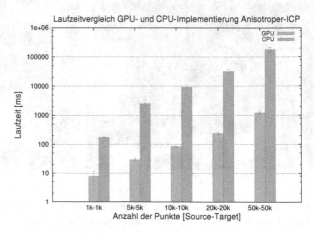

Tabelle 1. Durchschnittliche Laufzeit einer Iteration des GPGPU A-ICP in Millisekunden und (Geschwindigkeitsgewinn: ($\frac{T_{CPU}}{T_{GPU}}$)). Spalten/Zeilen: Anzahl Punkte der Target/Source Oberfläche. Mit x gekennzeichnete Einträge sind wegen Speichergrenzen nicht mehr berechenbar.

# Punkte	1.000	5.000	10.000	20.000	50.000	100.000	500.000
1.000	8(22)	19(23)	30(26)	50(28)	105(30)	200(31)	916(33)
5.000	8(110)	29(88)	48(92)	83(96)	189(95)	359(93)	1.615(99)
10.000	13(135)	47(112)	83(110)	150(110)	354(102)	694(97)	3.178(98)
20.000	19(196)	72(146)	129(142)	235(136)	548(128)	1.074(124)	5.147(119)
50.000	36(269)	148(176)	275(256)	515(155)	1.189(149)	2.378(140)	x
100.000	63(319)	270(197)	509(182)	959(166)	2.239(156)	x	x
500.000	249(451)	145(266)	234(234)	3.930(206)	x	x	x

Danksagung. Die vorliegende Studie wurde im Rahmen des DFG-geförderten Graduiertenkolleg 1126 Intelligente Chirurgie und des PD 15577 durchgeführt.

Literaturverzeichnis

1. Maier-Hein L, Franz AM, dos Santos TR, et al. Convergent iterative closest-point algorithm to accomodate anisotropic and inhomogenous localization error. IEEE Trans Pattern Anal Mach Intell. 2012;34(8):1520–32.
2. Maier-Hein L, Franz AM, Fangerau M, et al. Towards mobile augmented reality for on-patient visualization of medical images. Proc BVM. 2011; p. 389–93.
3. Heim E. GPGPU-Implementierung eines KD-Baums für die Visualisierung medizinischer Daten; 2012. Interdiziplinäres Projekt, Universität Heidelberg.
4. Horn BKP. Closed-form solution of absolute orientation using unit quaternions. J Opt Soc Am A. 1987;4(4):629–42.
5. Danilchenko A, Fitzpatrick JM. General approach to first-order error prediction in rigid point registration. IEEE Trans Med Imaging. 2011;30(3):679–93.
6. Kirk DB, Hwu WmW. Programming Massively Parallel Processors: A Hands-On Approach. 1st ed. San Francisco, CA, USA: Morgan Kaufmann Publishers Inc.; 2010.
7. Nolden M, Zelzer S, Seitel A, et al. The medical imaging interaction toolkit: challenges and advances. Int J Comput Assist Radiol Surg. 2013;8(4):607–20.
8. Seitel A, Yung K, Mersmann S, et al. MITK-ToF: range data within MITK. Int J Comput Assist Radiol Surg. 2012;7(1):87–96.
9. Hering J, Gergel I, Krömker S, et al. MITK-OpenCL: Eine Erweiterung für das Medical Imaging Interaction Toolkit. Proc BVM. 2011; p. 454–8.

Glomerular Filtration Rate Estimation from Dynamic Contrast-Enhanced MRI

Anna K. Trull[1], Benjamin Berkels[2], Jan Modersitzki[1]

[1]Institute of Mathematics and Image Computing, University of Luebeck
[2]AICES Graduate School, RWTH Aachen University
trull@mic.uni-luebeck.de

Abstract. The treatment of chronic renal diseases usually involves the estimation of the glomerular filtration rate (GFR). The GFR can be estimated in vivo without blood samples by pharmacokinetic methods. These models employ non-linear curve fitting techniques to obtain model parameters fitting the model to concentration curves extracted from 4D DCE-MRI data. However, currently proposed optimization strategies rely on the choice of the initial values. In this paper, we propose an improved optimization algorithm based on the analytical elimination of half of the parameters of the Sourbron model. This reduction vastly reduces the runtime of a parameter fit and essentially allows to eliminate the need to adjust the initialization to the input data using multiple fits on a uniform search space. With this approach, we are able to estimate the GFR in three of four clinical cases within 10% of the clinically measured GFR.

1 Introduction

Chronic renal dysfunctions are considered to be one of the most common causes of death in the western world. The glomerular filtration rate (GFR) is a quantitative coefficient in their diagnostics and treatment [1, 2, 3]. The clinical standard for the in vivo GFR measurement is iohexol clearance [4, 2] and requires multiple blood samples. Dynamic contrast-enhanced magnetic resonance imaging (DCE-MRI) is the basis for an alternative method for the GFR estimation without blood samples [5]. Prior to the 4D (3D + time) MRI acquisition, a gadolinium based contrast agent is injected as a bolus. In a data preprocessing step, concentration curves are extracted from the 4D DCE-MRI data and used as input data. The preprocessing step includes a registration of the DCE-MRI data over time and a segmentation of the region of interest in which the curve of the average tracer concentration is estimated. Unlike iohexol clearance, this method is also able to estimate the GFR for each kidney individually by choosing the region of interest accordingly [1]. Pharmacokinetic methods such as the separable compartment model [6] are designed to describe the behavior of the tracer concentration with a small number of parameters. The GFR is proportional to one of these parameters, so it can be estimated by fitting the parameters such that the concentration predicted by the model matches the measured concentration curve as closely as possible. In this paper, we focus on Sourbron's separable compartment model [6]. This model uses four parameters and the corresponding non-linear curve fitting leads to minimization problems with various local minima. The optimization methods proposed in [6] and thus the quality of the solution strongly depend on the initial values used for the minimization. The main contribution of this paper is an improved optimization approach that exploits the structure of the minimization problem and allows to eliminate half of the model parameters analytically, reducing the unknowns from four to two. This makes it feasible to eliminate the need for good initial values.

2   Materials and methods

2.1   Separable compartment model

The separable compartment model proposed by Sourbron [6] models the glomerular filtration and is more accurate than the Patlak model [6, 2]. It consists of two compartments, the plasma and the tubular space. The tracer concentrations therein are denoted by C_P and C_T respectively. The tracer concentration in the abdominal artery, called arterial input function (AIF), is denoted by C_A. A schematic illustration is given in Fig. 1. The plasma flow F_P carries the tracer into the organ and distributes it over the plasma volume V_P. The tubular flow F_T transports part of the tracer to the tubular volume V_T, the remaining tracer is filtered out of the tissue. By the central volume theorem [6] the mean transit time in plasma and tubular space, denoted by T_P and T_T respectively, fulfill the relations $F_P = \frac{V_P}{T_P}$ and $F_T = \frac{V_T}{T_T}$. Using this notation the total tracer concentration, in the organ, at time t can be expressed by the four parameters V_P, T_P, F_T and T_T as follows [6]

$$C[V_P, T_P, F_T, T_T](t) = V_P C_P[T_P](t) + F_T \left(\exp\left(-\frac{\cdot}{T_T}\right) * C_P[T_P] \right)(t) \quad (1)$$

Here, $\cdot$ is a placeholder for the variable of a function, e.g. $\exp(-\frac{\cdot}{T_T})(s) = \exp(-\frac{s}{T_T})$. Furthermore, $(f * g)(t) = \int_0^t f(s)g(t-s)\mathrm{d}s$ is a convolution and $C_P[T_P]$, the concentration of the tracer in the plasma space, is described by

$$C_P[T_P](t) = \frac{1}{T_P} \left(\exp\left(-\frac{\cdot}{T_P}\right) * C_A \right)(t) \quad (2)$$

The parameters are subject to the following physical constraints: $V_P \in [0,1]$, $T_P \in [0,\infty)$, $F_T \in [0,\infty)$ and $T_T \in [0,\infty)$. Once the optimal parameters are

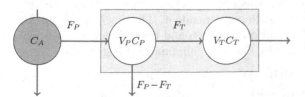

Fig. 1.   Schematic illustration of the separable compartment model.

determined, the GFR can be calculated by multiplying the obtained F_T with a known scaling constant [1].

2.2 Discretization

Since the tracer concentration is only measured for a certain time period, we confine to the interval $[0, T]$. Here, $T > 0$ denotes the measurement time length. Furthermore, we consider the equidistant discretization of $[0, T]$ given by $t_k = \frac{k-1}{K-1} T$ for $k = 1, \ldots, K$. Thereby, we use $T \approx 600\,\mathrm{s}$ and $K \approx 50$, where the exact choice depends on the input data. For the sake of simplicity, the input data that is given on a non-equidistant timeline is resampled on the chosen equidistant grid. For two discrete functions F, G on the equidistant grid, the convolution $*$ is discretized via $(F * G)(t_k) \approx \sum_{i=1}^{k} F(t_i) G(t_k - t_i)$. The measured AIF is denoted by the vector $\mathbf{C_A} := C_A(\mathbf{t}) := (C_A(t_1), \ldots, C_A(t_k)) \in \mathbb{R}^K$. Analogously, we define $\mathbf{C}[V_P, T_P, F_T, T_T]$ and $\mathbf{C_P}[T_P]$. Given the measured amount of contrast agent in the kidney $\mathbf{C_K} \in \mathbb{R}^K$ at the discrete time points, we need to find parameters minimizing the residual error $\|\mathbf{C}[V_P, T_P, F_T, T_T] - \mathbf{C_K}\|_2^2$. Using the Euclidean norm of the residual is a crucial ingredient for the parameter elimination:

2.3 Parameter elimination

The key observation to overcome most limitations of the optimization algorithm proposed for this problem so far is that the Sourbron model is linear in V_P and F_T. Thus, the residual error is quadratic in V_P and F_T, and the two minimizing parameters can be expressed analytically as a function of the remaining two parameters. The corresponding minimization problem is

$$\min_{V_P, F_T} \frac{1}{2} \|V_P \mathbf{a} + F_T \mathbf{b} - \mathbf{c}\|_2^2 \tag{3}$$

where $\mathbf{a}, \mathbf{b}, \mathbf{c} \in \mathbb{R}^K$ are given by $\mathbf{a} = \frac{1}{T_P} \exp(-\frac{\mathbf{t}}{T_P}) * \mathbf{C_A}$, $\mathbf{b} = \exp(-\frac{\mathbf{t}}{T_T}) * \mathbf{a}$ and $\mathbf{c} = \mathbf{C_K}$. Note that this problem is underdetermined in case $\mathbf{a}$ and $\mathbf{b}$ are linearly dependent. In this case, one can choose either V_P or F_T freely. Since V_P has more physical constraints than F_T, i.e. $V_P \in [0, 1]$ versus $F_T \in [0, \infty)$, we choose to prescribe V_P in the linear dependent case. This is done by adding the regularization term $\frac{\epsilon}{2} V_P^2$ resulting in the regularized minimization problem

$$\min_{V_P, F_T} \frac{1}{2} \|V_P \mathbf{a} + F_T \mathbf{b} - \mathbf{c}\|_2^2 + \frac{\epsilon}{2} V_P^2 \tag{4}$$

Here, $\epsilon > 0$ controls the strength of the regularization. In the linear dependent case, this leads to $V_P = 0$. Moreover, this regularization helps to avoid numerical problems arising if $\mathbf{a}$ and $\mathbf{b}$ are almost linear dependent. The downside is that the regularization slightly alters the solution in case $\mathbf{a}$ and $\mathbf{b}$ are linear independent.

The explicit solution (obtained by Gaussian elimination) is given by

$$\tilde{F}_T = \frac{(\|\mathbf{a}\|_2^2 + \epsilon)(\mathbf{c}^T \mathbf{b}) - (\mathbf{c}^T \mathbf{a})(\mathbf{b}^T \mathbf{a})}{\|\mathbf{b}\|_2^2(\|\mathbf{a}\|_2^2 + \epsilon) - (\mathbf{b}^T \mathbf{a})(\mathbf{b}^T \mathbf{a})} \quad \text{and} \quad \tilde{V}_P = \frac{\mathbf{c}^T \mathbf{a}}{\|\mathbf{a}\|_2^2 + \epsilon} - \frac{\mathbf{b}^T \mathbf{a}}{\|\mathbf{a}\|_2^2 + \epsilon} \tilde{F}_T \tag{5}$$

This explicit solution does not take into account the constraints $V_P \in [0,1]$ and $F_T \in [0,\infty)$. To this end, we introduce the restriction function $v_\delta : \mathbb{R} \to [0,\infty)$, where $x \mapsto 0$, if $x < -\delta$ and $x \mapsto x$ if $x > \delta$. Otherwise, x is mapped to $\frac{1}{4\delta}(x+\delta)^2$. Thereby, $\delta > 0$ denotes a regularization weight. We replace the explicit solution $\tilde{F}_T$ and $\tilde{V}_P$ by $F_T[T_P, T_T] := v_\delta(\tilde{F}_T)$ and $V_P[T_P, T_T] := 1 - v_\delta(1 - v_\delta(\tilde{V}_P))$ respectively. We have used the same regularization weights, i.e. $\epsilon = 10^{-4}$ and $\delta = 10^{-3}$, for all experiments. Due to the parameter reduction, the original problem simplifies to

$$\min_{T_P, T_T \geq 0} \| \mathbf{C}[V_P[T_P, T_T], T_P, F_T[T_P, T_T], T_T] - \mathbf{C_K} \|_2^2 \qquad (6)$$

Since v_δ is continuously differentiable, V_P and F_T are differentiable with respect to T_P and T_T. Thus, gradient based optimization methods can be used to solve this problem. In particular, we use MATLAB's Trust-Region algorithm [7] to solve the remaining constrained two parameter problem.

2.4   Clinical data

The 4D data was acquired with a 1.5 T Siemens Avanto MRI scanner at the University of Bergen using a TWIST-sequence (repetition time = 2.51 sec, echo time = 0.89 sec and flip angle = 15 deg). It has an isotropic voxel-resolution of $1.8 \times 1.8 \times 1.8$ mm, an acquisition matrix of 256×192 pixels and 52 transaxial slices at 49 non-equidistant time points. As contrast agent 4 ml multihance by Bracco were injected with a speed of 3 $\frac{ml}{sec}$. The data was motion corrected using a non-parametric registration with normalized gradients on a multi-level scheme and fixed point iterations [1]. Binary masks for the left and right kidney were determined using cropping and an automatic segmentation of the MRI data for a selected time point with the Mahalanobis distance to a training set of kidneys. Due to the difficulties of a reliable cortex segmentation, the whole kidney volume, i.e. cortex and medulla, was segmented [1]. Moreover, the original MRI intensities were converted to the gadolinium concentration. This concentration was then averaged separately over each kidney and each time point, resulting in an estimate of $\mathbf{C_K}$ for the each kidney at every time point. Finally, $\mathbf{C_A}$ was estimated analogously using a manual segmentation of the aorta. In total, we use four datasets of this type, denoted by D_1 to D_4, each with data for the left and the right kidney, for the evaluation.

3   Results

Fig. 2 depicts the curve obtained by the proposed parameter elimination based model for each dataset for the left kidney. Tab. 1 summarizes all results including the estimated GFR values and shows individual parameters for each kidney. The reduction of the unknowns reduces the runtime of a curve fit for a given set of initial parameters using MATLAB's Trust-Region algorithm approximately by a factor of two. The main advantage of the elimination lies in the enormous size reduction of the search space though. Instead of a four dimensional space, we only have to search a two dimensional one. Both, the original and the reduced minimization problem, suffer from non-convexity. Thus, the quality of the minimization results highly depends on the choice of the initial values. At worst, an improper initialization may lead to a local minimum indicating that the corresponding kidney is healthy although it has a renal dysfunction or vice versa. The reduction allows us to fit the parameters on a uniform set of initial values covering all physically meaningful ones. The best fit then is the one with the smallest residual error. This eliminates the need for a patient dependent initialization, which is a significant drawback of existing algorithms. Due to the larger dimension, this approach is computationally infeasible in the original four dimensional search space.

4   Discussion

We have proposed a novel optimization method to estimate the GFR from the separable compartment model. The key ingredient is the analytical elimination of two parameters. The proposed method provides a good curve fit (Fig. 2) without data dependent initialization and the estimated GFR is within 10% of the clinically measured GFR in three of the four evaluated clinical cases (Tab. 1). The overestimation of the GFR in D_2 is caused by the data that is highly affected by the partial volume effect. In comparison, the fit with the algorithm proposed in [6, 1] using the initial values given in the literature may lead to a substantial overestimation or an underestimation of the GFR for every dataset. As next step, we plan to validate the proposed method on a significantly larger amount of test cases. An angle to potentially improve the quality of the GFR estimation is the choice of the AIF. For instance, it could be chosen by Parker's method [8] or included as unknown in the optimization. With both of these approaches a manual segmentation of the aorta would be unnecessary, but the latter would require an adjustment of the model in order to avoid underdetermined optimization problems.

Fig. 2. Input concentration C_K (blue) and the curve obtained by our parameter elimination based model (green) for the left kidney on all datasets. From left to right, upper row: D_1 and D_2; lower row: D_3 and D_4.

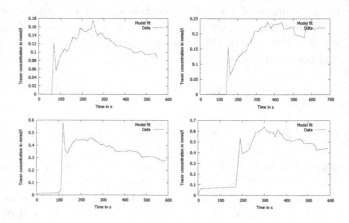

Table 1. Calculated GFR obtained by our proposed parameter elimination algorithm compared to the Iohexol clearance (IC) results. The computed parameters, the residual error and the GFR are listed for the left (upper row part) and right (lower row part) kidney for every dataset. The estimated GFR summed over both kidneys, the GFR of the IC test, and the deviation of the estimated GFR and the IC test are shown.

Data	V_P	T_P	F_T	T_T	Resid.	GFR	GFR $\sum$	IC GFR	Dev.
D_1	0	108.0830	0.0026	0.0031	0.0120	51	102	97	5%
	0.0503	152.8191	0.0025	0.0065	0.0189	51			
D_2	0.2927	135.2560	0.0036	0.0021	0.0204	62	193	127	52%
	0.3295	419.7976	0.0074	0.0015	0.0032	131			
D_3	0.5999	8.7426	0.0064	0.0074	0.0035	56	116	106	10%
	0.5320	8.1435	0.0048	0.0071	0.0402	60			
D_4	0.8165	99.3000	0.0004	0.0001	0.0501	11	98	101	3%
	1	68.6266	0.0041	0.0022	0.0031	87			

Acknowledgement. We thank the MR kidney function research group and Jarle Rørvik (MD, PhD) et al. from the Department of Radiology, Haukeland University Hospital, Bergen, Norway for providing this interesting data. In addition, we thank Antonella Zanna Munthe-Kaas (PhD) and Erlend Hodneland (PhD) form the Department for Mathematics and Biomedicine, University of Bergen, Norway for the interesting discussions.

References

1. Hodneland E, et al. In vivo estimation of glomerular filtration in the kidney using DCE-MRI. Proc Int Symp Image Signal Process Anal. 2011; p. 755–61.
2. Annet ML, et al. Glomerular filtration rate: assessment with dynamic contrast-enhanced MRI and cortical-compartment model in the rabbit kidney. J Magn Reson Imaging. 2004; p. 843–9.
3. Huang A, et al. MR imaging of renal function. Radiol Clin North Am. 2003;41:1001–17.
4. Bauer L, et al. Clinical appraisal of creatinine clearance as a measurement of glomerular filtration rate. Am J Kidney Dis. 1982;2:337–46.
5. Myers GL, et al. Recommendations for improving serum creatinine measurment: a report from the laboratory working group of the national kidney disease education program. Clin Chem. 2006; p. 5–18.
6. Sourbron PSP, et al. MRI-measurment of perfusion and glomerular filtration in the human kidney with a separable compartment model. Invest Radiol. 2008;43(1):40–8.
7. MATLAB. Version 7.10.0 (R2010a). Natick, MA: The MathWorks Inc.; 2010.
8. Parker GJ, et al. Automated arterial input function extraction for T1-weighted DCE-MRI. Proc Int Soc Magn Reson Med Sci Meet Exhib. 2003;1.

Reduction of Blind-Spot and Stripe Artifacts in 3D Digital Tomosynthesis

Yulia M. Levakhina, Thorsten M. Buzug

[1]Institute of Medical Engineering, University of Luebeck
levakhina@imt.uni-luebeck.de

Abstract. The limited-angle acquisition geometry of digital tomosynthesis (DT) provides incomplete projection datasets which leads inevitably to artifacts in reconstructed images. This work presents both an algorithmic and a hardware approach to reduce these artifacts and to improve the image quality. The algorithmic approach introduces a nonlinear weighted backprojector in the simultaneous algebraic reconstruction technique (ωSART). The hardware approach is based on an alternative dual-axis outside-the-arc geometry, where the acquisition is done by covering a spherical cap instead of an arc. The performance and artifact-reduction ability of the proposed app-roaches are evaluated based on real and simulated data using a three-dimensional reconstruction framework. It is shown that the weighting prevents the formation of stripe artifacts produced by high-density tissues while it preserves the true structures, which belong to the object. While reducing artifacts, this approach is unable to reduce the triangle-like shape distortion in the "blind"-spots. In turn, the outside-the-arc geometry reduces the degree of data incompleteness and the size of the "blind"-spots by capturing more singularities of the object. This reduces artifacts, particularly the shape distortion and results in images with better axial resolution. In practice, such geometry can be implemented without major mechanical modifications of existing tomosynthesis devices e.g. by using an object-tilting platform.

1 Introduction

Digital tomosynthesis (DT) is a limited angle three-dimensional tomographic technique. Nowadays it is being under intensive research and development as an attractive low dose high resolution alternative to CT in medical and industrial applications [1]. Fig. 1(a) shows schematically a DT geometry with an X-ray tube moving along an arc trajectory. Limited number of projections acquired over a limited angular range represents an incomplete dataset. Because of the data incompleteness, an accurate image reconstruction without artifacts turns into a challenging task [2, 3].

Typical DT artifacts appear as stripes and triangle-like shape distortions in z-slices. Stripe artifacts are produced along the rays which connect the object boundaries and the X-ray tube. They are especially pronounced when the number of projections is insufficient to provide adequate averaging during the backprojection process. These artifact in planar xy-slices might also be referred to as ripple or out-of-focus artifacts. The triangle-like shape distortion artifacts appear in a so-called "blind"-spots and hide the true appearance of the object. Information on the object shape in such a "blind"-spot cannot be stably recovered [4], because no projections tangential to object boundaries located in this area can be measured due to the limited arc. The size and orientation of the tomosynthesis arc defines the size and the orientation of the "blind"-spot, see the left and right circles in Fig. 1(b) and Fig. 1(c). In this example, a circle represents an object with singularities in all possible directions.

This work addresses the problem of the reduction of the DT artifacts and represents the summary of a PhD dissertation. Two approaches are discussed and summarized: an algorithmic approach based on the non-linear reconstruction [5] and a hardware approach based on the dual-axis outside-the-arc geometry [6].

2 Materials and methods

2.1 Non-linear backprojector ωBP and ωSART

In the n-th iteration of the simultaneous algebraic reconstruction technique SART [7] a forward projection **FP** of the estimated volume $\text{reco}^{(n)}$ is calculated and compared with the measured data proj. This results in an updating term, which is then backprojected into the volume using a backprojector **BP**

$$\text{reco}^{(n+1)} = \text{reco}^{(n)} - \mathbf{BP}\left[\text{proj} - \mathbf{FP}\left[\text{reco}^{(n)}\right]\right], \text{ for one view} \qquad (1)$$

If the object contains high-attenuation features such as bone and metal, the measured projection values along rays through these features will be relatively

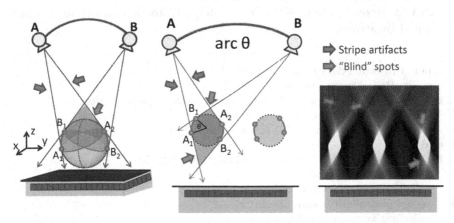

(a) DT acquisition in 3D   (b) DT acquisition in 2D   (c) reconstruction, z-cut

Fig. 1. Origin of the tomosynthesis artifacts is in the incomplete dataset. Stripe artifacts are produced along the rays. The shape distortion artifacts appears in the "blind"spots.

large. An updating term, calculated based on such values and homogeneously backprojected along the ray will produce stripes outside the high-attenuation feature. The proposed weighted backprojector ω**BP** uses a BP-space representation and a dissimilarity principle [5] to adaptively control the contribution of each updating term value into each voxel in the volume, Fig. 2 (Algorithm 1). If the value is too large, its contribution is reduced by the weighting $\omega \in (0, 1]$.

2.2 Outside-the-arc acquisition geometry

The set of directions of singularities to be stably reconstructed in the standard tomosynthesis geometry is limited by the size of the arc. The amount of stably reconstructed singularities of the object can be improved by acquiring more data of the object from different angular views [4]. To fulfill this requirement, additional projections must be acquired outside the original arc. Thus, the size of "blind"-spots can be reduced, Fig. 5(g), allowing more singularities to be reconstructed. In practice, such geometry can be implemented using a tiltable platform, which tilts the object in the direction perpendicular to the original arc, while the X-ray tube still moves over the original arc. This is geometrically equivalent to the acquisition which covers a spherical cup with the total number of projections $N_{proj} = N_{projx} * N_{projy}$.

3 Results

Fig. 3 demonstrates the dissimilarity and the weighting principle on real data of a hand: (a)-(d) show the xy-slice at $24\,$mm where the metacarpal bones marked by an ellipse) belong to the slice; (e)-(h) show the xy-slice at $35\,$mm where the thumb and the little finger belong to the slice. Fig. 4 shows a z-cut of SART and ωSART reconstruction of the hand, shape distortion and stripe artifacts highlighted by arrows.

1: Input: Projection data $p_\theta(u, v)$, $\theta \in \Theta$
2: Output: Reconstructed volume $V(x, y, z)$
3: **for all** $\theta \in \Theta$ {//construct BP-volume using a stack operator} **do**
4:     select $p_\theta(u, v)$ and use a stack operator
5:     add contribution into the BP-volume $h(x, y, z, \theta)$
6: **end for**
7: **for all** $(x, y, z) \in V$ {//introduce weighting into BP} **do**
8:     construct θ-vector $h_\theta(x, y, z)$
9:     calculate reference value $M_\theta(x, y, z)$
10:     assign dissimilarity degree $d_\theta(x, y, z)$
11:     calculate weighting coefficients $\omega_\theta(x, y, z)$
12:     $V(x, y, z) = V(x, y, z) + \omega_\theta(x, y, z) \cdot \mathbf{BP}(p_\theta(u, v))$
13: **end for**

Fig. 2. Algorithm: Weighted ω**BP**.

Fig. 3. Demonstration of dissimilarity and weighting images. (a)-(d) show the slice at 24 mm; (e)-(h) show the slice at 35 mm. It can be seen that the out-of-focus contributions from bones are reduced through the weighting, while in-focus bones are preserved.

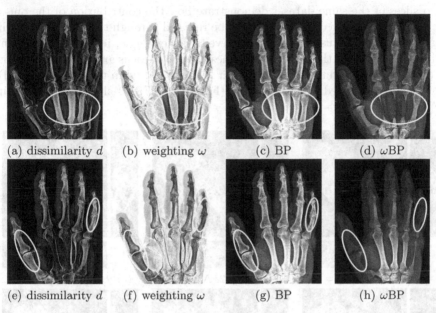

(a) dissimilarity d (b) weighting ω (c) BP   (d) ωBP

(e) dissimilarity d (f) weighting ω (g) BP   (h) ωBP

Fig. 5 represents the impact of acquisition parameters and the geometry on the obtained image quality of a simulated fingerbone dataset: (a)-(c) show reconstructed images for increasing the angular range in the single arc acquisition; (d)-(f) show reconstructed images for increasing the number of projections in the single arc acquisition; (g)-(i) show reconstructed images for the dual-axis outside the arc acquisition. In the images three orthogonal views are shown and regions of interest are highlighted by ellipses.

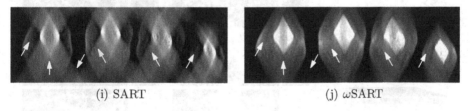

(i) SART   (j) ωSART

Fig. 4. Reconstruction of a hand, z-cut. White arrows point to artifacts. (a) artifacts are visible, (b) stripe artifacts are reduced, triangle-like distortion is still present.

4 Discussion

4.1 Stripe artifact reduction: ωSART

Two slices of the same dataset demonstrate how the contribution of the out-of-focus features (marked by ellipses) can be reduced through the proposed weighting, while the in-focus bones are preserved. For example, in the slice at 24 mm (Fig. 3(a)-Fig. 3(d)) the metacarpal bones are out-of-focus and their contribution in the resulting weighted backprojection ωBP is reduced in this slice (Fig. 3(d)), while being preserved in another slice (Fig. 3(h)). Fig. 4 shows that the stripe

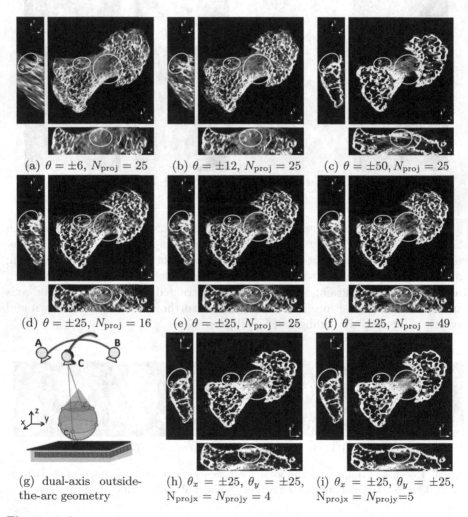

(a) $\theta = \pm 6$, $N_{proj} = 25$ (b) $\theta = \pm 12$, $N_{proj} = 25$ (c) $\theta = \pm 50$, $N_{proj} = 25$

(d) $\theta = \pm 25$, $N_{proj} = 16$ (e) $\theta = \pm 25$, $N_{proj} = 25$ (f) $\theta = \pm 25$, $N_{proj} = 49$

(g) dual-axis outside-the-arc geometry   (h) $\theta_x = \pm 25$, $\theta_y = \pm 25$, $N_{projx} = N_{projy} = 4$ (i) $\theta_x = \pm 25$, $\theta_y = \pm 25$, $N_{projx} = N_{projy} = 5$

Fig. 5. Influence of acquisition geometry on image quality. (a)-(c) increasing the angular range; (d)-(f) increasing the number of projections; (g)-(i) dual-axis outside the arc acquisition.

artifacts are reduced, when weighting is included into the SART reconstruction. At the same time, the triangle-like shape distortion of bones cannot be reduced by the weighting.

4.2   Shape distortion reduction: outside-the-arc

Simulated results show that an increasing the arc size θ (Fig. 5(a)-Fig. 5(c)) or the sampling density N_{proj} (Fig. 5(d)-Fig. 5(f)) reduces the size of "blind"-areas, recovering by this more singularities, see object boundaries in the regions of interest. This effect is especially visible in z-slices. However, an increase in those parameters above a certain threshold is not feasible due to the technical limitations or a patient dose issues. Acquiring projections outside the arc results in images with more boundaries recovered without a need to increase θ and N_{proj}, compare Fig. 5(e) and Fig. 5(i), both images are acquired using the same size of the original arc $\theta = \pm 25^o$ and the number of projections $N_{proj} = 25$. Moreover, the outside-the-arc acquisition allows for obtaining images with improved image quality even while using less projections, compare Fig. 5(e) (single arc, $N_{proj} = 25$) and Fig. 5(h) (outside the arc, $N_{proj} = 16$).

A practical validation of the simulation results can be easily performed using a tiltable platform, which can be attached to any existing tomosynthesis device without major mechanical modifications of the device. Potentially, the algorithmic and the geometry approaches should be considered together to combine the improvements introduced by each of them.

References

1. Dobbins J. Tomosynthesis imaging: at a translational crossroads. Med Phys. 2009;36(6):1956–67.
2. Sechopoulos I. A review of breast tomosynthesis. Part I. The image acquisition process. Med Phys. 2013;40(1).
3. Sechopoulos I. A review of breast tomosynthesis. Part II. Image reconstruction, processing and analysis, and advanced applications. Med Phys. 2013;40(1).
4. Quinto E. An introduction to X-ray tomography and radon transforms. Procs SAPM. 2006;63:1–23.
5. Levakhina YM et al. Weighted simultaneous algebraic reconstruction technique for tomosynthesis imaging of objects with high-attenuation features. Med Phys. 2013;40.
6. Levakhina YM et al. A hybrid dual-axis tilt acquisition geometry for digital musculoskeletal tomosynthesis. Phys Med Biol. 2013;58:4827–48.
7. Andersen A, Kak A. Simultaneous algebraic reconstruction technique (SART): a superior implementation of the ART algorithm. Ultrason Imag. 1984;6(1):81–94.

Evaluation of Spectrum Mismatching Using Spectrum Binning for Statistical Polychromatic Reconstruction in CT

Qiao Yang[1,2], Meng Wu[2], Andreas Maier[1,3], Joachim Hornegger[1,3],
Rebecca Fahrig[2]

[1]Pattern Recognition Lab, FAU Erlangen-Nürmberg
[2]Department of Radiology, Stanford University, Stanford, CA, USA
[3]Erlangen Graduate School in Advanced Optical Technologies (SAOT), Erlangen
qiao.yang@cs.fau.de

Abstract. In CT, the nonlinear attenuation characteristics of polychromatic X-rays cause beam hardening artifacts in the reconstructed images. Statistical algorithms can effectively correct beam hardening artifacts while providing the benefit of noise reduction. In practice, a big challenge for CT is the difficulty at acquiring accurate energy spectrum information, which hinders the efficiency of beam hardening correction approaches that require the spectrum as prior knowledge such as the statistical methods. In this paper, we used proposed energy spectrum binning approach for reducing prior knowledge from full spectrum to three energy bins to compare the results when applying parameters optimized for one spectrum to data measured using a different spectrum.

1 Introduction

In CT, beam hardening artifacts are caused by the polychromaticity of the X-ray source and the energy dependent attenuation coefficients of materials. Many beam hardening correction (BHC) algorithms have been developed for X-ray CT, both analytically [1] and iteratively [2, 3, 4]. De-Man et al. proposed a maximum likelihood based reconstruction algorithm [3] (IMPACT), in which the energy dependent attenuation coefficients of materials were decomposed into linear combinations of photoelectric and Compton scattering components. Another approach was proposed by Elbakri et al., which reconstructs a density map from pre-segmented base substance images [2]. Statistical algorithms can effectively correct beam hardening artifacts while providing the benefit of noise reduction from iterative reconstruction, and are very flexible with respect to various geometries, prior knowledge, noise statistics, etc. However, it is often the case that those approaches are very computationally intensive with respect to optimization, number of materials, and processing of the full X-ray spectrum.

Wu et al. have proposed a modified optimization problem for polychromatic statistical reconstruction algorithms, and simplified the algorithms with a spectrum binning method to reduce the full spectrum. From previous studies, it is

shown that a generalized spectrum binning algorithm using three energy bins
has an average to absolute error of logarithmic signal of less than 0.003. [5]

In practice, a big challenge for CT is the difficulty at acquiring accurate
energy spectrum information. This always hinders the efficiency of BHC approaches that require the spectrum as prior knowledge such as the statistical
methods. In this study, various spectra with different tube voltages or pre-
filtering are simulated, and evaluations of the spectrum binning methods with
mismatched spectra are carried out.

2   Materials and methods

2.1   Spectrum binning

In CT, emitted X-ray photons have varying energies and the detector response
is also energy dependent. According to Beer-Lambert's law, the measured detector signal of a polychromatic X-ray beam is the sum of the monochromatic
contributions from small energy bins

$$\bar{Y}_i = \int_{\varepsilon} b_i(\varepsilon) \exp\left(-\int_{L_i} \mu(\varepsilon)\mathrm{d}l\right) \mathrm{d}\varepsilon \tag{1}$$

where $b_i(\varepsilon)$ is the unattenuated scan signal of detector pixel i at energy ε, and
$\mu(\varepsilon)$ is the energy dependent attenuation coefficient of the object. Based on
the assumption of the Poisson measurement model and ignoring the electrical
noise, images can be reconstructed through minimizing the log-likelihood ob-
jected function [2, 3] as

$$\Psi = -\sum_{i=1}^{I}(Y_i \ln(\bar{Y}_i) - \bar{Y}_i) + \beta\mathbf{R}(\mu) \tag{2}$$

where $\mathbf{R}$ is the penalty function of image roughness.

Statistical polychromatic reconstruction assumes that for certain base substances k, the energy dependent attenuation coefficient can be approximated as
a linear combination of photoelectric and Compton scattering components [3]
(at low X-ray energies), such as

$$m_k(\varepsilon) = \phi_k\Phi(\varepsilon) + \theta_k\Theta(\varepsilon) \tag{3}$$

where $\Phi(\varepsilon)$ and $\Theta(\varepsilon)$ denote base functions of photoelectric and Compton scattering components, and ϕ_k and θ_k are the amount of two components for substances
k. Define ρ_j as the material density at spatial location j, and f_j^k is the fraction
of the kth material, then the measured signal from the detector from (1) can be
decomposed into two components

$$\mu_j(\varepsilon) = \sum_{k=1}^{K} m_k(\varepsilon)\rho_j f_j^k = \left(\Phi(\varepsilon)\sum_{k=1}^{K}\phi_k f_j^k + \Theta(\varepsilon)\sum_{k=1}^{K}\theta_k f_j^k\right)\rho_j \tag{4}$$

$$= (\phi_j\Phi(\varepsilon) + \theta_j\Theta(\varepsilon))\rho_j$$

Generally, the statistical reconstruction methods are computationally very expensive since they use prior knowledge about materials and energy spectrum. Wu et al. developed an optimal spectrum binning strategy, which uses the reduced number of energy bins instead of full spectrum information. A generalized spectrum binning approach that has freedoms in both the bin sizes and the values of Φ_s and Θ_s is proposed. The energy bin sizes only need to satisfy the following constrains

$$\sum_{s=1}^{S} B_s = \int_{\varepsilon_{\min}}^{\varepsilon_{\max}} b(\varepsilon) \mathrm{d}\varepsilon, \quad B_s > 0 \quad \text{for} \quad s = 1, 2, 3, \ldots, S \tag{5}$$

Therefore, the sum of all bins is identical to the integral over the spectrum. For two components (ϕ_t, θ_t), the true and approximated expected signals are

$$\bar{Y}^S(\phi_t, \theta_t; B_s, \Phi_s, \Theta_s) = \sum_{s=1}^{S} B_s \exp\left(-\Phi_s \phi_t - \Theta_s \theta_t\right) \tag{6}$$

Φ_s and Θ_s are the corresponding values of each bin. The optimal bin sizes, Φ_s and Θ_s are determined by optimizing

$$\operatorname*{argmin}_{B_s, \Phi_s, \Theta_s} \| \log(\bar{Y}^{\mathrm{full}}(\phi_t, \theta_t)) - \log(\bar{Y}^S(\phi_t, \theta_t, B_s, \Phi_s, \Theta_s)) \|_1 \tag{7}$$

where $\bar{Y}^S$ is computed by (6). The empirical result shows that the L_1 distance provides relatively good BHC results.

In a previous study, we compared our spectrum binning method with other reconstruction algorithms with respect to the effectiveness of beam hardening correction. In this paper, we examine the performance of optimized parameters applied to datasets with mismatch between assumed and actual spectra.

2.2   Experiments

In order to evaluate the stability of the spectrum binning method with respect to mismatched spectra, a digital phantom consisting of soft tissue and bone is used in the simulation. Each dataset consists of 640 projection images over an angular range of 360°, with a size of 512×512 pixels at an isotropic resolution of 0.8×0.8 mm. The image reconstruction was performed on a 320×320 voxel grid with spacing of 0.8×0.8 mm.

To perform the comparative analysis, datasets with different tube voltages and pre-filtration are simulated. We chose 120 kVp with 2 mm Al filter spectrum as reference, and applied the obtained optimized spectral binning parameters to other datasets for examination of influences on mismatched spectra.

3   Results

Fig. 1 shows spectra of different tube voltages Fig. 1(a) and spectra of different filters using the same voltage Fig. 1(b). A filtered back-projection reconstruction of the phantom is illustrated, where the cupping and streak artifacts can be observed. Denote $C_t = f(P_t)$ as the correct reconstruction for tube voltage t, where P are parameters obtained from spectrum t. $M_t = f(P_g)$ is the reconstruction of datasets with tube voltage t using mismatched parameters obtained from voltage g. We used the 120kVp including 2mm Al filter spectrum g as reference. Then, the optimal parameters B_g, Φ_g and Θ_g from the reference spectrum are applied to datasets simulated with other spectra. Fig. 2 shows the resulting reconstructions from various spectrum setups in three aspects: reconstructed slices using mismatched parameters M_t, difference images between C_t and M_t, and corresponding center line profiles. Two sets of comparisons are carried out: with different tube voltages, and with various filters applied at identical voltage. From the reconstructed images, it can be seen that beam hardening artifacts are sufficiently suppressed even though the applied parameters are from unmatched spectra. The difference images show that an increase in distance between real and reference spectra results in larger differences, e.g. 80 kVp vs. 100 kVp, and 1 mm Al & 1 mm Ti vs. 1 mm Al & 0.5 mm Cu. We plot line profiles from the uncorrected reconstructions and from the reconstruction corrected by using matched and mismatched parameters for binning with two and three energy bins, respectively. As discussed previously, three bins generally achieve better results than an optimization using 2 bins.

In Tab. 1, quantitative comparisons of the mismatched spectra with correct spectra parameters are listed. The binning parameters obtained from the reference spectrum (120 kVp & 2 mm Al) are applied to other spectra datasets. Root mean square error (RMSE) is used for illustration. As observed from the difference images in Fig. 2, the more the spectra deviate from the reference spectrum, the larger the RMSE value.

4   Discussion

In this work, energy spectrum binning approach is used for reducing prior knowledge from full spectrum to three energy bins in statistical polychromatic reconstruction. A simulation study was carried out that compared the results when applying parameters optimized for one spectrum to data measured using a different spectrum. The quantitative results indicate, using RMSE, that the spectrum

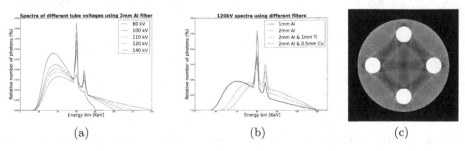

Fig. 1. Simulated spectra and reconstruction of the phantom using filtered backprojection.

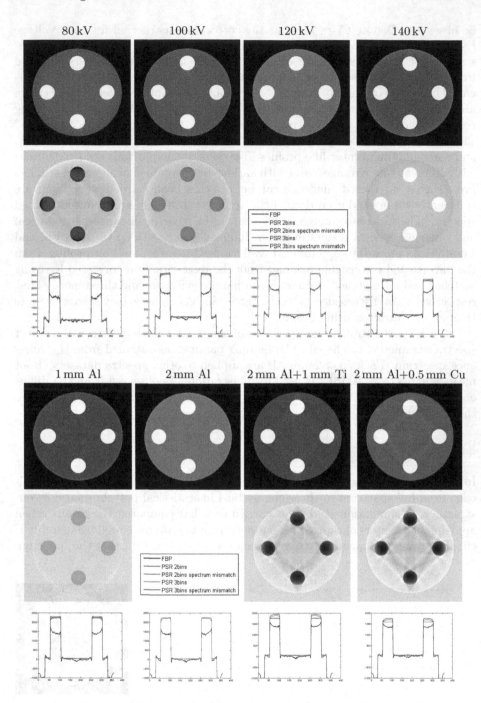

Fig. 2. Results of reconstructed images from mismatched spectral binning parameters and corresponding line profiles. Reconstructed images are displayed with window $[-200, 400]$ HU.

Table 1. Spectrum binning results for reference and test spectra, and RMSE of reconstructions between matched and mismatched spectrum binning parameters.

Spectrum	**120 kVp**	80 kVp	100 kVp	140 kVp	120 kVp	120 kVp	120 kVp
	2 mm Al	2 mm Al	2 mm Al	2 mm Al	1 mm Al	2 mm Al	2 mm Al
							1 mm Ti	0.5 mm Cu
B_s (norm.)	**0.40**	0.65	0.56	0.46	0.50	0.37	0.35
	0.45	0.22	0.29	0.36	0.34	0.41	0.35
	0.15	0.13	0.15	0.18	0.16	0.22	0.30
Φ_s	**3.5754**	1.8080	2.2787	3.3056	2.6732	2.6816	2.3862
	0.7658	0.5013	0.5640	0.7895	0.6676	0.9424	1.1076
	0.2021	0.2719	0.2490	0.2155	0.2302	0.3351	0.4128
Θ_s	**1.0601**	1.0245	1.0369	1.0595	1.0468	1.0528	1.0546
	0.9886	0.9673	0.9705	0.9865	0.9780	0.9965	1.0120
	0.9008	0.9345	0.9229	0.9033	0.9126	0.9303	0.9359
RMSE(HU)	0	**0.0165**	**0.0075**	**0.0056**	**0.0033**	**0.0113**	**0.0116**
RMSE(HU)	0	**76.814**	**29.205**	**17.415**	**11.430**	**33.429**	**31.688**

mismatch does not significantly degrade the correction results, with a maximum additional RMSE of 76.814 HU when compared to the corrected image generated using the spectrum for which the optimum parameters were calculated.

Acknowledgement. This work was supported by the Research Training Group 1773 "Heterogeneous Image Systems", funded by the German Research Foundation (DFG). The authors gratefully acknowledge funding of the Erlangen Graduate School in Advanced Optical Technologies (SAOT) by the German Research Foundation (DFG) in the framework of the excellence initiative.

References

1. Joseph P, Spital R. A method for correction bone induced artifacts in computed tomography scanners. J Comput Assist Tomogr. 1978.
2. Elbakri IA, Fessler JA. Statistical image reconstruction for polyenergetic X-ray computed tomography. IEEE Trans Med Imaging. 2002;21(2):89–99.
3. De Man B, Nuyts J, Dupont P, et al. An iterative maximum-likelihood polychromatic algorithm for CT. IEEE Trans Med Imaging. 2001;20(10):999–1008.
4. Van Gompel G, Van Slambrouck K, Defrise M, et al. Iterative correction of beam hardening artifacts in CT. Med Phys. 2011;38(7):36.
5. Wu M, Yang Q, Maier A, et al. A practical statistical polychromatic image reconstruction for computed tomography using spectrum binning. SPIE Med Imaging. 2014.

Region of Interest Reconstruction from Dose-Minimized Super Short Scan Data

Yan Xia[1,2], Andreas Maier[1], Martin Berger[1], Joachim Hornegger[1,2]

[1]Pattern Recognition Lab, FAU Erlangen-Nürnberg
[2]Erlangen Graduate School in Advanced Optical Technologies (SAOT), FAU Erlangen-Nürnberg
yan.xia@cs.fau.de

Abstract. In this paper, we investigate an ROI image reconstruction in super short scan. The redundant rays in such scan are further shielded by using dynamic collimation. The acquired data coming with an extremely minimized radiation dose are sufficient for image reconstruction. For compensating resulting truncation, we apply a recently proposed algorithm – Approximated Truncation Robust Algorithm for Computed Tomography (ATRACT). The evaluation with two clinical datasets demonstrates that high image quality is achieved using this super short scan, with more dose reduction compared to a standard short scan.

1 Introduction

For many interventional procedures in neuroradiology, changes of the examined patient are often restricted to a small part of the full field of view (FOV). A restriction of the X-ray beam to only that area would significantly reduce radiation dose. In this paper we investigate an ROI image reconstruction in a novel acquisition scan coming with an extremely minimized radiation dose to the patient. Let us consider the 2D fan-beam geometry. Assume that the object support is a disk of radius R and the X-ray source rotates on the a circular trajectory $\boldsymbol{\alpha}(\lambda) = (D\cos\lambda, D\sin\lambda)^T$, where λ is the rotation angular range and D is the radius of circle. It is known that reconstruction is possible from projections acquired over an angular range $\Lambda_s = [0, \pi + 2 \cdot \arcsin(R/D)]$. Such a projection interval is referred to as the short scan. The question is whether this short scan range can be relaxed when only a ROI is required to be reconstructed.

Noo et al. [1] reformulated a 2D FBP-type reconstruction of a ROI from X-ray fan-beam projections and showed that an exact reconstruction of the ROI can be achieved on an angular range less than a short scan. In this work, we adapt this concept into an ROI reconstruction. One advantage of our data acquisition is that the acquired projections can be truncated so that only the ROI is irradiated by X-rays. In order to compensate the resulting truncation artifacts, we apply the recently proposed truncation correction algorithm – Approximated Truncation Robust Algorithm for Computed Tomography (ATRACT) [2, 3]. Although the algorithm is not mathematically exact, the shift-invariant feature is preserved and reconstruction of high image quality can be achieved [2].

To even further reduce radiation dose, we also adopt our prior work to the new data acquisition method. That is to deploy the dynamic collimation to shield the redundant rays during data acquisition [4]. The new data acquisition method, together with the truncation robust ATRACT algorithm, has various potential benefits, such as higher temporal resolution, lower patient dose, and reduced computational requirements.

2 Materials and methods

2.1 Asymmetric collimation with fixed distance

In many clinical applications, the position of the ROI may not be located exactly around the iso-center of the patient, as illustrated in Fig. 1a. Dependent on the location of the ROI, the position of the collimator blades may vary from one angulation to the other (i.e. $u_1 \neq u_1'$ and $u_2 \neq u_2'$) while the distance between the blades does not change, i.e. $u_2 - u_1 = u_2' - u_1'$. We refer to this collimation as Asymmetric Collimation with Fixed Distance (ACFD). Such collimation can be generally applied for ROI imaging with off-center ROIs within the patient.

2.2 Asymmetric collimation with changeable distance

It is known that a short scan measures data once in some views while twice in other views due to the fan-beam. The redundant data are weighted by a smooth weighting function, e.g. the Parker weights [5] before the filtering. In Ref. [4], we investigated the possibility to block redundant rays during short scan acquisition by successively moving the collimator into the ray path at the beginning of the scan. One requirement is the distance between the two collimator blades varies during the angulation, i.e. $u_2 - u_1 \neq u_2' - u_1'$, as illustrated in Fig. 1b. We

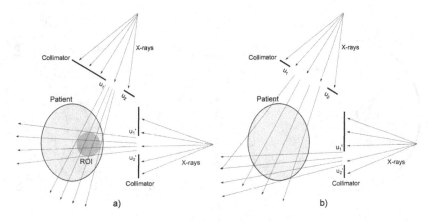

Fig. 1. Illustration of dynamic collimation: a) Asymmetric collimation with fixed distance (ACFD) and b) asymmetric collimation with changeable distance (ACCD).

investigate in this work an Asymmetric Collimation with Changeable Distance (ACCD) to block redundant rays in super short scans. Again, such collimation provides minimal complete data for reconstruction without redundancy, suggesting no weighting function is needed and further dose reduction is possible.

2.3 Super short scan acquisition

Conventionally, a short scan acquisition is used when the entire object is to be reconstructed. However, the angular interval can be further reduced when only the ROI is required to be irradiated and reconstructed. Let us first consider the off-center ROI case in Fig. 2a and the corresponding short scan sinogram in Fig. 2b. When using the ACFD collimation to get the truncated projections to reconstruct the specific ROI, we will only obtain the curved band (including dashed curves) in the sinogram. Then, let us consider the data redundancy. We know that a short scan measures some redundant rays at the beginning and at the end of data acquisition in a fan-beam geometry and these redundant rays follow the relation $g(\beta, \alpha) = g(\beta + \pi + 2\alpha, -\alpha)$. This reflects on the sinogram: The data in the triangle area ABC are redundant to the data in $A'B'C'$, which means only one must be required to reconstruct the object. Therefore, the short scan angular range can be reduced and the acquisition can start at the point where the line AC intersects the ROI sinogram boundary since the scan segment below the intersect (shown in the dashed band) will be measured again at the area $A'B'C'$. This enables the reconstruction of the ROI over an angular range less than a short scan, i.e. super short scan.

The data acquisition is divided into two stages: 1) using ACCD to acquire the data corresponding triangle area 1 and 2) using ACFD to acquire the rest (area 2). It is important to note that the super short scan, together with dynamic collimation, is able to minimize the dose to the patient while acquiring non-redundant data for reconstruction. The angular interval for super short scan,

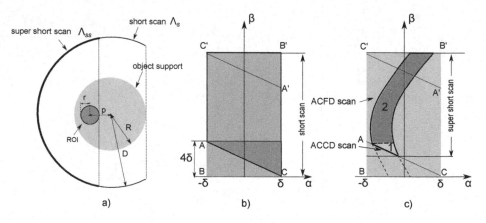

Fig. 2. a) Illustration of the short scan and the super short scan, b) and c) the corresponding sinograms.

i.e. $\Lambda_{ss} = [0, \vartheta]$, can be determined by the radius r and location p of the ROI

$$\vartheta = \pi - 2 \cdot \arcsin\left(\frac{p - r}{D}\right) \tag{1}$$

With increasing distance from the isocenter and decreasing ROI radius, the angular interval decreases. Note that when the ROI is located at the iso-center ($p = 0$) and the radius of the ROI is equal to the object support ($r = R$), the interval above extends to the short scan range Λ_s. The dose reduction can be approximated by computing the ratio between the short scan range and the difference of short scan and super short scan range plus half of the angular range to acquire the area 1 (since it is a triangle)

$$\gamma = \frac{2 \cdot \arcsin\left(\frac{R}{D}\right) + \arcsin\left(\frac{p-r}{D}\right) + \arcsin\left(\frac{p+r}{D}\right)}{\pi + 2 \cdot \arcsin\left(\frac{R}{D}\right)} \tag{2}$$

For instance, for an off-centered ROI with radius $r = 22.5\,\mathrm{mm}$ and location $p = 30\,\mathrm{mm}$ acquired from a C-arm CT system with the standard configuration $D = 750\,\mathrm{mm}$, $\arcsin(R/D) = 10°$. The potential dose reduction is $\gamma = 12.2\%$.

2.4   ATRACT algorithm

Both ACCD and ACFD collimation will result in truncation in all projections, which is not compatible to conventional reconstruction algorithms. Hence, we apply a truncation robust algorithm to deal with truncation problem [2, 3]. The idea behind ATRACT is to adopt the FDK (Feldkamp, Davis, and Kress) algorithm [6] by decomposing the 1D ramp filter into two successive filter steps. Thus, the algorithm can be preformed as follows: 1) Cosine and Parker weighting of projection data; 2) 1D Laplace filtering of the pre-weighted data; 3) 1D convolution-based filtering with a kernel $\ln|u|$ to get the filtered projection data; 4) standard backprojection with a distance weighting to obtain the final volume.

2.5   Experimental setup

We applied two clinical datasets of human head to validate and evaluate the proposed method. The datasets were acquired on a C-arm system with 496 projection images (1240 × 960 px) at the resolution of 0.308 mm / px.

Two experimental configurations were considered. In configuration 1, no collimation was applied, yielding the non-truncated short scan data. In the second one, the datasets were virtually cropped onto the centered and off-centered ROI, with $r = 22.5\,\mathrm{mm}$. The angular range of the super short scan is $\Lambda_{ss} = [0, 184°]$ for the centered ROI, and $\Lambda_{ss} = [0, 179°]$ for the off-centered ROI.

All clinical data were reconstructed onto a volume of 512 × 512 × 350 with an isotropic voxel size of 0.45 mm³. The standard FDK reconstruction of configuration 1, i.e. short scan non-truncated data were used as reference in each clinical case. The truncated datasets with super short scan were reconstructed by the ATRACT and FDK algorithm. To quantify retained accuracy obtained by the proposed algorithm, two quantitative metrics were used: the relative Root Mean Square Error (rRMSE) and the correlation coefficient (CC).

Table 1. Summary of quantitative analysis in two ROI cases (SS: short scan).

ROI	Metrics	Super SS FDK	SS ATRACT	Super SS ATRACT
Centered	rRMSE	42.1 %	4.66 %	4.84 %
	CC	0.14	0.96	0.96
Off-centered	rRMSE	38.4 %	4.71 %	4.96 %
	CC	0.20	0.96	0.95

3   Results

The reconstructed results are presented in Fig. 3, 4 and the summary of quantitative analysis is tabulated in Tab. 1. As expected, the FDK algorithm can not handle the data acquired from configuration 2. Two types of artifacts are observed: a bright ring artifact at the border of the ROI and streaking artifacts within the ROI. The reasons for these artifacts are data truncation caused by ACFD and ACCD, respectively. An rRMSE of as large as 42.1% confirms this observation. In contrast, the ATRACT reconstructions from configuration 2 are able to achieve high image quality. No significant difference within the ROI is found when comparing the reference to short scan and super short scan ATRACT reconstruction. The rRMSE is reduced to 4.84% for truncated super short scan ATRACT, which is closer to its short scan counterpart (4.66 %). Both methods yield high CC values. This demonstrates that with the ATRACT algorithm, an ROI acquisition with a super short scan achieves reconstructions of high quality, while minimizing the radiation dose to the patient.

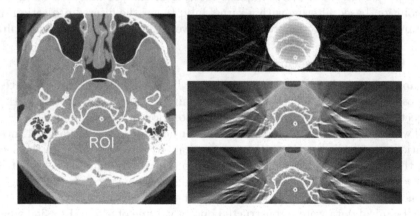

Fig. 3. Reconstructed results of the centered ROI dataset by the different algorithms. Left: the FDK reconstruction of non-truncated data; right from top to bottom: the super short scan FDK , the short scan ATRACT and super short scan ATRACT reconstruction.

Fig. 4. Reconstructed results of the off-centered ROI dataset by the different algorithms. From left to right: the FDK reconstruction of super short scan data, the short scan ATRACT, the super short scan ATRACT and reference FDK reconstruction.

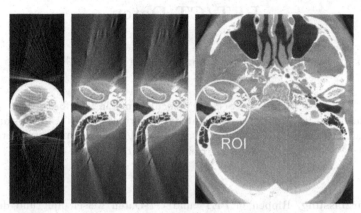

4 Discussion

In this paper we presented a new ROI acquisition method that acquires data in a super short scan using different types of dynamic collimation. A major advantage of this super short scan is that the acquired data satisfy both data sufficiency and non-redundancy with minimized dose to the patient. A limitation of the method is that it is only extended to the fan-beam geometry. For a circular cone beam scan, the extension is not straightforward due to two reasons: the relation $g(\beta, \alpha) = g(\beta + \pi + 2\alpha, -\alpha)$ will not be held for the slices away from the mid-plane; discontinuous behavior of the dynamic collimation to the cone-beam data. Future work involves investigating these issues and extending the method to a cone-beam geometry.

References

1. Noo F, Defrise M, Clackdoyle R, et al. Image reconstruction from fan-beam projections on less than a half scan. Phys Med Biol. 2002;47:2525–46.
2. Dennerlein F, Maier A. Approximate truncation robust computed tomography: ATRACT . Phys Med Biol. 2013;58:6133–48.
3. Xia Y, Maier A, Dennerlein F, et al. Efficient 2D filtering for cone-beam VOI reconstruction. Proc IEEE NSS/MIC. 2012;2415–20.
4. Xia Y, Berger M, Riess C, et al. Dose reduction achieved by dynamically collimating the redundant rays in fan-beam and cone-beam CT. Proc IEEE NSS/MIC. 2013; p. To appear.
5. Parker DL. Optimal short scan convolution reconstruction for fan-beam CT. Med Phys. 1982;9:254–7.
6. Feldkamp LA, Davis LC, Kress JW. Practical cone beam algorithm. J Opt Soc Am. 1984;1(6):612–9.

Multimodale Bildregistrierung für die effiziente Beurteilung von Rippenläsionen in PET/CT-Daten

Marcin Kopaczka[1,3], Andreas Wimmer[2], Peter Faltin[3], Günther Platsch[1], Jens N. Kaftan[1]

[1]Siemens Healthcare Sector, Molecular Imaging, Oxford, UK
[2]Siemens Healthcare Sector, Computed Tomography, Forchheim, Germany
[3]Institute of Imaging & Computer Vision, RWTH Aachen University, Germany
jens.kaftan@siemens.com

Kurzfassung. Rippen in PET- und CT-Daten weisen aufgrund der Atembewegung des Patienten selbst bei Aufnahme in kombinierten PET/CT-Geräten oft unterschiedliche Positionen auf. Dies verringert die diagnostische Aussagekraft der Aufnahmen, da zur korrekten Befundung eine genaue Überlappung von Auffälligkeiten in beiden Modalitäten notwendig ist. Um dies zu erreichen, wird hier ein neuartiges Registrierungsverfahren vorgestellt, welches die präzise Registrierung von Rippen in PET/CT-Aufnahmen erlaubt. Das Verfahren benutzt die automatisch aus den CT-Aufnahmen extrahierten Mittellinien der Rippen sowie Matched Filter, um eine separate rigide Transformation jeder Rippe zu bestimmen. Die registrierten Daten werden in einer kombinierten Ansicht dargestellt, welche gleichzeitig die PET- und CT-Aufnahmen aller Rippen eines Patienten präsentiert und somit die effiziente Beurteilung von Auffälligkeiten erlaubt. Das Verfahren wurde anhand von 20 PET/CT-Aufnahmen validiert. Die Ergebnisse zeigen, dass die rigide Methode eine präzise Registrierung der Rippen ermöglicht, welche nicht durch außerhalb der Rippen liegende Bildinhalte beeinflusst wird. Unter Berücksichtigung klinisch relevanter Grenzwerte konnte der Anteil der Rippenachsenpunkte mit guter Überlappung von 60.6% auf 87.7% nach Registrierung gesteigert werden. Qualitativ konnte die klinische Verwertbarkeit für alle 20 Fälle gesteigert werden.

1 Einleitung

Rund 70% der mit einem Primärtumor der Lunge, Brust, Prostata, Nieren oder der Schilddrüse diagnostizieren Patienten bilden Knochenmetastasen [1]. Diese Krebsarten machen etwa 50% der neu diagnostizierten Primärtumore aus, was in Deutschland jährlich etwa 200 000 Fällen entspricht [2].

Knochenmetastasen unterschiedlicher Tumorentitäten können mit nuklearmedizinischen Untersuchungen sehr gut nachgewiesen werden, wobei die Präsenz von Metastasen die Einstufung des Krebsstadiums und damit auch die zur Verfügung stehenden Therapieoptionen beeinflussen kann. Zur Detektion von osteoblastischen Knochenläsionen, wie z.B. beim Prostatakarzinom, hat sich insbesondere PET/CT mit ^{18}F-NaF als Radiotracer mit Sensitivitäten und Spezifitäten nahe der 100% als besonders genau und empfindlich erwiesen [3].

Für die effiziente Lokalisierung und anatomische Beschreibung von Rippenläsionen in CT-Bildern haben Kiraly et al. ein Verfahren vorgestellt, welches basierend auf den Mittelachsen der Rippen eine aufgefaltete Ansicht des Brustkorbs ermöglicht [4]. Die klinische Aussagekraft der so aufgearbeiteten anatomischen CT-Daten könnte durch eine Kombination mit gleichzeitig gewonnenen funktionellen ^{18}F-NaF PET-Daten erheblich gesteigert werden. Allerdings führt die Atembewegung des Patienten aufgrund der wesentlich längeren Aufnahmedauer der PET-Daten im Vergleich zu den CT-Daten zur Verfälschung der Position der Rippen zwischen den Datensätzen. Die unterschiedlichen Positionen der Rippen in beiden Modalitäten haben zur Folge, dass klinische Auffälligkeiten der einen Modalität nicht eindeutig im korrespondierenden Bild der anderen Modalität lokalisiert werden können. Abb. 1a zeigt diesen Effekt am Beispiel einer fusionierten aufgefalteten Ansicht des Brustkorbs bei Nutzung der intrinsischen Registrierung beider Modalitäten. Es ist zu sehen, wie z.B. eine Läsion der Rippe $R06$ basierend auf den CT-Daten (Position A) in den fusionierten PET-Daten auf der Rippe $R05$ erscheint (Position A').

Zur Lösung dieses Problems wird hier eine Methode zur Registrierung der Rippen in CT- und PET-Datensätzen unter Berücksichtigung der anatomischen Mittelachsen vorgestellt. Die Mittelachsen der Rippen in CT-Daten werden mit einem automatischen Verfahren detektiert [5]. Im Vergleich zu traditionellen, typischerweise nicht-rigiden Registrierungsansätzen zur Kompensation von atmungsbedingten Ausrichtungsartefakten wie z.B. [6], ermitteln wir die optimale Position der Mittelachse jeder individuellen Rippe in dem korrespondierenden PET-Datensatz über ein rigides Transformationsmodell. Die separate Registrierung hat den Vorteil, dass bei der Visualisierung der fusionierten Datensätze in einer aufgefalteten Ansicht der Rippen die nicht-rigiden atmungsbedingten Ausrichtungsartefakte kompensiert werden können (Abb. 1b), ohne die PET-Daten zusätzlich verformen zu müssen. Hierdurch wird eine Verfälschung der Tumorvolumina und weiterer quantitativer Kennzahlen wie z.B. dem Standardized Uptake Value (SUV) minimiert.

2   Material und Methoden

Als Vorverarbeitungsschritt wird zunächst das PET-Volumen mit Hilfe eines Algorithmus zur Verringerung des Einflusses des Aufnahmeprotokolls vorgefiltert [7], was die Verwendung protokollunabhängiger Registrierungsparameter ermöglicht. Anschließend wird das in Abschnitt 2.1 beschriebene Verfahren benutzt, um die aus dem CT-Datensatz gewonnenen Mittellinien optimal mit der Mitte der korrespondierenden Rippen des PET-Datensatzes in Übereinstimmung zu bringen. Die Registrierung wird mit der intrinsischen Ausrichtung der obersten Rippe initialisiert und bestimmt nacheinander die Transformation für die darauffolgenden Rippen, wobei ab der zweiten Rippe das Ergebnis der Registrierung der vorausgehenden Rippe zur Initialisierung des Verfahrens benutzt wird. Dies erhöht die Robustheit des Verfahrens gegenüber größeren Unterschieden in der Position der Rippen in beiden Datensätzen und verringert die Gefahr des Konvergierens zu einer falschen Rippe.

2.1 Registrierung einzelner Rippen mit einem Matched Filter

Eine optimierbare Bewertungsfunktion E, welche den Grad der Übereinstimmung einer CT-Mittellinie A mit der Mittelachse der Rippe im PET-Bild angibt, wird über Matched Filter definiert. Hierzu wird zunächst unter der Annahme einer ideal knochenspezifischen Radionuklidverteilung und einer nicht idealen Übertragungsfunktion des Scanners die Intensitätsverteilung senkrecht zur Rippe im PET-Bild durch eine mittelwertfreie Gaußsche Normalverteilung mit der Varianz σ^2 modelliert. Diese wird genutzt, um eine eindimensionale Filterfunktion h_σ zu definieren, die an jedem Punkt einer Rippe $\mathbf{p} \in A$ mit dem dort vorgefundenen Intensitätsprofil $I(\mathbf{p}, \mathbf{v})$ des PET-Bildes entlang des Vektors $\mathbf{v}$ senkrecht zur Rippe gefaltet wird und somit angibt, wie gut der Punkt $\mathbf{p}$ mit dem Mittelpunkt einer idealen Rippe übereinstimmt. Zur Erhöhung der räumlichen Präzision der Registrierung werden an jedem Punkt mehrere Filter in verschiedene Richtungen $\mathbf{v}_i$ mit $i \in [1, N]$ senkrecht zur Mittelachse ausgewertet. Um den Einfluss lokaler Intensitätsmaxima entlang der Rippe auf das

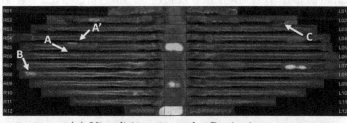

(a) Visualisierung vor der Registrierung

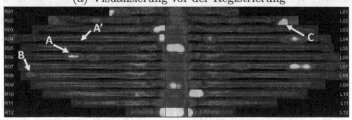

(b) Visualisierung nach der Registrierung

Abb. 1. Beispiel einer fusionierten aufgefalteten Ansicht des Brustkorbs. Ohne Anwendung des vorgestellten Verfahrens können Läsionen auf der falschen Rippe erscheinen (Position A, A') oder sogar gar nicht dargestellt werden (Position B). Für vereinzelte Rippen kann sich die Ausrichtung aber auch verschlechtern was neue Artefakte einführen kann (Position C), was sich in diesem Fall durch Ungenauigkeiten der CT-basierten Mittellinie der Rippe $R02$ erklären lässt.

Gesamtergebnis zu begrenzen und die Teilergebnisse vergleichbarer zu gestalten, wird weiterhin die Summe der Filterantworten an jedem Punkt $\mathbf{p}$ durch den an diesem Punkt festgestellten maximalen Intensitätswert $I_{\max}(\mathbf{p}) = \max_i I(\mathbf{p}, \mathbf{v}_i)$ normalisiert. Die Gesamtfunktion lautet somit

$$E(A) = \sum_{\mathbf{p} \in A} \frac{1}{I_{\max}(\mathbf{p})} \sum_{i=1}^{N} I(\mathbf{p}, \mathbf{v}_i) * h_\sigma \tag{1}$$

E wird als Optimierungskriterium zur Bewertung der Transformationsgüte in einem iterativen Registrierungsframework eingesetzt. Die Umsetzung mit dem Insight Segmentation and Registration Toolkit (ITK, www.itk.org) benutzt zur Optimierung das ableitungsfreie Powell-Verfahren und einen linearen Interpolator zur Ermittlung der benötigten Intensitätswerte I des PET-Volumens.

2.2 Material und Evaluationsmethodik

Zur Validierung des vorgestellten Verfahrens wurden in der Summe 24 ^{18}F-NaF PET/CT Datensätze von verschiedenen Kliniken berücksichtigt. Der Schichtabstand der CT-Bilder variierte zwischen 1.5 und 5.0 mm. Die Mittellinien der Rippen wurden mit dem Verfahren von Wu et al. [5] detektiert und in zwei Fällen grobe Fehler im Detektionsergebnis manuell korrigiert. Die PET-Aufnahmen wiesen Voxelgrößen zwischen $4.07 \times 4.07 \times 3.00$ mm^3 und $5.31 \times 5.31 \times 5.00$ mm^3 sowie verschiedene Rekonstruktionsprotokolle auf. Darüber hinaus wurden die Mittellinien der Rippen in den PET-Daten halbautomatisch bestimmt. Hierbei wurden manuell Markierungen entlang der Rippe gesetzt und editiert, welche anschließend durch eine Spline-Interpolation nach dem Catmull-Rom-Verfahren verbunden wurden. Um daraus Referenztransformationen zu definieren, die optimal die u.U. fehlerbehafteten CT-Mittellinien mit den manuell definierten PET-Mittellinien in Übereinstimmung bringen, wurde ferner jede CT-Mittellinie geometrisch mittels des Iterative Closest Point (ICP)-Algorithmus [8] zu ihrem PET-Gegenstück registriert.

Von den 24 Datensätzen wurden 4 zur empirischen Optimierung der Registrierungsparameter benutzt. Das Verfahren wurde anschließend auf den verbleibenden 20 Fällen mit insgesamt 476 detektierten Rippen und ca. 250 000 Rippenpunkten erprobt. Weiterhin wurden in Zusammenarbeit mit einem Nuklearmediziner klinisch relevante Grenzwerte für die akzeptable Registrierungsgenauigkeit erarbeitet. Ein Abstand zur Referenz von unter 4.5 mm wurde als gut, ein Abstand unter 9.0 mm als mäßig und ein Abstand darüber als nicht akzeptabel definiert. Zusätzlich wurden Verschiebungen entlang der Mittellinie geringer gewichtet ($0.5 \times d_\parallel$) als Verschiebungen orthogonal zur Mittellinie ($d_\perp$), da im letzteren Fall die Wahrscheinlichkeit wesentlich größer ist, dass eine Läsion im resultierenden aufgefalteten Bild auf der falschen Rippe oder sogar gar nicht dargestellt wird. Die gewichtete l^2-Norm von $d_\parallel$ und $d_\perp$ wird im Folgenden durch die Einheit [nmm] repräsentiert.

3   Ergebnisse

Die Ergebnisse können auf Punkt-, Rippen- und Patientenebene interpretiert werden. Der mittlere Abstand der Punkte aller Mittellinien zu ihren Referenzpunkten konnte durch die Registrierung von 4.6 nmm auf 2.6 nmm verringert werden. Das entspricht einem Anteil von Punkten mit guter Registrierung von 87.7% (vorher: 60.6%) und einem Anteil von mindestens mäßiger Registrierung von 97.7% (vorher: 93.3%) (Abb. 2a). Die mittlere Distanz zur Referenz auf Rippenebene wurde um 60.4% von 4.8 nmm auf 2.9 nmm verbessert. Wie Abb. 3 zeigt, konnte die Position der Rippen in den meisten Fällen (81.1% aller Rippen) verbessert werden. Dabei konnte beobachtet werden, dass die Ausrichtung der mittleren und damit längeren Rippen eine höhere Genauigkeit aufweist. Auf Patientenebene ergibt sich daraus eine Verbesserung des Medians für insgesamt 19 der 20 Testdatensätze (Abb. 2b). Eine qualitative Inspektion der Ergebnisse ergab ebenfalls, dass die klinische Verwertbarkeit der aufgefalteten fusionierten Visualisierung für alle 20 Fälle verbessert worden ist. Während Läsionen in mehreren Fällen vor der Registrierung gar nicht oder stark verschoben dargestellt wurden, konnten nach der Registrierung alle Läsionen, die auch für die Referenzausrichtung zu sehen waren, mit akzeptabler Präzision dargestellt werden.

4   Diskussion

Das vorgestellte Verfahren ermöglicht die Registrierung von Rippen in PET/CT-Datensätzen, die aufgrund der durch die Atembewegung verursachten Verschiebung notwendig wird. Die exklusive Fokussierung auf Rippen durch Benutzung automatisch detektierter Mittellinien des CT-Bildes ermöglicht eine hohe Genauigkeit bei gleichzeitig geringer Anfälligkeit für Störungen durch außerhalb der Rippen liegende Bildelemente. Die vorgestellte Methode ist robust gegenüber

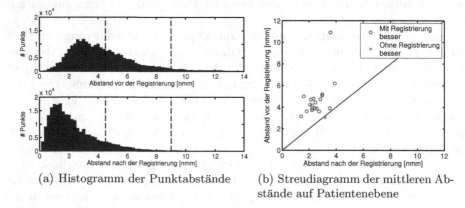

(a) Histogramm der Punktabstände   (b) Streudiagramm der mittleren Abstände auf Patientenebene

Abb. 2. Abstand aller Mittellinien zu ihren Referenzlinien auf (a) Punkt- bzw. (b) Patientenebene. Die klinisch relevanten Grenzwerte zur Kategorisierung der Ergebnisse in gut, mäßig und schlecht sind im Histogramm durch vertikale Linien gekennzeichnet.

Abb. 3. Boxplot der Differenzen der mittleren Rippenabstände pro Datensatz vor und nach der Registrierung. Eine negative Abstandsdifferenz entspricht hier einer Verringerung des Abstands zur Referenz und damit einer Verbesserung der Ausrichtung.

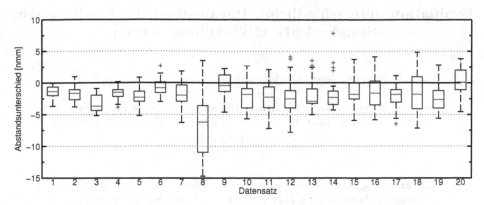

Ungenauigkeiten der automatisch extrahierten Mittellinien sowie Variationen der PET-Rekonstruktionsparameter. Die Kombination der Information aus PET- und CT-Daten in einer Ansicht, die alle Rippen gleichzeitig präsentiert, erlaubt eine effiziente Beurteilung von Auffälligkeiten. Das vorgestellte Verfahren wurde weiterhin bereits erfolgreich auf ersten ^{99m}Tc MDP-SPECT/CT-Datensätzen angewendet, was in der Zukunft näher untersucht werden soll.

Literaturverzeichnis

1. Jacofsky DJ, Frassica DA, Frassica FJ. Metastatic disease to bone. Hosp Physician. 2004;40(11):21–8.
2. Kaatsch P, Spix C, et al.. Krebs in Deutschland 2007-2008. Robert-Koch-Institut und die Gesellschaft der epidemiologischen Krebsregister in Deutschland e.V.; 2012.
3. Even-Sapir E, Metser U, et al. The detection of bone metastases in patients with high-risk prostate cancer: 99mTc-MDP Planar bone scintigraphy, single- and multi-field-of-view SPECT, 18F-fluoride PET, and 18F-fluoride PET/CT. J Nucl Med. 2006;47(2):287–97.
4. Kiraly AP, Qing S, Shen H. A novel visualization method for the ribs within chest volume data. Proc SPIE. 2006; p. 614108–1–8.
5. Wu D, Liu D, et al. A learning based deformable template matching method for automatic rib centerline extraction and labeling in CT images. Proc IEEE. 2012; p. 980–7.
6. Mattes D, Haynor DR, et al. PET-CT image registration in the chest using free-form deformations. Proc IEEE. 2003;22(1):120–8.
7. Kelly M, Declerck J. SUVref: reducing reconstruction-dependent variation in PET SUV. EJNMMI Res. 2011;1(1):16.
8. Besl PJ, McKay ND. A method for registration of 3-D shapes. Proc IEEE. 1992;14(2):239–56.

Klassifikation des Verschlussgrades der Epiphyse der proximalen Tibia zur Altersbestimmung

Evaluation unterschiedlicher Parameter auf Grundlage von Standard 3D-MRT-Bildsequenzen

Dennis Säring[1], Markus auf der Mauer[1], Eilin Jopp[2]

[1]Institut für Computational Neuroscience, Universtätsklinikum Hamburg-Eppendorf
[2]Institut für Rechtsmedizin, Universitätsklinikum Hamburg-Eppendorf
d.saering@uke.de

Kurzfassung. Die Altersbestimmung von lebenden Individuen ist ein wichtiger Teil des Asyl- und Strafrechts. Ein Anhaltspunkt für die Altersbestimmung ist der Ossifikationsprozesses in den Wachstumsfugen. Die nicht-invasive Magnetresonanztomographie ermöglicht die strahlenfreie Beurteilung dieses Prozesses. Ziel dieser Arbeit ist die Entwicklung eines Workflows zur automatischen Klassifikation des Epiphysenverschlusses im Knie auf Basis von MRT-Bilddaten. Dazu wurden aus einer Studie zur Altersbestimmung 21 MRT-Datensätze von jungen Männern (Alter zwischen 15 und 19 Jahren) zur Verfügung gestellt für die jeweils eine visuelle Einordnung der Epiphysenfuge in offen, zentral geschlossen und geschlossen existiert. Der entwickelte Workflow besteht aus mehreren aufeinander aufbauenden Methoden zur Segmentierung, Vorverarbeitung der Daten, Analyse und Klassifikation der vorliegenden MRT-Sequenzen. Die Klassifikation erfolgt mittel Support-Vector-Regression (SVR) auf Grundlage des prozentualen Auftretens sowie der Verteilung eines neuen Parameters p. Bei der Evaluation konnten 20 Datensätze richtig klassifiziert werden. Die Ergebnisse zeigen, dass das neue Verfahren eine automatische Bestimmung des Epiphysenverschlusses ermöglicht. Der Workflow erlaubt erstmals eine schnelle Klassifizierung von großen Datenkollektiven und bildet somit die Grundlage zur Beantwortung der forensischen Fragestellung der Altersbestimmung.

1 Einleitung

1.1 Forensische Problemstellung

Die Altersbestimmung von lebenden Individuen insbesondere die Abgrenzung von Jugendlichem- zum Erwachsenenalter ist ein wichtiger Teil des Asyl- und Strafrechts. Hierzu werden körperlichen Untersuchungen, Handradiographien sowie odontologische Untersuchungen durchgeführt. Allerdings dürfen radiologische Untersuchungen nur in einem Strafverfahren angewendet werden. Nicht-invasive Bildgebungsverfahren, wie die Magnetresonanztomographie (MRT), ermöglichen die strahlenfreie Beurteilung des Ossifikationsprozesses in den Wachstumsfugen. Dabei wird der Prozessverlauf des Verschlusses mit dem Lebensalter korreliert. Der Status des Verschlusses wird häufig visuell auf einer repräsentativen 2D-MRT-Schicht in 3 Klassen (I: offen, II: zentral geschlossen, III: geschlossen) eingeteilt (Abb. 1). Dies ist auf Grund der Interaktion zeitaufwendig und nicht immer eindeutig, so dass es bei den Ergebnissen zu Benutzerabhängigkeit und Fehlklassifikationen kommen kann. Bislang ist keine Studie bekannt die Methoden der Bildverarbeitung einsetzt, um die Altersbestimmung bzw. die Klassifikation des Verschlussgrades zu automatisieren und so eine robuste Auswertung großer Datenkollektive zu ermöglichen.

Ziel dieser Arbeit ist die Entwicklung und Evaluation eines Workflows zur automatischen Klassifikation des Epiphysenverschlusses im Knie auf Basis von MRT-Bilddaten. Es sollen neue Verfahren entwickelt werden, die den Status des Verschlusses unter Berücksichtigung von 3D-Bildinformationen bestimmt. Das Verfahren soll die Grundlage für eine automatische Altersbestimmung bei Lebenden bilden.

1.2 Stand der Forschung

Da sich die knorpelige Struktur der Epiphysenfuge im MRT besonders gut von knöchernen Strukturen unterscheiden lässt, und diese Technik eine strahlenfreie Beschreibung der Ossifikationsprozesse in den Wachstumsfugen von Langknochen zulässt, wird in einigen Arbeiten die MRT-Diagnostik bei der Beurteilung des Epiphysenwachstums verwendet [1]. Die einzelnen Zonen der knorpeligen Epiphysenfuge lassen sich jedoch auch im MRT nicht unterscheiden [2]. Bislang haben sich daher nur wenige Autoren der bildgebenden MRT-Technik zur Beantwortung der Frage nach der altersveränderlichen Entwicklung von Wachstumsfugen im Kniebereich und der Altersbestimmung bei Menschen bedient. In der Regel werden retrospektive Untersuchungen mittels strahlenintensiver Röntgenbilder durchgeführt [3, 4, 5]. Darüber hinaus diente die MRT-Diagnostik in klinischen Studien vor allem der Visualisierung normaler und pathologischer Entwicklungen im Bereich der Epiphysenfugen im Knie und basiert häufig auf Tiermodellen [6].

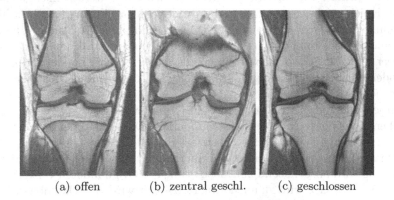

(a) offen   (b) zentral geschl.   (c) geschlossen

Abb. 1. Mittleres koronales 2D-MRT-Schichtbild.

Aktuelle Verfahren zur computerbasierten forensischen Altersbestimmung basieren in der Literatur auf unterschiedlichen Bildmodalitäten. Line Eikvil et al. (2012) haben eine Übersichtsarbeit zum Thema Altersbestimmung veröffentlicht und dort u.a. die Bildmodalitäten und die etablierten manuellen und computergestützten Methoden zusammengetragen [7]. Die meisten verfügbaren Toolboxen wie beispielsweise BoneXpert (Dänemark, [8] oder Maturos 4.0 (Frankreich) fokussieren auf die Analyse von Handknochen in Röntgenaufnahmen. Das Sunlight BonAge System (Israel) ermöglicht die Analyse von Ultraschall Aufnahmen.

Für die Auswertung von Epiphysenfugen im Knie auf Basis von MRT wurde bislang nur eine vorläufige Studie von Dedouit et al (2012) veröffentlicht [9]. Für den Verschluss der Epiphyse wurden hier entgegen den häufig verwendeten 3 allerdings 5 Klassen definiert und im Rahmen der Studie jeder Patient qualitativ auf einer 2D-Schicht einer dieser Klassen zugeordnet. Eine automatische Stufenzuordnung durch einen Algorithmus wurde dort nicht verwendet. Die Ergebnisse zeigen eine moderate bis gute Interobserver-Reproduzierbarkeit. Insbesondere die visuelle Zuordnung im Bereich der proximalen Tibia zeigte größere Unterschiede. Alle 290 Datensätze wurden manuell ausgewertet. Dennoch bestätigt diese Studie dass eine Altersbestimmung auf Basis von MRT-Bildsequenzen möglich ist [3].

2   Material und Methoden

Für die Entwicklung und Evaluation der Verfahren wurden aus einer Studie zur Altersbestimmung 21 von 80 MRT-Datensätzen von jungen Männern (Alter zwischen 15 und 19 Jahren) zur Verfügung gestellt. Der Status des Epiphysenverschlusses wurde von Radiologen visuell auf Basis einer mittleren koronalen 2D-MRT-Schicht in 3 Klassen unterteilt. Die 21 Datensätzen wurden so gewählt, dass für jede Klasse (I,II,III) jeweils 7 Datensätze vorlagen. Die MRT-Aufnahmen erfolgten mit Hilfe eines 1,5T-MRT (Privatpraxis) und eines 3T-MRT (Radiologie / Klinikum). Es wurde eine T1 gewichtete Turbo-spin-echo- (TSE-)MRT-Sequenz mit folgenden typischen Parametern eingesetzt (TR = 600 ms, TE = 15 ms, Kippwinkel von 90 Grad). Dabei wurden der Unterschenkelknochen sowie der Kniebereich in koronaler und sagitaler Schichtführung (ca. 24 Schichten mit 3 mm Schichtdicke) aufgenommen. Mit einer in-plane Auflösung von 0,4 mm x 0,4 mm können somit Wachstumsveränderungen im mm-Bereich erfasst werden. Der entwickelte Workflow besteht aus mehreren aufeinander aufbauenden Methoden zur Segmentierung, Vorverarbeitung, Analyse und Klassifikation der vorliegenden MRT-Sequenz.

Für jeden Datensatz wird zunächst auf Grundlage eines zuvor generierten statistischen Atlas die proximale Tibia segmentiert. Dabei wird der jeweilige MRT-Datensatz linear mit dem Atlas registriert und die zuvor bestimmten Grenzen der Tibia aus dem Atlas auf die Daten übertragen. Die daraus resultierende Segmentierung wird anschließend zur Maskierung der Originaldaten verwendet. Der maskierte Datensatz wird dann normiert. Hierzu wird der Datenbereich oberhalb und unterhalb des Tibiakopfes beschränkt und so die dargestellte Länge des Schaftes in Relation zur Position des Kopfes festgelegt (Abb. 2(a)). Für den nächsten Schritt wurde eine 3D-region-of-interest (3D-ROI) im Atlas derart definiert, dass der Bereich der Epiphysenfuge komplett überdeckt ist. Durch die Variabilität der Position und der Orientierung der Epiphysenfuge wurde die Region mit $150 \times 40 \times 70 \, mm^3$ ausreichend groß gewählt (Abb. 2(b)). Auf Grundlage der 3D-ROI werden dann Intensitätsverläufe in axialer Richtung extrahiert und analysiert. In Abb. 2(c) sind je 20 charakteristische Intensitätsverläufe für die 3 Klassen dargestellt. Im Falle einer offenen Epiphysenfuge lässt sich ein negativer Peak erkennen, dessen Minimum im unteren Drittel der Intensitäten liegt. Bei einer zentral geschlossenen Fuge tritt dieser negative Peak nur bei wenigen Verläufen und abgeschwächt auf. Die Kurven der geschlossenen Fuge schwanken im Bereich des Bildrauschens und der technisch bedingten Bildinhomogenitäten von MRT-Daten. Resultierend aus diesen Beobachtungen wurde für jeden Verlauf ein Parameter p berechnet, der über den Richtungswechsel von starken Gradienten bestimmt wird. Dabei wird für jeden Datenpunkt zweimal eine lineare Regression, auf Basis der fünf Datenwerte vor und nach dem Punkt, berechnet (Abb. 2(d)). Der Parameter ($p(x, y) \in 0, 1$) gibt an, ob innerhalb des Intensitätsverlaufs die Richtung der berechneten Regressionsgeraden für einen beliebigen Datenpunkt wechselt und somit ein negativer Peak vorliegt. Analog zu einer Projektionsabbildung werden die berechneten Parameter in eine axiale 2D-Map (Abb. 3) eingetragen und das prozentuale Auftreten sowie die Verteilung von p quantitativ erfasst. Für die Berechnung der Verteilung wird das Bild in 2 Regionen (A, B) unterteilt. Die Region A wird über Schwerpunkt- und Abstandsberechnung als innerer Kern automatisch definiert, B repräsentiert die äußere Schale um den Kern. Ziel dieser Einteilung ist eine verbesserte Differenzierung zwischen den Klassen II und III. In der Literatur sind bislang keine automatischen Verfahren zur Klassifikation des Verschlussstatus der Epiphysenfuge (proximale Tibia) bekannt. Daher wird für die Evaluation eine Support-Vector-Regression (SVR: lineares Modell, leave-one-out) durchgeführt und deren Ergebnis mit der manuell bestimmten Klassifikation verglichen.

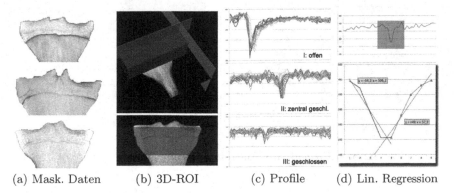

(a) Mask. Daten   (b) 3D-ROI   (c) Profile   (d) Lin. Regression

Abb. 2. Workflow: Teilschritte zur Berechnung und Analyse von p.

Abb. 3. Axiale 2D-Map für den Parameter p.

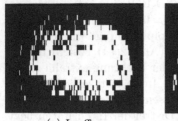 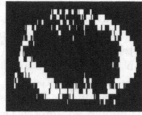 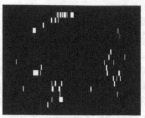

(a) I: offen   (b) II: zentral geschl.   (c) III: geschlossen

3 Ergebnisse

In Abbildung 4 sind das prozentuales Auftreten sowie die Verteilung von p dargestellt. Das prozentuale Auftreten (Gesamt [%]) zeigt für Daten der Gruppe I (offen) die größten Werte und somit eine Vielzahl an Intensitätsverläufen mit Charakteristika für eine offene Fuge. Diese Werte sind für die Klassen II (zentral geschl.) und III (geschlossen) geringer. Die Verteilung von p auf die innere Region A (Kern) und die äußere Region B (Schale) zeigen in der Klasse II die höchsten Differenzen. Wobei für die Klassen I und III das Verhältnis größtenteils ausgeglichen ist. In Abbildung 4 sind die beiden Messwerte (x: Gesamt [%]; y: Differenz $(A - B)$ [%]) dargestellt. Auf Grundlage des prozentualen Auftretens sowie der Verteilung p konnten mittels SVR 20 von 21 Datensätze korrekt klassifiziert werden. Dabei wurde eine Abweichung des SVR-Wertes vom Klassenwert (1(offen),2(zentral geschl.),3(geschlossen)) $< 0,5$ als korrekt definiert.

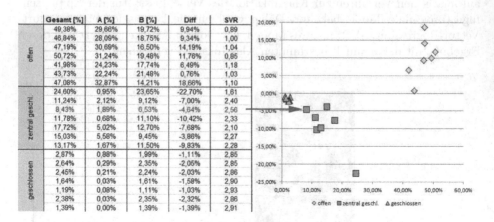

	Gesamt [%]	A [%]	B [%]	Diff	SVR
offen	49,38%	29,66%	19,72%	9,94%	0,89
	46,84%	28,09%	18,75%	9,34%	1,00
	47,19%	30,69%	16,50%	14,19%	1,04
	50,72%	31,24%	19,48%	11,76%	0,85
	41,98%	24,23%	17,74%	6,49%	1,18
	43,73%	22,24%	21,48%	0,76%	1,03
	47,08%	32,87%	14,21%	18,66%	1,10
zentral geschl.	24,60%	0,95%	23,65%	-22,70%	1,61
	11,24%	2,12%	9,12%	-7,00%	2,40
	8,43%	1,89%	6,53%	-4,64%	2,56
	11,78%	0,68%	11,10%	-10,42%	2,33
	17,72%	5,02%	12,70%	-7,68%	2,10
	15,03%	5,58%	9,45%	-3,86%	2,27
	13,17%	1,67%	11,50%	-9,83%	2,28
geschlossen	2,87%	0,88%	1,99%	-1,11%	2,85
	2,64%	0,29%	2,35%	-2,05%	2,85
	2,45%	0,21%	2,24%	-2,03%	2,86
	1,64%	0,03%	1,61%	-1,58%	2,90
	1,19%	0,08%	1,11%	-1,03%	2,93
	2,38%	0,03%	2,35%	-2,32%	2,86
	1,39%	0,00%	1,39%	-1,39%	2,91

Abb. 4. Prozentuales Auftreten und die Verteilung von p.

4 Diskussion

Auf Grundlage des prozentualen Auftretens sowie der Verteilung p konnten mittels SVR 20 Datensätze korrekt klassifiziert werden. Bei einem Datensatz war der Verschluss bereits weit fortgeschritten und wurde daher mit $2, 56$ knapp als geschlossen klassifiziert. Die Ergebnisse zeigen, dass es möglich ist den Status des Epiphysenverschlusses automatisch bestimmen zu können, allerdings müssen noch weitere Parameter (z.B. 3D-Krümmungsmaße) bei der SVR berücksichtigt werden. Aufbauend darauf kann die forensische Fragestellung der Altersbestimmung jetzt in großen Kollektiven untersucht und durch die Verwendung einer SVR weitere Informationen (u.a. Körpermasse) integriert werden. In Zukunft soll zunächst für ein eng definiertes Probandenkollektiv erforscht werden, ob und welche Parameter für die Bestimmung der Volljährigkeit relevant sind.

Literaturverzeichnis

1. Laor T, Jaramillo D. MR imaging insights into skeletal maturation: what is normal? Radiology. 2009;250(1):28–38.
2. Cartilaginous epiphysis and growth plate: normal and abnormal MR imaging findings. AJR Am J Roentgenol. 1992;158(5):1105–10.
3. Cameriere R, Cingolani M, Giuliodori A, et al. Radiographic analysis of epiphyseal fusion at knee joint to assess likelihood of having attained 18 years of age. Int J Legal Med. 2012;126(6):889–99.
4. Cardoso HFV. Epiphyseal union at the innominate and lower limb in a modern Portuguese skeletal sample, and age estimation in adolescent and young adult male and female skeletons. Am J Phys Anthropol. 2008;135(2):161–70.
5. O'Connor JE, Bogue C, Spence LD, et al. A method to establish the relationship between chronological age and stage of union from radiographic assessment of epiphyseal fusion at the knee: an Irish population study. J Anat Physiol. 2008;212(2):198–209.
6. Disler DG, Recht MP, McCauley TR. MR imaging of articular cartilage. Skeletal Radiol. 2000;29(7):367–77.
7. Eikvil L, Kvaal SI, Teigland A, et al. Age estimation in youths and young adults: a summary of the needs for methodological research and development. SAMBA/52/12. 2012.
8. Thodberg HH, Kreiborg S, Juul A, et al. The bonexpert method for automated determination of skeletal maturity. IEEE Trans Med Imaging. 2009;28(1):52–66.
9. Age assessment by magnetic resonance imaging of the knee: a preliminary study. Forensic Sci Int;217(1-3):232.e1–7.

Epiphyses Localization for Bone Age Assessment Using the Discriminative Generalized Hough Transform

Ferdinand Hahmann[1], Gordon Böer[1], Thomas M. Deserno[2], Hauke Schramm[1]

[1]Institute of Applied Computer Science, University of Applied Sciences Kiel
[2]Department of Medical Informatics, Uniklinik RWTH Aachen
ferdinand.hahmann@fh-kiel.de

Abstract. This paper presents the Discriminative Generalized Hough Transform (DGHT) as a robust and accurate method for the localization of epiphyseal regions in radiographs of the left hand. The technique utilizes a discriminative training approach to generate shape models with individual positive and negative model point weights for the Generalized Hough Transform. The framework incorporates a multi-level approach which reduces the searched region in two zooming steps, using specifically trained DGHT shape models. In addition to the standard method, a novel landmark combination approach is presented. Here, the N-best lists of individual landmark localizations are combined with anatomical constraints to achieve a globally optimal localization result for all 12 considered epiphyseal regions of interest. The technique has been applied to extract 12 epiphyseal regions of interest for a subsequent automatic bone age assessment. It achieved a localization success rate of 98.1% on a corpus with 412 left hand radiographs covering the age range from 3 to 19 years.

1 Introduction

Bone Age Assessment (BAA) is an important method in diagnostic radiology which is used for evaluating the skeletal maturity to diagnose growth disorders in children and adolescents. Since manual BAA techniques (e.g. Tanner & Whitehouse (TW) [1]), are time consuming, subjective and require expert opinion from a physician a number of automatic methods have been developed in recent years. Many of these approaches follow the basic concept of TW to classify only certain extracts from the radiograph since this substantially reduces the complexity of the classification problem. However, an important prerequisite for all these techniques is the availability of a reliable and robust object detection method to enable the extraction of the required region-of-interest.

Object detection problems in medical image analysis are often solved by individually adjusted methods, which make heavy use of expert knowledge about the shape and neighborhood of the searched object. [2], for example, analyzes image lines to assign the maxima in the vertical stripe pattern of a hand radiograph to the individual phalanges. The localization approach in [3] is based on the same idea using an arc scanning procedure to generate a gray value matrix whose maximal column sums refer to the phalanges. A more general approach has been presented in [4] where an active appearance model is used for bone reconstruction. This method can also be used for epiphysis localization but requires a high number of manually defined shaped points for the training process. [5] presents another segmentation approach used for epiphysis localization. Here, a graph-based structural prototype, representing the phalanges and metacarpal bones, is registered to the image and successfully provides the epiphyseal regions on 77% of 137 images.

There are only a few general object detection techniques which have shown a good performance in the field of medical image analysis. Marginal space learning [6] trains probabilistic boosting trees and gradually estimates the translation, rotation and scaling parameters of the searched object. The technique has successfully been applied to a number of anatomical objects but requires a large number of training images which are difficult to obtain in the field of medical imaging. Another general object detection approach is described in [7] where random forests are used to map image patches to Hough space votes for possible target point location. The work of [8] is based on the same idea but utilizes so called regression forests.

In this paper, the Discriminative Generalized Hough Transform (DGHT) is introduced as a robust method for the detection of epiphyseal regions of interest (eROI), located around the finger joints (Fig. 2.2a), in hand radiographs. The DGHT is a general object localization approach, which has been successfully applied to the localization of anatomical structures in medical images and several non-medical tasks [9]. To assure a reasonable combination of the localization results for all visible eROIs the technique is applied in conjunction with some simple geometrical constraints taken from the hand anatomy.

2   Materials and methods

In this contribution, the DGHT is used in the first step to generate a ranked list of localization candidates for each searched landmark (Sect. 2.1). The obtained set of lists is searched for an optimal combined solution for all eROI positions. This solution must meet a number of predefined constraints derived from the hand anatomy (Sect. 2.2).

2.1   Discriminative generalized Hough transform

The technique extends the well-known Generalized Hough Transform (GHT) by an iterative and discriminative training approach for the generation of optimal shape models with individually weighted model points [9]. The availability of models compensating moderate target object variability is crucial due to the expected anatomical variability. Apart from the object's translation no additional GHT transformation parameters are considered in this work, since we follow the idea of learning medium variability into the model.

The DGHT training procedure starts with the generation of an initial shape model which is extracted from a set of training images by overlaying their edge features inside a predefined region-of-interest with respect to a target point. The individual contributions of each initial model point to the Hough space are combined in a Maximum Entropy Distribution. This step introduces model point specific weights which are optimized in the next step using a Minimum Classification Error (MCE) training approach [10]. The optimized weights reflect the importance of each individual model point for supporting the correct localization and suppressing votes at similar but false structures. The latter aspect is possible since model point weights may also have negative values. After the model point weights in the initial shape model have been optimized with the described procedure, points with low absolute weights may be eliminated since their influence on the localization result is negligible.

The optimized and thinned initial model is further enhanced by an iterative procedure. This technique evaluates the model on the training images and extends it with image features from the target region and confusable areas in training images with high localization error. The procedure is repeated until the localization error on all training images is below some given threshold.

In addition to the model optimization procedure the applied framework uses a coarse-to-fine localization strategy to split different levels of anatomical detail into different localization models. This technique may also speed-up the processing in case of high resolution images. In this work, only two zooming steps are applied since the confusability of individual fingers in intermediate levels is quite high. In zoom level 0, showing the whole hand, the resolution is reduced to one-eight and a specifically trained DGHT model is used to obtain a coarse localization result. An image extract of size 192×256 with the original resolution is cut around the localized point and used for a precise eROI detection in zoom level 1 with a specific and more detailed DGHT model.

2.2   Constrained localization

To avoid the confusion of eROIs, which is a frequent source of error, the individual eROI localization results are combined with 133 simple anatomical constraints obtained from the hand anatomy. These describe (1) the minimum distance of eROIs (50 pixels), (2) the positioning of the fingers with respect to other fingers (e.g. index finger is right to middle finger), and (3) the positioning of eROIs inside a single finger with respect to the other eROIs in this finger (e.g. metacarpophalangeal is below proximal interphalangeal).

To derive a confidence measure from these requirements, each of the 12 considered eROI localization hypotheses (Fig. 2.2a) is assigned an individual error score which is determined by the number of unmet conditions. With this score the localization hypotheses are corrected in the following iterative manner: First, the eROI localization hypothesis with the highest error score is identified. Second, the hypothesis is rejected and replaced by a concurrent one from the 10-best list. The replacement is selected to have at least 95% of the GHT votes of the best hypothesis and the smallest error score of all remaining 10-best entries.

Third, the error score is recalculated using the replacement hypothesis and the next iteration is started. The iteration stops if the error scores of all eROIs are zero or if all landmarks have been changed. If it is not possible to fulfill all constraints, the system may ask the user for manual correction.

2.3 Experimental setup

The aim of this contribution is to set up a framework for localizing the 12 eROIs labelled in Fig. 2.2a. Since these regions are extracted for later usage in an automatic BAA system [11] it is necessary that the complete epiphysis is visible inside the identified image fragment. Due to the anatomy of the epiphyseal region the image extract chosen here is a narrow upright rectangle. Consequently, the applied error distance for measuring the success of the localization is asymmetric and tolerates a larger deviation from the target point in vertical direction than in horizontal direction. Thus, the localization is defined as being successful if the localized point differs less than 50 / 100 pixels in horizontal / vertical direction from the given target point. This assures the containment of the eROI inside the resulting image extract and therefore allows for a subsequent BAA classification step. An alternative error measure for eROI detection has been given in [5]. Here, it was stated that a human observer may accept a localization error of 6 pixel for hand radiographs with a height of 256 pixel. Below we will also refer to this error mesasure as "Fischers measure" for better comparability with the literature.

For training and test of the described framework an inhouse corpus from the University Hospital Aachen, consisting of 812 unnormalized hand radiographs with an average size of 1185 × 2066 pixel ranging from 3 to 19 years, has been used. Note that radiographs of children younger than 3 years were not considered since only little data with low image quality, especially with respect to contrast

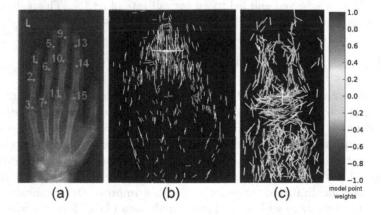

Fig. 1. Location and ID of eROIs (a) and examples of the global DGHT localization model of zoom level 0 (b) and zoom level 1 (c) with color-coded weights of the model points.

Table 1. Success rates in % for eROI localization using (1) the standard DGHT, (2) the method of constrained localization (Const.), and (3) two zooming-levels (Zoom). Results are provided for the considered 12 eROIs defined in Fig. 2.2a. The average error is given in pixels.

eROI	1	2	3	5	6	7	9	10	11	13	14	15	All	Error
DGHT	94.9	94.9	96.6	98.1	96.1	96.8	95.4	98.3	98.8	93.9	96.6	97.8	**96.3**	23.2
Const.	96.4	98.1	97.6	98.8	98.5	98.5	96.4	99.0	99.8	95.4	98.6	98.1	**97.8**	20.1
Zoom	96.6	98.3	98.5	98.8	98.5	98.8	96.8	99.0	99.8	95.4	98.1	98.5	**98.1**	11.4

and hand positioning, was available. The corpus, which contained target point annotations for all eROIs, was split into 400 randomly selected training and 412 evaluation images. For each eROI a single DGHT localization model was trained for both genders and the complete age range from 3 to 19 years.

3   Results

With the standard procedure using a global DGHT model (Fig. 2.2b) an overall localization success rate of 96.3% was obtained for all eROIs (Tab. 1). The average localization error for this experiment was 23 pixel corresponding to about 1% of the image height. This result could be significantly improved to an overall success rate of 97.8% by applying the constrained localization method (Sect. 2.2). The technique also improved the average localization error to about 20 pixel. A much more exact localization with an average error of only 11 pixel could be achieved with a second zooming step utilizing a refined model, specifically trained on small image extracts around the eROI. This model has been optimized to represent fine details instead of global characteristics and is therefore much more exact than the global model (Fig. 2.2c). An additional gain of the success rate of 0.3% was achieved and led to an overall rate of 98.1%. This value is only slightly decreased to 97.6% when using the stricter Fischers measure.

4   Discussion and conclusion

The experimental results show that the DGHT can be used as a robust and accurate method for the localization of epiphyseal regions of interest in radiographs of the left hand. The high localization rates of the basic technology can be substantially improved by the introduced novel landmark combination approach. It utilizes a set of simple anatomical constraints and successfully identifies globally optimal eROI localization results from the N-best lists of the individual DGHT-based localizations. In order to further improve the localization accuracy a zoom-in strategy with a specialized high-detail DGHT model was applied which nearly halved the average localization error to about 11 pixel.

Considering the few remaining errors of the system nearly two-thirds can be identified by unfulfilled anatomical conditions (2.2) which allows for eliminating those results in a subsequent BAA classification step. Since the applied BAA framework requires only a subset of eROIs, the elimination of single regions from the combined decision is probably not critical for the overall classification success. It is additionally expected that the influence of isolated undetected localization errors on the BAA result is low since several eROIs are utilized for the final decision.

The experiments were performed on radiographs of the complete age range from 3 to 19 years and both genders. The achieved high localization rates demonstrate that most of the resulting large object variability could be successfully trained into a single weighted DGHT shape model. An important source of variability for this task is, however, the spreading of fingers which lead to a clear error rate increase in the upper eROIs (especially No. 1, 9, and 13 in Fig. 2.2a). Although this specific kind of shape variability might in general be learned by the training process it is not sufficiently represented in the used training corpus and therefore lead to a substantial amount of the remaining errors.

For the addressed BAA task, the achieved localization accuracy is sufficient. A combination of the presented DGHT based localization framework with the Classifying GHT for bone age assessment [11] will be addressed in the next step of the investigations.

References

1. Tanner J, Healy M, Goldstein H, et al. Assessment of Skeletal Maturity and Prediction of Adult Height (TW3); 2001.
2. Pietka E, Gertych A, Pospiech S, et al. Computer-assisted bone age assessment: image preprocessing and epiphyseal/metaphyseal ROI extraction. IEEE Trans Med Imaging. 2001;20:715–29.
3. Hsieh C, Jong T, Tiu C. Bone age estimation based on phalanx information with fuzzy constrain of carpals. Med Biol Eng Comput. 2007;45:283–95.
4. Thodberg H, Kreiborg S, Juul A, et al. The BoneXpert method for automated determination of skeletal maturity. IEEE Trans Med Imaging. 2009;28:52–66.
5. Fischer B, Brosig A, Deserno T, et al. Structural scene analysis and content-based image retrieval applied to bone age assessment. Proc SPIE. 2009;7260:726004–1.
6. Zheng Y, Georgescu B, Comaniciu D. Marginal space learning for efficient detection of 2D/3D anatomical structures in medical images. Inf Process Med Imaging. 2009;21:411–22.
7. Gall J, Yao A, Razavi N, et al. Hough forests for object detection, tracking, and action recognition. IEEE Trans Pattern Anal Mach Intell. 2011;33:2188–202.
8. Criminisi A, Shotton J, Robertson D, et al. Regression forests for efficient anatomy detection and localization in CT studies. Med Comput Vis. 2011.
9. Ruppertshofen H. Automatic Modeling of Anatomical Variability for Object Localization in Medical Images. Ph.D. thesis, University Magdeburg; 2013.
10. Juang BH, Katagiri S. Discriminative learning for minimum error classification. IEEE Trans Image Process. 1992;40:3043–54.
11. Hahmann F, Berger I, Ruppertshofen H, et al. Bone age assessment using the classifying generalized hough transform. Pattern Recognit. 2013; p. 313–22.

Kombination von Atemsignalen zur Optimierung der Prädiktion komplexer atmungsbedingter Organ- und Tumorbewegungen

Jonas Ortmüller[1], Matthias Wilms[1], René Werner[2], Heinz Handels[1]

[1]Institut für Medizinische Informatik, Universität zu Lübeck
[2]Institut für Computational Neuroscience, Universitätsklinikum Hamburg-Eppendorf
jonas.ortmueller@miw.uni-luebeck.de

Kurzfassung. Für eine präzise Bestrahlung abdominaler und thorakaler Tumoren ist eine Kompensation der Atembewegung notwendig. Moderne Systeme zur Bewegungskompensation werden häufig mithilfe externer Atemsignale und patientenspezifischer Korrespondenzmodelle gesteuert. Diese Modelle ermöglichen die Prädiktion der internen Bewegung auf Basis des Atemsignals. Durch die Komplexität bzw. Variabilität der Atembewegung werden für eine präzise Bewegungsprädiktion in der Regel mehrdimensionale Atemsignale benötigt, welche z.B. durch die Kombination verschiedener eindimensionaler Signale (Spirometer, Bauchgurt,...) generiert werden können. In diesem Beitrag wird ein Verfahren zur automatischen Auswahl patientenindividuell optimaler Kombinationen von (eindimensionalen) Atemsignalen für die modellbasierte Bewegungsprädiktion vorgestellt. Das Verfahren wird anhand von 12 Lungentumorpatienten und 6 simulierten Atemsignalen evaluiert und mit anderen Methoden zur Generierung mehrdimensionaler Atemsignale (u.a. hochdimensionale Tiefenbilddaten) verglichen. Die Ergebnisse zeigen, dass durch Kombination einfacher 1D Signale die Prädikationgenauigkeit signifikant erhöht werden kann. Durch eine optimale Signalkombination können letztlich zu einer hochdimensionalen Tiefenabtastung gleichwertige Ergebnisse erzielt werden.

1 Einleitung

Bei der Strahlentherapie thorakaler und abdominaler Tumoren führen atmungsbedingte Bewegungen zu Unsicherheiten hinsichtlich der Position therapierelevanter Strukturen während der Behandlung. Deshalb wurden verschiedene Methoden zur Bewegungskompensation, wie Gating oder Tumortracking, entwickelt [1]. Deren Steuerung erfolgt zumeist durch externe Atemsignale in Verbindung mit patientenspezifischen Korrespondenzmodellen, die eine Prädiktion der internen Bewegung auf Basis des externen Atemsignals (Surrogat) ermöglichen [2]. In der klinischen Praxis werden häufig 1D Surrogatsignale, wie Spirometriedaten oder Bauchgurtsignale, eingesetzt [1]. Mit Korrespondenzmodellen, die durch ausschließliche Berücksichtigung der 1D Signalinformationen parametrisiert werden, ist allerdings eine Beschreibung komplexer Atemmuster (z.B. Hystereseverhalten) nicht möglich [2]. Hierfür werden in der Regel mehrdimensionale Atemsignale benötigt, die grob in drei Gruppen unterteilt werden können [2]:

1. Aus 1D Signalen abgeleitete mehrdimensionale Signale (z.B. 1D Signal+zeitliche Ableitung),
2. Durch Kombination verschiedener (1D) Signale generierte mehrdimensionale Signale [3] und
3. Durch die Aufnahmetechnik direkt erzeugte mehrdimensionale Signale, z.B. hochdimensionale Abtastung der Körperoberfläche durch Tiefenbildgebung [4].

Während bei der direkten Aufnahme eines hochdimensionalen Signals mittels Tiefenbildgebung die Dimension nur durch die Sensorauflösung begrenzt wird, ist u.a. wegen des Patientenkomforts und zur Vereinfachung der Datenaufnahme bei der Kombination verschiedener Surrogatsignale die Auswahl einer möglichst kleinen, aber optimalen Teilmenge möglicher Signalen erstrebenswert. Deshalb wird in diesem Beitrag „unter Verwendung eines diffeomorphen Frameworks zur Korrespondenzmodellierung und Techniken zur bildbasierten Simulation von Surrogatesignalen" ein automatisches Verfahren zur Auswahl patientenindividuell optimaler Signalkombinationen vorgestellt. Die Nutzung anhand von 4D-Bilddaten simulierter Surrogatsignale für die Bestimmung der optimalen Signalkombinationen eröffnet hierbei die Möglichkeit, auch Surrogate bzw. Surrogatpositionen (z.B. verschiedene Bauchgurtpositionen) zu berücksichtigen, ohne für diese vorher aufwendig Daten aufnehmen zu müssen. In einer Evaluation anhand von 12 4D-CT-Datensätzen wird die Präzision der modellbasierten Bewegungsprädiktion mithilfe der generierten optimalen mehrdimensionalen Surrogatsignale untersucht. Die Ergebnisse werden mit denen verglichen, die für die einzelnen 1D Signale, 2D Signale (1D+Ableitung) resultieren. Als alternatives mehrdimensionales Signal werden zudem Tiefenbilddaten betrachtet.

2 Material und Methoden

2.1 Diffeomorphes Framework zur Korrespondenzmodellierung

Im Folgenden wird kurz das genutzte diffeomorphe Framework zur Korrespondenzmodellierung vorgestellt. Für zusätzliche Informationen sei auf [5] verwiesen. Für jede Atemphase j eines 4D-CT-Datensatzes $(I_j)_{j \in \{1,\ldots,n_{opt}\}} : \Omega \to R \ (\Omega \subset R^3)$ liegen jeweils korrespondierende n_{sur}-dimensionale Surrogatsignalmessungen $(\xi_j)_{\in \{1,\ldots,n_{opt}\}}$ mit $\xi_j \in R^{n_{sur}}$ vor. Informationen über die Bewegungen von internen Strukturen zwischen einer Referenzatemphase I_{ref} und den restlichen Atemphasen I_j werden mit Hilfe diffeomorpher Registrierung ermittelt und durch nicht-lineare Transformationen $\varphi_j : \Omega \to \Omega$ repräsentiert. Diese Transformationen werden mittels stationärer Geschwindigkeitsfelder v_j mit $\varphi_j = \exp(v_j)$ beschrieben. Die Surrogatsignalmessungen ξ_j und die Geschwindigkeitsfelder v_j

werden nun als Zufallsvariablen $Z_j \equiv \xi_j$ und $V_j \in R^{3m}$ (m = Anzahl Bildvoxel) aufgefasst. Das diffeomorphe Korrespondenzmodell ist dann durch

$$\hat{V} = \bar{V} + B(\hat{Z} - \bar{Z}) \tag{1}$$

mit $\bar{V} = 1/n_{opt} \sum_{j=1}^{n_{opt}} V_j$ und $\bar{Z} = 1/n_{opt} \sum_{j=1}^{n_{opt}} Z_j$ gegeben und beschreibt, wie aus dem gemessenem Surrogatsignal $\hat{Z}$ das korrespondierende Geschwindigkeitsfeld $\hat{V}$ bestimmt werden kann. Die Koeffizienten der Schätzmatrix B werden mittels multivariater linearer Regression bestimmt.

2.2 Simulation von Surrogatsignalen

Für diesen Beitrag werden exemplarisch die folgenden klinisch relevanten (1D) Surrogatsignale auf Basis von 4D-CT-Datensätzen bildbasiert simuliert.

– *Spirometer:* Spirometer-basierte Messungen des Atemzugvolumens werden mittels bildbasierter Analyse des Luftinhalts der Lunge simuliert [6].
– *Bauchgurt:* Bauchgurte messen die atmungsbedingte Expansion/Kontraktion des Körpers. Die Simulation eines Bauchgurtsignals erfolgt durch Messung des Körpervolumens anhand einer Körpersegmentierung. Hierzu werden auf Höhe der gewählten Gurtposition in einer geringen Anzahl von Schichten die Körpervoxel gezählt, sodass ungefähr 1 cm der Oberfläche abgedeckt ist.
– *Zwerchfellverfolgung:* Die Bewegung des Zwerchfells, in der Praxis bestimmbar z.B. mit Fluoroskopie, wird aus der mittleren Bewegung beider Zwerchfellkuppeln in cranio-caudaler Richtung bestimmt. Die Bestimmung der Zwerchfellkuppelpositionen erfolgt subvoxelgenau mittels Kantendetektion.
– *Tiefenbildgebung:* Tiefenbildgebende Systeme (Lasersysteme, Time-of-Flight-Kameras, ...) können genutzt werden, um die atmungsbedingte Bewegung des Körpers in anterior-posteriorer Richtung zu erfassen. Hierzu wird, wie in [4] vorgeschlagen, ein virtueller Sensor oberhalb des Patienten platziert und mittels Strahlverfolgung die Körperoberfläche subvoxelgenau abgetastet. Auf diese Weise können sowohl ein- als auch mehrdimensionale Signale erzeugt werden.

2.3 Auswahl optimaler Signalkombinationen

Gegeben ein 4D-CT-Datensatz mit n_{opt} Atemphasen und eine Menge S von n_{sig} simulierten Surrogatsignalen, dann soll patientenindividuell eine Teilmenge $T_{opt} \subseteq S$ bestimmt werden, die am besten zur modellbasierten Bewegungsprädiktion nach (1) geeignet ist. Um auf Basis nur eines 4D-CT-Datensatz die Eignung einer Teilmenge U zu untersuchen, wird eine Leave-One-Out-Kreuzvalidierung durchgeführt. D.h., es werden n_{opt} Modelle erstellt, die jeweils auf Basis von n_{opt}-1 Atemphasen trainiert wurden und anschließend eingesetzt werden, um die Geschwindigkeitsfelder zwischen I_{ref} und der jeweils ausgelassenen Phase I_j vorherzusagen. Als Evaluationskriterium wird der quadratische Abstand $||V_j - \hat{V}_j^U||_2^2$ zwischen vorhergesagtem Geschwindigkeitsfeld $\hat{V}_j^U$ und dem mittels

Registierung bestimmten Geschwindigkeitsfeld V_j genutzt. Die Abstände für alle Modelle einer getesteten Teilmenge werden addiert. Das Optimierungsproblem lässt sich dann als

$$T_{\text{opt}} = \arg\min_{U \in \mathcal{P}(S)} \sum_{j=1}^{n_{\text{opt}}} ||V_j - \hat{V}_j^U||_2^2 \qquad (2)$$

schreiben, wobei $\mathcal{P}(S)$ die Potenzmenge von S ist. Als Optimierungsverfahren wird hier, wie in [7] vorgeschlagen, Sequential Forward Selection eingesetzt.

2.4 Bilddaten und Experimente

Für die Evaluation des vorgestellten Verfahrens werden 12 thorakale 4D-CT-Datensätze von Lungentumorpatienten (10-14 Atemphasen, $512 \times 512 \times 270$ Voxel, Voxelgröße ca. $1 \times 1 \times 1.5$ mm) genutzt. Es werden 6 verschiedene Surrogatsignale simuliert: Spirometer, Zwerchfellverfolgung, 3 verschiedenen Bauchgurtpositionen (oberhalb des Xiphoids (1), auf Höhe des Xiphoids (2) , unterhalb des Xiphoids (3)) und eine Punktabtastung mittels Tiefenbildgebung auf Höhe des untersten Bauchgurtes. Zu Vergleichszwecken werden aus diesen 6 1D Signalen zusätzlich 6 abgeleitete 2D Signale generiert (1D Signal+zeitliche Ableitung) und außerdem eine flächenweise Abtastung der Körperoberfläche mit 100 Samplingpunkten mittels Tiefenbildgebung simuliert. Insgesamt werden in diesem Beitrag 15 verschiedene Surrogate bzw. Surrogatkombinationen auf ihre Eignung für die Bewegungsprädiktion hin untersucht (6 1D Signale, 6 2D Signale, opt. Kombination der 1D Signale, opt. Kombination der 2D Signale, 100 Oberflächenpunkte).

Da pro Patient jeweils nur ein 4D-CT-Datensatz zur Verfügung steht, werden für alle zu testenden Surrogate bzw. Surrogatkombinationen mittels Leave-Out-Strategie drei Testszenarien gebildet, um die Präzision der Bewegungsprädiktion zu evaluieren. Für ein Extrapolationsszenario ist die Lungenbewegung zwischen maximaler Ein- (EI) und Ausatmung (EE) zu bestimmen, wobei EI als Referenzphase dient und die Phasen EE, EE+1 und EE-1 beim Modelltraining nicht berücksichtigt werden. Analog dazu werden für die zwei Interpolationsszenarien Modelle trainiert, um die Lungenbewegung zwischen EI und den Phasen der mittleren Einatmung (MI) bzw. der mittleren Ausatmung (ME) zu bestimmen. Hierfür wird entsprechend die MI-Phase/ME-Phase nicht für das Modelltraining genutzt. Zur quantitativen Beurteilung der Prädikationsgenauigkeit wird der Target-Registration-Error (TRE) basierend auf manuellen Landmarkenkorrespondenzen innerhalb der Lunge ermittelt (ca. 70 Landmarken pro Patient).

3 Ergebnisse

Die Ergebnisse der Experimente sind in Tab. 1 dargestellt. Die einzelnen 1D Signale liefern im Mittel sehr ähnliche Ergebnisse. Die meisten Unterschiede zwischen den 1D Signalen sind nicht statistisch signifikant (zweiseitiger, gepaarter t-Test mit Signifikanzniveau $p < 0.05$). Gleiches gilt auch für die Unterschiede zwischen den 2D Signalen. Eine Erhöhung der Dimensionalität von 1D auf 2D

Tabelle 1. Prädiktionsergebnisse der verschiedenen Surrogate und der automatisch generierten Kombination für die gesamte Lunge (TRE) in mm. Siehe Text für Erläuterungen. Die Ergebnisse sind gemittelt über alle Patienten angegeben als $\mu \pm \sigma$.

Phase	TRE für EE	TRE für MI	TRE für ME
ohne Bewegungsschätzung	6.59 ± 1.70	4.72 ± 1.10	2.46 ± 0.53
Intrapatienten-Registierung	1.35 ± 0.16	1.55 ± 0.12	1.49 ± 0.16
Surrogatbasierte Bewegungsprädiktion mittels 1D Signal:			
1) Spirometer	1.89 ± 0.41	2.03 ± 0.28	1.72 ± 0.20
2) Zwerchfellbewegung	1.90 ± 0.25	2.03 ± 0.29	1.78 ± 0.25
3) Bauchgurt(1)	2.52 ± 1.26	2.23 ± 0.53	1.89 ± 0.45
4) Bauchgurt(2)	2.85 ± 1.59	2.31 ± 0.70	2.10 ± 0.83
5) Bauchgurt(3)	1.85 ± 0.28	2.05 ± 0.28	1.85 ± 0.28
6) Oberflächenpunkt	1.86 ± 0.34	2.05 ± 0.28 '	1.81 ± 0.18
opt. Kombination vom 1D Signalen	1.85 ± 0.28	1.80 ± 0.22	1.73 ± 0.26
Surrogatbasierte Bewegungsprädiktion mittels 2D Signal (1D+Ableitung):			
1) Spirometer + Ableitung	1.86 ± 0.39	1.82 ± 0.16	1.66 ± 0.14
2) Zwerchfellbewegung + Ableitung	1.86 ± 0.24	1.80 ± 0.16	1.70 ± 0.16
3) Bauchgurt(1) + Ableitung	2.47 ± 1.16	2.28 ± 0.75	2.15 ± 1.08
4) Bauchgurt(2) + Ableitung	2.49 ± 1.20	2.02 ± 0.64	1.92 ± 0.45
4) Bauchgurt(3) + Ableitung	1.84 ± 0.28	1.77 ± 0.13	1.70 ± 0.16
5) Oberflächenpunkt + Ableitung	1.84 ± 0.33	1.79 ± 0.16	1.68 ± 0.13
opt. Kombination von 2D Signalen	1.85 ± 0.34	1.72 ± 0.13	1.69 ± 0.17
Bewegungsprädiktion mittels hochdimensionaler Oberflächenabtastung:			
100 Oberflächenpunkte	1.72 ± 0.28	1.75 ± 0.24	1.67 ± 0.16

durch Nutzung der zeitlichen Ableitung führt für alle Signale außer Bauchgurt (1) und (2) zu statistisch signifikant besseren Ergebnissen bei den Interpolationsszenarien. Für die optimalen Signalkombinationen wurden bei den 1D Signalen/2D Signalen durchschnittlich 3 Surrogate/2 Surrogate kombiniert. Durch Nutzung der kombinierten Surrogatsignale ergeben sich in den meisten Fällen im Durchschnitt (leicht) verbesserte Ergebnisse, verglichen mit den Ergebnissen der 1D und 2D Einzelsignale. Allerdings ist nur das für die optimale Kombination von 1D Signalen angegebene Ergebnis des Interpolationsszenarios MI statistisch signifikant besser als die Ergebnisse aller Einzelsignale. Für die Interpolationsszenarien sind die Ergebnisse der optimalen Surrogatsignale und die mittels Abtastung von 100 Oberflächenpunkten erreichten Ergebnisse gleichwertig (Unterschiede nicht stat. signifikant). Bezogen auf einzelne Patienten lassen sich auch weitere signifikante Unterschiede zwischen Einzelsignalen und kombinierten Signalen feststellen. Weiterhin lässt sich feststellen, dass die automatische Signalauswahl zwischen den drei Testszenarien unterschiedliche Surrogatteilmengen als optimale Kombination zurückliefert für Patient 11 wurden z.B : 1,3 (EE); 1,5 (MI); 1,2,5,6 (ME) ausgewählt (Nummerierung der Surrogate siehe Tab. 1).

4   Diskussion

In diesem Beitrag wurde eine Verfahren zur automatischen Auswahl patienten-individuell optimaler Kombinationen von (1D) Signalen verschiedener Surrogate zu mehrdimensionalen Atemsignalen für die modellbasierte Prädiktion atmungsbedingter Bewegungen vorgestellt und mit anderen Methoden zur Generierung mehrdimensionaler Atemsignale (abgeleitete Signale und hochdimensionale Tiefenbilddaten) verglichen. Die Ergebnisse bestätigen Erkenntnisse anderer Arbeiten [3, 4], dass durch die Nutzung mehrdimensionaler statt eindimensionaler Atemsignale eine signifikante Verbesserung der Bewegungsprädiktion möglich ist. Zwischen den Ergebnissen der drei verglichenen Methoden zur Generierung mehrdimensionaler Atemsignale haben sich zumeist nur geringe Unterschiede gezeigt. Bezogen auf das Potenzial des hier vorgestellten Kombinationsverfahrens lässt sich festhalten, dass durch die Kombination von durchschnittlich drei 1D Surrogatsignalen zumeist Ergebnisse erreicht werden konnten, die denen einer Prädiktion mittels hochdimensionaler Tiefenbilddaten gleichwertig sind. Die beobachteten Unterschiede in der optimalen Surrogatauswahl für die drei pro Patient getesteten Szenarien zeigen allerdings, dass weitere Untersuchungen auch im Hinblick auf die verwendete Auswahlmetrik notwendig sind. Durch die auftretenden Unterschiede zwischen den drei Szenarien bei der Surrogatauswahl lassen sich keine Surrogatkombinationen benennen, die in der Praxis grundsätzlich zur Prädiktion gewählt werden sollten. Zusätzliche Untersuchungen (mit realen Signalen) sind nötig, um weitere Aussagen bezüglich möglicher Unterschiede der drei verglichenen Methoden treffen zu können.

Danksagung. Die Arbeit wurde von der DFG gefördert (HA 2355/9-2). ·

Literaturverzeichnis

1. Keall PJ, Mageras GS, Balter JM, et al. The management of respiratory motion in radiation oncology report of AAPM Task Group 76. Med Phys. 2006;33:3874–900.
2. McClelland JR, Hawkes DJ, Schaeffter T, et al. Respiratory motion models: a review. Med Image Anal. 2012; p. 19–42.
3. Savill F, Schaeffter T, King AP. Assessment of input signal positioning for cardiac respiratory motion models during different breathing petterns. Proc ISBI. 2011; p. 1698–701.
4. Blendowski M, Wilms M, Werner R, et al. Simulation und Evaluation tiefenbildgebender Verfahren zur Prädiktion atmungsbedingter Organ- und Tumorbewegungen. Proc BVM. 2012; p. 350–5.
5. Werner R, Wilms M, Ehrhardt J, et al. A diffeomorphic MLR framework for surrogate-based motion estimation and situation-adapted dose accumulation. Proc MICCAI. 2012; p. 42–9.
6. Lu W, Parikh PJ, Naqa IME, et al. Quantitation of the reconstruction quality of a four-dimensional computed tomography process for lung cancer patients. Med Phys. 2005;32:890–901.
7. Wu Q, Chung AJ, Yang GZ. Optimal sensor placement for predictive cardiac motion modeling. Proc MICCAI. 2006; p. 512–9.

Comparison of Super-Resolution Methods for HD-Video Endoscopy

M. Häfner[1], M. Liedlgruber[2], A. Uhl[2]

[1]Department for Internal Medicine, St. Elisabeth Hospital, Vienna
[2]Department of Computer Sciences, University of Salzburg, Austria
mliedl@cosy.sbg.ac.at

Abstract. The main question we try to answer in this work is whether it is feasible to employ super-resolution (SR) algorithms to increase the spatial resolution of endoscopic high-definition (HD) images in order to reveal new details which may have got lost due to the limited endoscope magnification of the HD endoscope used (e.g. mucosal structures).
For this purpose we compare the quality achieved of different SR methods. This is done on standard test images as well as on images obtained from endoscopic video frames. We also investigate whether compression artifacts have a noticeable effect on the SR results.
We show that, due to several limitations in case of endoscopic videos, we are not consistently able to achieve a higher visual quality when using SR algorithms instead of bicubic interpolation.

1 Introduction

Throughout the past years different approaches aiming at the classification of colonic polyps have been developed. Most of these works are based on traditional endoscopes. But there also exists work based on zoom-endoscopes equipped with an optical zoom [1]. Such endoscopes are advantageous as they allow to inspect the colonic mucosa in a magnified manner, revealing the fine surface structure of the mucosa and small lesions. However, throughout the past few years high-definition (HD) endoscopes got more and more popular. While providing a roughly four times higher image resolution as compared to many zoom-endoscopes, they are often not equipped with an optical zoom.

One possible way to unveil more details from such HD images is to use super-resolution (SR) algorithms. There already exists a work in which an SR method is applied to wireless capsule endoscopy video frames [2]. In this work the authors test their algorithm on low-resolution (LR) images generated from a single video frame by shifting it into different directions and downscaling the shifted frames. But this does not reflect a realistic application scenario.

Hence, the main question we try to answer in this work is whether it is feasible to use SR algorithms to increase the resolution of endoscopic HD images and reveal new details. Fig. 1 shows two tubulovillous adenoma, one captured with a zoom-endoscope and one captured with an HD endoscope without zoom. The dramatic difference between these images in terms of visible details is obvious.

While we can not expect high-resolution (HR) images generated by SR methods to be comparable to the ones obtained with zoom-endoscopes, we at least hope to be able to increase the level of detail in HD images. For this purpose we evaluate a set of SR methods on real-world HD endoscopy videos. Since these are compressed, they also suffer from compression artifacts. Thus, we also investigate the impact of such artifacts on the SR quality of the algorithms evaluated using deblocking on the video sequences. We also carry out experiments using uncompressed videos.

Throughout literature many SR algorithms are evaluated on artificially generated LR images only. That is, although real-world video test sequences are available, the respective sequences are subject to blur and downsampling to generate LR frames [2]. These frames are then used to reconstruct an HR image. While this is a practical way to assess if an algorithm works (i.e. an accurate quality assessment is possible since the HR ground truth is available), this hardly matches real-world scenarios.

Since our aim is to reveal new details in endoscopy videos, it is not meaningful to evaluate SR algorithms on artificially generated LR frames. We thus apply SR algorithms to HD videos frames. Doing so, we face different problems:

– Compression artifacts: Although there exists work which specifically aims at SR for videos [2], these algorithms are quite often evaluated only on uncompressed sequences. Since HD videos would require a fairly high amount of storage if stored uncompressed, they are usually compressed. This comes at the price of sometimes clearly noticeable compression artifacts (e.g. 8 × 8 DCT blocks). To get an idea of how these artifacts influence the SR reconstruction quality, we also carry out experiments with sequences which have been deblocked using the method described in [3].

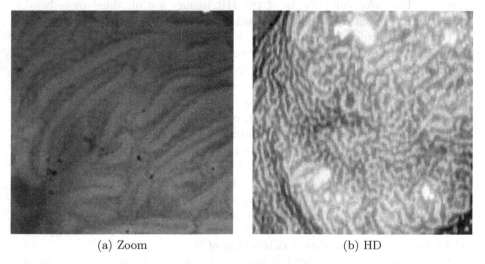

(a) Zoom   (b) HD

Fig. 1. Illustration of the difference between two different imaging modalities.

- Lack of aliasing artifacts: The images we used in this work show a lack of aliasing artifacts. One reason for this is that the videos are compressed. To investigate whether SR algorithms produce better results on uncompressed videos we will also examine different algorithms on endoscopic videos sequences which have not been compressed.

  In addition, since in endoscopic images there are usually no sharp edges (i.e. high frequency content) which may result in aliasing artifacts due to undersampling, it is clear that our images do not expose clearly noticeable aliasing. Another cause may be the presence of noise and blur, caused by the sensor and small camera movements.

- Complex motion: Since in endoscopic videos we are facing highly complex motion (e.g. position-variant transformations) simple motion models fail to describe the motion between successive HD endoscopy video frames.

  As a consequence we use an optical flow method [4]. Such methods are more versatile when it comes to the estimation of arbitrary complex motion between images. This is mainly due to the fact that optical flow methods allow to estimate local motion, while simpler methods usually work well only with global motion. In our case this task is hindered to some extent by compression artifacts and a lack of aliasing artifacts.

2 Materials and methods

To be able to assess whether SR with endoscopy images is feasible, we carried out experiments using different SR methods. These are Shift-and-Add (S&A) [5], regularized super-resolution (ROB) [6], iterated back-projection (IBP) [7], and robust super-resolution (ROBZ) [8]. Although the LR images used are color images, we apply the SR algorithms only to the intensity component in the CIELAB color space since this channel usually contributes most to textural features. The color components of the HR images are obtained by a bicubic upscaling of the first frame of the respective LR sequence.

For our experiments we evaluated the SR algorithms on two different sets of LR image sequences: widely used sequences and sequences extracted from endoscopic videos. For all sequences we always use eight LR frames and an upscaling factor of two for the SR algorithms. The endoscopic sequences are based on successive frames of videos acquired during colonoscopy sessions between the years 2011 and 2012 at the Department for Internal Medicine (St. Elisabeth Hospital, Vienna) using an HD colonoscope (Pentax HiLINE HD+ 90i Colonoscope) with a resolution of 1280 × 1024 pixels. To reduce the computational demand for the SR methods we chose positions from which we manually extracted 256 × 256-pixel patches which serve as LR images (the position remained the same in case of a single sequence). Details on the LR sequences used can be found in Tab. 1. As we notice from this table, experiments with two endoscopy videos without compression have also been conducted (U1 and U2). Furthermore, the sequences D1-D5 have been obtained by a deblocking of E1-E5.

Due to the lack of reference HR images in case of endoscopic images, we use two reference-free quality metrics. The first metric used is called BRISQUE [9].

Table 1. Details on our LR image sets used ("Compr." and "Debl." indicate the sequences which are compressed and subject to deblocking, respectively).

Name	ID	Color	Compr.	Debl.	Name	ID	Color	Compr.	Debl.
Carphone	R1	Y	N	N	Endoscopy 5	E5	Y	Y	N
City	R2	Y	N	N	Endoscopy 6	D1	Y	Y	Y
Container	R3	Y	N	N	Endoscopy 7	D2	Y	Y	Y
Garden	R4	Y	N	N	Endoscopy 8	D3	Y	Y	Y
Mobile	R5	Y	N	N	Endoscopy 9	D4	Y	Y	Y
Endoscopy 1	E1	Y	Y	N	Endoscopy 10	D5	Y	Y	Y
Endoscopy 2	E2	Y	Y	N	Endoscopy 11	U1	Y	N	N
Endoscopy 3	E3	Y	Y	N	Endoscopy 12	U2	Y	N	N
Endoscopy 4	E4	Y	Y	N					

It is a so-called natural scene statistics-based approach, which computes statistical features based on edge responses at different scales. Based on the features for the training set, support vector regression (ϵ-SVR) is used to learn a mapping from feature space to quality scores. The learned model is then used to predict the quality score for a new image with an unknown quality. For the training we generated a different set of sequences (similar to the ones in Tab. 1). This set has been rated by eight human raters. Based on these ratings, the differential mean opinion score (DMOS) was computed (using the median instead of the mean to be resistant against outlier ratings), which is used for the training.

The second metric measures the entropy within an image for different directions [10]. This is done by first computing the discrete Pseudo-Wigner distribution for an image. Then, an approximate PDF is computed, for which the pixel-wise Rény-entropy is computed. By repeating these computations for different directions and taking the mean over all entropy values for each direction considered, an anisotropic entropy measure for an image is obtained.

For both metrics a higher score indicates a higher quality. For BRISQUE the score is usually in the range 0 to 100 (some scores may leave this range due to SR reconstruction results not represented appropriately in the training set).

To assess whether the SR methods produce useful results, we also create an upscaled image from the first image of each sequence using bicubic interpolation, for which we also compute quality scores.

3   Results

Tab. 2 shows the results obtained. The anisotropic scores have been multiplied by 10^4 due to the small values originally yielded. According to these scores, the methods IBP and ROBZ almost always produce results of higher quality than INT. For sequences R1-R5 all SR methods are able to improve the visual quality. In case of sequences E1-E5, the methods S&A and ROB sometimes yield a score below the INT score. The overall picture is very similar for the deblocked

Table 2. Detailed metric results for the SR algorithms (INT denotes interpolation).

	Anisotropic					BRISQUE			
ID	INT	S&A	IBP	ROB	ROBZ	INT	S&A	IBP	ROB	ROBZ
---	---	---	---	---	---	---	---	---	---	---
R1	25.8	55.4	61.8	46.7	59.8	51.3	45.0	62.0	52.4	65.5
R2	10.6	21.6	31.2	19.8	29.9	32.6	47.1	40.3	26.5	42.8
R3	39.6	106.7	67.2	97.7	67.0	28.6	12.8	36.0	-9.3	37.5
R4	59.2	86.3	109.7	69.8	103.0	52.4	48.6	23.5	14.6	30.3
R5	37.8	49.9	66.3	39.8	63.0	38.2	52.1	23.4	-13.7	25.3
E1	75.0	68.7	105.4	117.8	94.1	49.2	45.9	31.1	32.9	41.9
E2	14.0	15.8	23.9	15.2	22.4	48.4	35.5	24.3	37.5	36.1
E3	10.1	7.7	18.9	9.4	16.7	49.8	49.0	25.1	51.4	29.3
E4	40.2	32.0	68.2	36.3	59.9	49.3	52.7	26.6	56.5	37.0
E5	90.2	86.6	124.8	83.3	118.1	51.2	36.8	28.9	41.3	37.4
D1	66.1	62.6	92.8	118.6	84.1	49.1	46.0	31.9	23.8	41.9
D2	12.9	14.4	21.1	14.1	20.5	50.2	36.0	26.3	36.8	40.6
D3	8.8	6.8	16.1	7.9	14.5	47.9	47.8	24.9	49.3	32.0
D4	34.7	29.5	59.6	32.6	51.7	48.7	51.4	28.1	56.6	39.1
D5	85.7	83.1	120.9	80.2	111.5	52.9	38.8	30.4	41.2	41.8
U1	18.1	12.8	30.8	17.9	27.2	50.6	46.3	28.9	15.6	30.6
U2	47.5	39.5	105.8	57.5	80.6	53.7	48.3	37.6	27.1	41.6

sequences D1-D5. The combinations of SR methods and sequences, showing an improvement over INT, highly correlate with the respective combinations in case of sequences E1-E5. Interestingly, deblocking almost always lowers the scores (in case of INT as well as in case of the SR methods). For the uncompressed videos the SR algorithms sometimes yield a higher score than INT, but not always.

The BRISQUE scores are quite different. Comparing the scores for the SR results with the INT scores shows that SR rarely improves the image quality. This accounts to all image sequences. Regarding E1-E5, we observe a higher score for SR in three cases only. These are the same combinations of SR methods and sequences for which a higher score is yielded by BRISQUE as compared to INT in case of the sequences D1-D5. While deblocking sometimes lowers the scores, this happens not as often as in case of the anisotropic metric. The SR scores for sequences U1-U2 are always below the scores for INT.

The bottom line is that the scores yielded by the metrics are quite different. While the anisotropic measure seems to detect an improvement by SR methods as compared to INT quite often, this is not the case for BRISQUE. According to the anisotropic measure, at least the IBP and ROBZ methods are always able to produce high quality SR results. For BRISQUE such a trend is not observable. When using deblocking the metrics behave slightly different. While the anisotropic metric almost always shows a lowered score, in case of BRISQUE about 30%

of the combinations yield a higher score. Moreover, the ROBZ method always yields a higher BRISQUE score after deblocking.

4 Discussion

Our experimental results indicate that it highly depends on the quality metric used for image quality assessment whether SR algorithms seem to deliver a higher quality than a bicubic interpolation. We have also shown that a deblocking in case of endoscopic videos – at least for the sequences used in this work – has no positive impact on the visual quality of the SR outcomes. In contrast, we have shown, that the deblocking consistently lowers the quality. This may be attributed to a lack of aliasing artifacts in endoscopic images, which gets even worse when deblocking is applied (due to an additional smoothing of details). This is also supported by the fact that even in case of uncompressed videos SR algorithms seldom deliver a higher quality as compared to an interpolation.

In future work we therefore plan to conduct a study with physicians, routinely performing endoscopy, to perform subjective tests. This will provide a solid basis to assess the real quality of the SR results obtained. We will also investigate how SR algorithms affect diagnostic performance.

Acknowledgement.   This work is partially funded the Austrian Science Fund (FWF) under Project No. TRP-206.

References

1. Tischendorf JJW, Gross S, Winograd R, et al.   Computer-aided classification of colorectal polyps based on vascular patterns: a pilot study.   Endoscopy. 2010;42(3):203–7.
2. Duda K, Zieliński T, Duplaga M. Computationally simple super-resolution algorithm for video from endoscopic capsule. Proc ICSES. 2008; p. 197–200.
3. List P, Joch A, Lainema J, et al. Adaptive Deblocking Filter. IEEE Trans Circuits Syst Video Technol. 2003;13(7):614–9.
4. Liu C. Beyond pixels: exploring new representations and applications for motion analysis [dissertation]. Massachusetts Institute of Technology; 2009.
5. Elad M.   A fast super-resolution reconstruction algorithm for pure translational motion and common space-invariant blur.   IEEE Trans Image Process. 2001;10(8):1187–93.
6. Farsiu S, Robinson D, Elad M, et al. Advances and challenges in super-resolution. Int J Imaging Syst Technol. 2004;14(2):47–57.
7. Irani M, Peleg S. Improving resolution by image registration. Comp Vis Graph Image Process. 1991 Apr;53(3):231–9.
8. Zomet A, Rav-Acha A, Peleg S. Robust super-resolution. Proc IEEE. 2001;1:645–50.
9. Mittal A, Moorthy AK, Bovik AC. No-reference image quality assessment in the spatial domain. IEEE Trans Image Process. 2012;21(12):4695–708.
10. Gabarda S, Cristóbal G. Blind image quality assessment through anisotropy. J Opt Soc Am A. 2007;24(12):B42–51.

Outlier Detection for Multi-Sensor Super-Resolution in Hybrid 3D Endoscopy

Thomas Köhler[1,2], Sven Haase[1], Sebastian Bauer[1], Jakob Wasza[1],
Thomas Kilgus[3], Lena Maier-Hein[3], Hubertus Feußner[4], Joachim Hornegger[1,2]

[1]Pattern Recognition Lab, FAU Erlangen-Nürnberg
[2]Erlangen Graduate School in Advanced Optical Technologies (SAOT)
[3]Division of Medical and Biological Informatics, DKFZ Heidelberg
[4]Research Group Minimally-invasive Interdisciplinary Therapeutical Intervention,
TU München
thomas.koehler@fau.de

Abstract. In hybrid 3D endoscopy, range data is used to augment photometric information for minimally invasive surgery. As range sensors suffer from a rough spatial resolution and a low signal-to-noise ratio, subpixel motion between multiple range images is used as a cue for super-resolution to obtain reliable range data. Unfortunately, this method is sensitive to outliers in range images and the estimated subpixel displacements. In this paper, we propose an outlier detection scheme for robust super-resolution. First, we derive confidence maps to identify outliers in the displacement fields by correlation analysis of photometric data. Second, we apply an iteratively re-weighted least squares algorithm to obtain the associated range confidence maps. The joint confidence map is used to obtain super-resolved range data. We evaluate our approach on synthetic images and phantom data acquired by a Time-of-Flight/RGB endoscope. Our outlire detection improves the median peak-signal-to-noise ratio by 1.1 dB.

1 Introduction

In hybrid 3D endoscopy, photometric information is augmented with 3D data provided by range imaging (RI) sensors, e.g. based on Time-of-Flight (ToF) imaging [1]. While range data is essential for robotic-based interventions, photometric data provides color and texture of tissue to enhance an intuitive representation of the underlying scene. However, a serious issue towards clinical applications is the limited spatial resolution and the low signal-to-noise ratio (SNR) of todays range sensors. Super-resolution algorithms reconstruct a high-resolution (HR) image from multiple low-resolution (LR) frames by exploiting subpixel displacements present in an image sequence [2]. This approach has recently been introduced to RI in image-guided surgery [3]. For an improved reconstruction, Köhler et al. [4] proposed a super-resolution framework for a multi-sensor setup. In this approach, photometric data is utilized for optical flow estimation to derive displacement fields for the associated range images.

Due to the increased accuracy of motion estimation on photometric data this yields accurate super-resolved range data. However, the method relies entirely on optical flow estimation and is susceptible to mis-registration in difficult scenarios such as large displacements caused by sizable non-rigid deformations of tissue or independent moving objects. Additionally, range data is disturbed by outliers, e.g. due to specular highlights. There are two strategies to deal with such outliers: (i) Error models accounting for outliers can be utilized for super-resolution. This results in an optimization problem involving robust error norms [5]. (ii) Outliers can be removed before super-resolution is performed. This can be achieved using image similarity metrics to identify outliers caused by erroneous motion estimation [6].

Both approaches focus on a single modality without exploiting additional guidance by different modalities in hybrid imaging. To overcome this issue, we propose outlier detection for multi-sensor super-resolution. Our method identifies outliers in displacement fields as well as in LR range data. For robust super-resolution, we derive confidence maps using image similarity and an iterative scheme to assign less weights to imputed outliers. The performance of our method is demonstrated in hybrid 3D endoscopy to super-resolve range data.

2 Materials and methods

Super-resolution is applied to range images $y^{(1)}, \ldots, y^{(K)}$ where each $y^{(k)} \in \mathbb{R}^M$ is represented as a vector. Due to movements of the camera or motion in the underlying scene, each $y^{(k)}$ is related to a reference frame $y^{(r)}$ by a geometric transformation. For each range image $y^{(k)}$, there exists an optical image $z^{(k)}$ acquired simultaneously to encode photometric information in a hybrid imaging setup.

2.1 Multi-sensor super-resolution

The objective of multi-sensor super-resolution is to reconstruct a super-resolved range image $\hat{x} \in \mathbb{R}^N$ with $N > M$ from $y^{(1)}, \ldots, y^{(K)}$ according to

$$\hat{x} = \arg\min_{x} \sum_{i} \beta_i \, |r_i(x)|^p + \lambda R(x) \tag{1}$$

where $r : \mathbb{R}^N \to \mathbb{R}^{KM}$ denotes a residual term employed in the underlying error model based on the L_p norm and $\beta \in \mathbb{R}^{KM}$ is a confidence map to weight the residual element-wise. For the regularizer $R(x)$ with weight $\lambda > 0$, the edge-preserving Huber prior is employed. We set $r(x) = (r^{(1)}, \ldots, r^{(K)})^\top$ and the residual of the kth frame $y^{(k)}$ is given as

$$r^{(k)} = y^{(k)} - \gamma_m^{(k)} W^{(k)} x - \gamma_a^{(k)} 1 \tag{2}$$

where $W^{(k)}$, $\gamma_m^{(k)}$ and $\gamma_a^{(k)}$ denote the system matrix and the associated range correction factors for the kth frame and $1 \in \mathbb{R}^M$ is the all-one vector. In a multi-sensor approach, $W^{(k)}$ encodes downsampling, the range sensor point spread

function (PSF) and 2D geometric displacements derived from optical flow estimated on photometric data. The parameters $\gamma_m^{(k)}$ and $\gamma_a^{(k)}$ are determined by a
range correction scheme to account for out-of-plane motion [4].

2.2 Outlier detection

The confidence map $\boldsymbol{\beta}$ in (1) is composed element-wise as $\beta_i = \beta_{r,i} \cdot \beta_{z,i}$. Here,
$\boldsymbol{\beta}_r$ is chosen to suppress outliers in range data. The confidence map $\boldsymbol{\beta}_z$ weights
outliers in the associated displacement fields. The confidence maps are derived
by image similarity analysis and an iterative outlier detection procedure.

We detect outliers in displacement vector fields provided by optical flow in the
domain of the photometric data. Therefore, the reference frame $\boldsymbol{z}^{(r)}$ is aligned
with each frame $\boldsymbol{z}^{(k)}$ according to the estimated displacements. Afterwards, we
analyze the similarity between the warped reference $\tilde{\boldsymbol{z}}^{(r)}$ and each frame $\boldsymbol{z}^{(k)}$.
In this paper, we employ the normalized cross-correlation (NCC) as similarity
metric patch-wise to derive the confidence map $\boldsymbol{\beta}_z$ according to

$$\beta_{z,i} = \frac{\sum_{v \in \mathcal{N}(u_i)} (z^{(k)}(v) - \bar{z}^{(k)})(\tilde{z}^{(r)}(v) - \bar{z}^{(r)})}{\sqrt{\sum_{v \in \mathcal{N}(u_i)} (z^{(k)}(v) - \bar{z}^{(k)})^2} \sqrt{\sum_{v \in \mathcal{N}(u_i)} (\tilde{z}^{(r)}(v) - \bar{z}^{(r)})^2}} \tag{3}$$

where $\mathcal{N}(u_i)$ denotes the local neighborhood formed by the set of pixels in the
photometric data associated with the ith pixel u_i in the range images, and $\bar{z}^{(k)}$
and $\bar{z}^{(r)}$ are the local means in $\mathcal{N}(u_i)$ for the kth frame and the reference,
respectively. For $\beta_{z,i} < \varepsilon_z$, we set $\beta_{z,i} = 0$ to reject u_i as an outlier where ε_z
is adjusted to the noise level of photometric data. The confidence map $\boldsymbol{\beta}_z$ is
transformed to the domain of LR range data. This approach is similar to [6],
whereas in our work outliers are detected in photometric data instead of using
LR data directly.

While displacement outliers are removed based on photometric data exploited
as guidance, outliers in depth data must be detected in range images directly.
Therefore, we propose an iterative re-weighted least squares (IRLS) scheme [7] to
derive the confidence map $\boldsymbol{\beta}_r$. Let $\boldsymbol{x}^{(0)}$ be the super-resolved image as solution
of (1) using the confidence maps $\boldsymbol{\beta}_r^{(0)} = 1$ and $\boldsymbol{\beta}_z$ determined according to (3).
For $p = 2$, this is done by common least squares optimization such as a scaled
conjugate gradient (SCG) algorithm. Then, the residual $\boldsymbol{r}^{(0)} = r(\boldsymbol{x}^{(0)})$ given by
(2) is used to derive the range confidence as

$$\beta_{r,i}^{(0)} = \begin{cases} 1 & \text{if } |r_i^{(0)}| \leq \varepsilon_r \\ \frac{\varepsilon_r}{|r_i^{(0)}|} & \text{otherwise} \end{cases} \tag{4}$$

We set $\varepsilon_r = \sigma_r$ for the residual standard deviation σ_r. Therefore, we employ
the robust estimator $\sigma_r = 1.4826 \cdot \text{MAD}$ based on the median absolute deviation
$\text{MAD} = \text{Median}_i(|r_i - \text{Median}_i(r_i)|)$. The confidence map $\boldsymbol{\beta}_r$ and the super-
resolved data $\boldsymbol{x}$ are iteratively updated in IRLS:

1. Initialize range confidence map $\beta_{r,i}^{(0)} = 1$ for $i = 1, \ldots, KM$ and $t = 0$.
2. Determine residual term $r^{(t)} = r(x^{(t-1)})$ according to (2).
3. Set $\beta_i^{(t)} = \beta_{r,i}^{(t)} \cdot \beta_{z,i}$ with β_z according to (3) and $\beta_r^{(t)}$ according to (4).
4. Solve for $x^{(t)}$ with $p = 2$ according to (1) using SCG optimization $x^{(t)} = \arg\min_x \left\{ \sum_i \beta_i^{(t)} r(x)^2 + \lambda R(x) \right\}$
5. Set $t \leftarrow t + 1$ and proceed with step 2 until convergence.

2.3 Experiments

We compared the proposed multi-sensor super-resolution (MSR) to the approach using the L_2 norm model introduced in [4]. Additionally, we evaluated MSR based on L_2 norm with outlier detection on LR data [6] and MSR using a robust L_1 norm model [5]. Motion estimation and regularization was realized analogous to [4]. $K = 31$ frames were used to achieve a magnification of 4. We approximated the PSF as a Gaussian of width $\sigma = 0.2$. For outlier detection, we set $\varepsilon_z = 0.8$. Supplementary material for our experiments is available on our web page[1].

First, RGB images (640×480 px) and LR range data (64×48 px) were obtained from a laparoscopic model using an RI simulator. Range data was affected by distance-dependent Gaussian noise (max. $\sigma_n = 10$ mm) and Gaussian blur ($\sigma_b = 3$ mm). Perlin noise was induced to simulate invalid ToF measurements caused by specular highlights. We simulated flying pixels in range data by randomly flipping 20% of all edge pixels. In terms of motion, we generated four data sets (S1 – S4): Small random motion of the virtual camera was used to simulate a jitter of a hand-held endoscope (S1). The endoscope was displaced to slightly different viewing directions (S2). Surgical tools were shifted (S3). Organ surfaces were moved to simulate respiratory motion (S4). Super-resolved data was assessed by comparison to a ground truth using the peak-signal-to-noise ratio (PSNR) and structural similarity (SSIM). Second, we measured a liver phantom with a ToF/RGB endoscope prototype manufactured by Richard Wolf GmbH, Knittlingen, Germany. Image data was captured with a frame rate of 30 Hz in the same spatial resolution as synthetic data. During acquisition the endoscope was moved relative to the liver and tools were moved due to a jitter of the hand.

3 Results

Qualitative results for synthetic data is presented in Fig. 1. If no outlier detection was employed, super-resolved data contained artifacts due to mis-registrations. PSNR and SSIM was evaluated for ten sequences per data set using sliding window processing and is shown as boxplot in Fig. 2. We obtained median values of 33.4 dB for PSNR and 0.94 for SSIM in the absence of outlier detection. The proposed method improved the median PSNR (SSIM) by 1.1 dB (0.01). Our

---

[1] http://www5.cs.fau.de/research/data/

Fig. 1. Synthetic RGB (a) and range data (b): Multi-sensor super-resolution (MSR) using L_2 norm model without (c) and with outlier detection (d), based on L_1 norm model (e) and our method (f) compared to the ground truth (g).

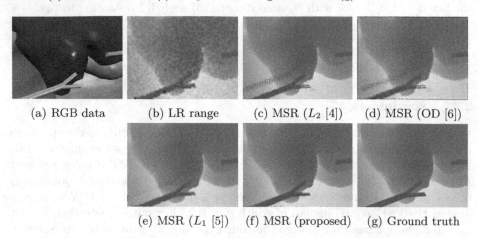

(a) RGB data   (b) LR range   (c) MSR (L_2 [4])   (d) MSR (OD [6])

(e) MSR (L_1 [5])   (f) MSR (proposed)   (g) Ground truth

approach also outperformed outlier detection on LR data and L_1 norm based super-resolution. For phantom data, super-resolved range images are presented in Fig. 3. In our experiments, mis-registrations for endoscopic tools caused artifacts in the super-resolved image if outlier detection was not employed. These artifacts were still present in case of outlier detection on LR data and the L_1 norm approach but well suppressed using the proposed method.

4   Discussion

In this work, we proposed an outlier detection scheme for robust multi-sensor super-resolution. Our approach detects outliers in range data and the associated displacement fields to obtain reliable range data for hybrid 3D endoscopy. The proposed method outperforms outlier detection based on LR data only and exploits photometric data as guidance. Compared to super-resolution using an L_1

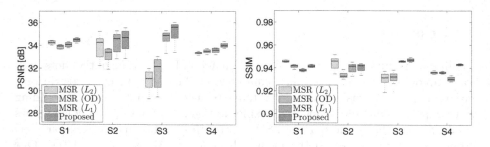

Fig. 2. Boxplots of peak-signal-to-noise ratio (PSNR) and structural similarity (SSIM) created for ten sequences per data set using sliding window processing.

Fig. 3. RGB (a) and range data (b) obtained from a liver phantom with the results of multi-sensor super-resolution (MSR) using L_2 norm model without (c) and with outlier detection (d), based on L_1 norm model (e) and our method (f).

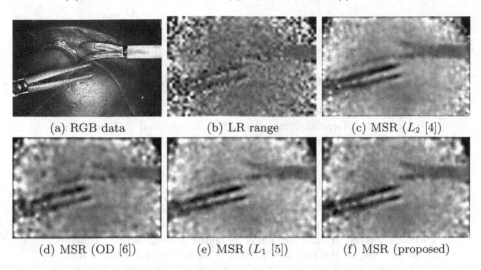

(a) RGB data   (b) LR range   (c) MSR (L_2 [4])

(d) MSR (OD [6])   (e) MSR (L_1 [5])   (f) MSR (proposed)

norm model, our method achieves improved robustness under real conditions on phantom data and improved results in terms of PSNR and SSIM on synthetic data. Future work will focus on the integration of different weighting schemes to our outlier detection and a combination of IRLS with L_1 norm optimization.

Acknowledgement. This work is supported by the Graduate School of Information Science in Health (GSISH), the TUM Graduate School, the German National Science Foundation (DFG-HO 1791/7-1), and Metrilus GmbH.

References

1. Haase S, Forman C, Kilgus T, et al. ToF/RGB sensor fusion for 3-D endoscopy. Curr Med Imaging Rev. 2013;9:113–9.
2. Park SC, Park MK, Kang MG. Super-resolution image reconstruction: a technical overview. IEEE Signal Process Mag. 2003;20(3):21–36.
3. Wetzl J, Taubmann O, Haase S, et al. GPU-Accelerated time-of-flight super-resolution for image-guided surgery. Proc BVM. 2013; p. 21–6.
4. Köhler T, Haase S, Bauer S, et al. ToF meets RGB: novel multi-sensor super-resolution for hybrid 3-D Endoscopy. Proc MICCAI. 2013;8149:139–46.
5. Farsiu S, Robinson MD, Elad M, et al. Fast and robust multiframe super resolution. IEEE Trans Image Process. 2004;13(10):1327–44.
6. Zhao W, Sawhney HS. Is super-resolution with optical flow feasible? Proc ECCV. 2002;2350:599–613.
7. Scales JA, Gersztenkorn A. Robust methods in inverse theory. Inverse Probl. 1988;4(4):1071–91.

Temporal Non-Local-Means Filtering in Hybrid 3D Endoscopy

Tobias Lindenberger[1], Sven Haase[1], Jakob Wasza[1], Thomas Kilgus[3],
Lena Maier-Hein[3], Hubertus Feußner[4], Joachim Hornegger[1,2]

[1] Pattern Recognition Lab, Friedrich-Alexander-Universität Erlangen-Nürnberg
[2] Erlangen Graduate School in Advanced Optical Technologies (SAOT)
[3] Div. Medical and Biological Informatics Junior Group: Computer-assisted
Interventions, German Cancer Research Center (DKFZ) Heidelberg
[4] Minimally Invasive Therapy and Intervention, Technical University of Munich
sven.haase@fau.de

Abstract. Time-of-Flight (ToF) cameras are a novel and fast developing technology for acquiring 3D surfaces. In recent years they have gathered interest from many fields including 3D endoscopy. However, preprossessing of the obtained images is absolutely mandatory due to the low signal-to-noise ratio of current sensors. One possibility to increase image quality is the non-local-means (NLM) filter that utilizes local neighborhoods for denoising. In this paper we present an enhanced NLM filter for hybrid 3D endoscopy. The introduced filter gathers the structural information from an RGB image that shows the same scene as the range image. To cope with camera movements, we incorporate a temporal component by considering a sequence of frames. Evaluated on simulated data, the algorithm showed an improvement in range accuracy of 70% when compared to the unfiltered image.

1 Introduction

Endoscopes are an important and widely established part of modern medicine due to the many advantages they provide for clinicians and patients, e.g. less stress and infection risk. Although conventional endoscopes are common instruments, the loss of intuitive orientation complicates navigation. Here, 3D endoscopy assists the surgeon by providing metric range data of the operation site. This information can serve as input data to build applications for tool localization or risk avoidance [1, 2]. One possibility for the acquisition of 3D range data are Time-of-Flight (ToF) cameras as it was introduced by Penne et al. [3] for minimally invasive surgery. These cameras are capable of acquiring range images with constant resolution in real-time and thus show important advantages compared to other range measuring technologies like structured light [4] or stereo vision [5]. In hybrid 3D endoscopy besides conventional color information additional range data is acquired as proposed in [6]. Here, the approach of Penne et al. [3] is enhanced by a RGB imaging sensor and a beam splitter within the optical system of the endoscope to separate the color and ToF signal.

Thus both sensors acquire images from the exact same scene that can be aligned via calibration [6]. However, as modern ToF cameras still show a low signal-to-noise ratio (SNR), data preprocessing is absolutely mandatory. Here, one established technique is the non-local-means (NLM) filter. It denoises a pixel by a weighted average of pixels with a similar neighborhood. The filter shows great potential in removing noise from natural images while preserving fine details and strong edges [7]. However, the original algorithm leads to insufficient results when applied on range data due to the low SNR. In this paper, we introduce two extensions to the NLM filter that make it suitable to denoise endoscopic range data in a hybrid imaging setup. First, the computation of weights is extended to neighborhoods in the color image that correspond to those in the range image, resulting in additional color weights. Huhle et al. [8] have shown that color weights allow a more robust NLM filter output for conventional ToF range images. Second, we extend the concept of the algorithm into the temporal domain. This has the advantage that a pixel can be denoised by its representations over time.

2   Materials and methods

The workflow of the algorithm is illustrated in Fig. 1. The algorithm computes weights for the neighborhood of every pixel in every range and color image pair in a sequence. In this paper, $\tilde{r}_i$ denotes a denoised pixel for position i, r_i a pixel in the original range image and c_i a pixel in the registered color image.

2.1   The non-local-means filter

The NLM filter exploits the repetitiveness in images by averaging pixels weighted by the similarity of their neighborhood [7]. A pixel is then computed by

$$\tilde{r}_i = \sum_{j \in N_i} w(i,j) r_j \tag{1}$$

where N_i is the search window around position i and $w(i,j)$ are the weights computed by comparing the neighborhoods of i and j. Since the weights are the essential part of the algorithm, their quality is crucial for the result.

2.2   Extension by color weights

Due to the low SNR of endoscopic ToF data the original algorithm is error-prone to incorrect weights computed on the noisy range images. This can be tackled by incorporating color weights due to the better SNR of RGB images. A pixel is then denoised by including these weights into the denoising process with a parameter α that controls their effect on the result as

$$\tilde{r}_i = \sum_{j \in N_i} \alpha w^c(i,j) r_j + (1-\alpha) w^r(i,j) r_j \tag{2}$$

where $w^c(i,j)$ are the weights computed from the color image and $w^r(i,j)$ the weights computed from the range image. The color weights are generated from the greyscale converted RGB image by

$$w^c(i,j) = \frac{1}{k_i^c}\exp\left(-\frac{1}{h}\sum_{j'\in N'}\exp\left(-\frac{\|i-j'\|_2}{\sigma^2}\right)|c_{i+j'}-c_{j+j'}|^2\right) \quad (3)$$

where N' is the similarity window and j' a pixel offset. k_i^c denotes a normalizing constant, h is the filtering parameter and σ the standard deviation of the Gaussian function. The range weights w^r are computed equivalent to (3).

2.3   Extension in the temporal domain

In a second step, we incorporate a time component. Instead of one single pair of range and color image, a sequence of pairs is used for the denoising process. Therefore, we denoise a pixel not by similar pixels in its neighborhood but by its representation in the other images. Thereby, it is assumed that the representations of the actual pixel over time shows the most similar neighborhood and thus the highest weights when compared to the actual pixel. Due to movements of the endoscope during the intervention temporal denoising has to consider moving corresponding pixels in subsequent frames. To track this movement, the search window is shifted according to the weights. The search window on the previous image of the sequence is moved to the position that shows the highest similarity with the reference position in the current image and thus has the highest weights

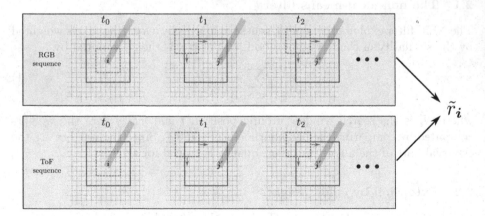

Fig. 1. Workflow of the NLM filter on image sequences with color weights. The three images for each sensor are corresponding image pairs for time step t_0, t_1 and t_2. Red marks the search window, blue the similarity window around i and green the similarity windows of the neighborhood pixels j. Note that because of the movement of the endoscopic tool between t_0 and t_1 the search window is shifted for the next frame. $\hat{j}^c$ and $\hat{j}^r$ denote the maximum similarity measurements for other time steps in the color and the range domain, respectively.

according to (3). A pixel in the denoised image is then computed based on the concept of hybrid NLM filtering according to (2) by

$$\tilde{r}_i = \frac{1}{k_i^h} \sum_{t \in S} \alpha w_t^c(i, \hat{j}^c) \mathrm{r}_{\hat{j}^c}^t + (1 - \alpha) \mathrm{w}_t^r(i, \hat{j}^r) \mathrm{r}_{\hat{j}^r}^t \tag{4}$$

where S is the sequence of images for the denoising process, t denotes a time position in the sequence and k_i^h is a normalizing constant considering all pixel weights calculated on the hybrid temporal NLM. The weights $w_t^c(i, \hat{j}^c)$ and $w_t^r(i, \hat{j}^r)$ are the maximum weights that were found inside the search window for the image at position t in the sequence and $r_{\hat{j}^c}^t$ and $r_{\hat{j}^r}^t$ are the corresponding pixel values in the range image. The color and range weights are computed analogue to (3). This approach results in a denoised image that incorporates for each time step t for each pixel i only the corresponding pixel with the highest similarity.

2.4 Experiments

For the evaluation of the algorithm, real endoscopic data and artificial data was generated. The real data was acquired with a 3D ToF/RGB endoscope prototype with a resolution of 64×48 px for range and 640×480 px for RGB images and with an exposure rate of 30 Hz, using porcine organs. Two livers and a gallbladder were positioned in a box simulating the human abdomen. 12 data sets were obtained with different organ positions, camera movements and endoscopic instruments. The artificial data is generated from meshes extracted from CT data and textures from real human organs and thus provide realistic 3D structures of the inner human body. This leads to very realistic images, suitable for the evaluation of the algorithm. The complex noise that occurs in real ToF images is modeled by adding Gaussian noise. However this is just an approximation and can not cover the noise behavior of the ToF sensor completely. The parameters for our experiments were found by a grid search on a separate dataset. For all evaluations they were kept fixed with $h = 0.1$, $\alpha = 1$, $\sigma = 1$, N as a square with edge length 11 and N' as a square with edge length 5.

3 Results

A comparison of our approach with the original NLM algorithm and a version that only applies color weights on a simulated dataset is given in Fig. 2. Note that the filter is capable of effectively denoising the image while preserving sharp edges. In comparison to the color weighted NLM we do not copy texture information in the final result. Qualitative results of our method for real data are given in Fig. 3. A comparison of distance errors between the ground truth and the filtered images is given in Fig. 4. Note that even though the median error of the final approach is slightly higher, the mean error is 10% less.

4   Discussion

In this paper we introduced a temporal NLM filter for hybrid 3D endoscopy. The filter shows promising results on both, simulated and real endoscopic data created from porcine organs. We clearly improved image quality by removing noise while preserving edges in the images. The simulated data showed an average distance error of 4.8 mm before denoising. The error was reduced to 3.7 mm for the original algorithm, to 1.6 mm for the approach using color weights and to 1.4 mm for our temporal NLM filter. This leads to an improvement of 70% for our method.

Future work will be facing the run-time of the algorithm that is currently not suited for real time applications as they are required for endoscopic interventions. Therefore, an efficient GPU implementation of the algorithm that parallelizes the weight computation for every pixel is mandatory. Also, a removal of specular

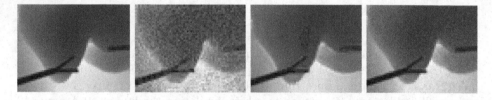

Fig. 2. Illustration of the algorithm on simulated data. From left to right: Ground truth data, result of original NLM algorithm, result of NLM algorithm with color weights, result of temporal NLM algorithm with color weights.

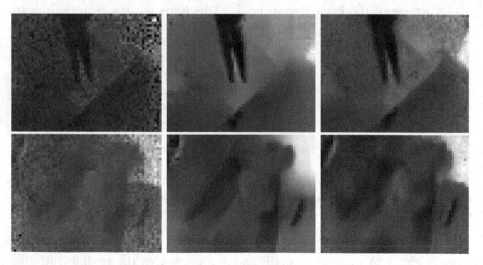

Fig. 3. Illustration of the algorithm on real data of a porcine liver. From left to right: Raw range data, result of NLM algorithm with color weights and result of temporal NLM algorithm with color weights.

Fig. 4. Comparison of the absolute errors in boxplots. From left to right: Error without filtering, error after original NLM filter, error after NLM filter with color weights and error after temporal NLM filter with color weights. The blue crosses mark the mean error. Note that the final approach has a lower mean error due to fewer outliers.

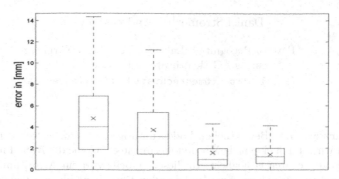

highlights before the filtering would be a benefit since they cause invalid data in both, the color and range image.

Acknowledgement. The authors gratefully acknowledge funding of the Erlangen Graduate School in Advanced Optical Technologies (SAOT) by the German National Science Foundation (DFG) in the framework of the excellence initiative and the support by the DFG under Grant No. HO 1791/7-1. This research was funded by the Graduate School of Information Science in Health (GSISH) and the TUM Graduate School. We thank the Metrilus GmbH for their support.

References

1. Haase S, Wasza J, Kilgus T, et al. Laparoscopic instrument localization using a 3-D Time-of-Flight/RGB endoscope. Proc IEEE Workshop Appl Comput Vis. 2013; p. 449–54.
2. Speidel S, Sudra G, Senemaud J, et al. Recognition of risk situations based on endoscopic instrument tracking and knowledge based situation modeling. Proc SPIE. 2008;6918:1–8.
3. Penne J, Höller K, Stüurmer M, et al. Time-of-flight 3-D endoscopy. Proc MICCAI. 2009;5761:467–74.
4. Schmalz C, Forster F, Schick A, et al. An endoscopic 3D scanner based on structured light. Med Image Anal. 2012;16(5):1063–72.
5. Röhl S, Bodenstedt S, Suwelack S, et al. Real-time surface reconstruction from stereo endoscopic images for intraoperative registration. Proc SPIE. 2011;7964:1–13.
6. Haase S, Forman C, Kilgus T, et al. ToF/RGB Sensor Fusion for 3-D Endoscopy. Curr Med Imaging Rev. 2013;9(2):113–9.
7. Buades A, Coll B, Morel JM. A non-local algorithm for image denoising. Proc IEEE Comput Soc Conf Comput Vis Pattern Recognit. 2005;2:60–5.
8. Huhle B, Schairer T, Jenke P, et al. Robust non-local denoising of colored depth data. Proc IEEE Comput Soc Conf Comput Vis Pattern Recognit Workshops. 2008; p. 1–7.

Approximation der Projektionsmatrizen einer C-Bogen 3D-Fahrt anhand der Odometriedaten

Daniel Stromer[1,2], Andreas Maier[1]

[1]Pattern Recognition Lab, FAU Erlangen-Nürnberg
[2]Siemens AG Healthcare H IM AX R&D SC
daniel.stromer@medtech.stud.uni-erlangen.de

Kurzfassung. Bei aktuellen boden-montierten C-Bogen Röntgengeräten wird durch eine neue Motorsteuerungstechnologie die Aufnahme der Odometriedaten ermöglicht. In dieser Arbeit wird ein Algorithmus beschrieben, der anhand einer bestehenden Datenbank, die mit Geometrie-Kalibrierungen und deren synchron aufgenommenen Odometriedaten, die Projektionsmatrizen für eine spätere Rekonstruktion approximiert. Nachdem Gütekriterien für eine 3D-Fahrt ausgewählt wurden, wird ein Algorithmus vorgestellt, der die am besten passenden Projektionsmatrizen für die jeweilig durchgeführte Fahrt annähert. Die Genauigkeit der berechneten Matrizen wird dann anhand der Originalmatrizen überprüft. Die Auswertung ergab eine durchschnittliche Fehlerreduzierung um bis zu 30.7%. Dies wird auch in den resultierenden Rekonstruktionen ersichtlich.

1 Problemstellung

Für C-Bogen Röntgensysteme müssen 3D-Fahrten exakt reproduzierbar sein, da im Falle einer Störung (z.B. leichte Kollision) eine Rekonstruktion unmöglich wird. In diesem Falle wäre ein Patient der applizierten Strahlendosis umsonst ausgesetzt gewesen. Bisherige C-Bogen Röntgengeräte waren nicht in der Lage Abweichungen in einer Fahrt festzustellen. Eine neue Generation der Antriebssteuerung (Sinumerik, 840 d sI [1]), ermöglicht bei aktuellen Systemen die Aufnahme der Odometriedaten einer Fahrt. Aus diesen Fahrtdaten kann nun auftretender Verschleiß oder eine Hindernisüberwindung anhand von Antriebsparametern analysiert werden um bei deren Auftreten mit Korrekturmaßnahmen zu reagieren. Ziel dieser Arbeit ist es, einen Algorithmus vorzustellen, der die Odometriedaten einer 3D-Fahrt analysiert und anhand einer angelegten Datenbank, die berechnete Projektionsmatrizen und deren Odometriedaten beinhaltet, die am besten zur Fahrt passenden Projektionsmatrizen approximiert. Durch diese Maßnahme soll die Rekonstruktion genauer und anpassungsfähiger für Abweichungen, wie beispielsweise Komponentenverschleiß, werden.

2   Methoden

2.1   Gütekriterien

Um bewegungsspezifische Fehler bei der Geometrie-Kalibrierung feststellen zu können, müssen zuerst Variablen der Sinumerik gefunden werden, die die Identifizierung von Odometrieabweichungen in einer 3D-Fahrt ermöglichen. Da bei einer 3D-Fahrt lediglich die C-Bogen Rotationsachse verfahren wird, müssen nur Parameter dieser Achse überwacht werden. Als erster Parameter wurde die aktuelle Ist-Geschwindigkeit der Achse ausgewählt. Ein weiteres aussagekräftiges Gütekriterium der Fahrt ist der drehmomentbildende Ist-Strom dieser Achse. Treten äußere Einwirkungen auf die Achse auf, so wird über diesen Parameter die Geschwindigkeit sofort nachgeregelt. Abweichungen im Vergleich zu störfreien Fahrten werden durch diese Variable sofort durch markante Sprünge ersichtlich.

2.2   Generieren der Datenbank

Für den vorliegenden Testzweck wird ein Drive Trace eingerichtet, der die festgelegten Gütekriterien jede 5 ms aufzeichnet. Als Start-Trigger wird eine manuelle Tastenbetätigung mit einer Zeitdauer von 10 s konfiguriert. Im Strahlengang wird das PDS-2 Phantom [2] positioniert und bei jeder Fahrt zusätzlich zum Drive Trace eine Bilderserie aufgenommen, um daraus später die benötigten Projektionsmatrizen der Geometriekalibrierung berechnen zu können [3]. Es wurden fünf korrekte 3D-Fahrten und fünfzehn störbehaftete Fahrten durchgeführt. Als Störquelle werden Latexbänder (Thera-Band®, Dornburg) verschiedener Stärken (stark, spezial stark, extra stark) am Detektorschlitten der Rotationsachse und am Boden mit Klebeband fixiert (Abb. 1(a)), die bei maximaler Dehnung an der jeweiligen Position reißen und einen Ruck in der Fahrt verursachen.

2.3   Approximationsalgorithmus

Nach Aufruf der während der 3D-Fahrt akquirierten Odometriedatei O_{app}, glättet ein Mittelwert Filter (Filterbreite 35 ms) eine Strom-Istwert Kurve (D_F). Der Wert wird gewählt, da bei 133 Bildern in einem Aufnahmelauf von fünf Sekunden die Abtastrate 35 ms beträgt. Später wird dann das Ergebnisfeld an jedem Projektionswinkel λ abgetastet und der Wert gespeichert. Um Störeinflüsse der Fahrt zu erkennen, wird ein Ableitungsfilter auf die gefilterte Kurve angewandt und die Ergebnisse erneut Mittelwert gefiltert abgelegt (D_A). Eine Abweichung wird durch eine zeitabhängige Schwellwertüberschreitung der Ableitungskurve detektiert. Im Bereich konstanter Geschwindigkeit wird im Falle einer Abweichung stärker nachgeregelt und die Odometriedatei als störbehaftet erkannt. Als Ausgangsdaten für die Approximation werden die Mittelwert gefilterten Odometriedaten und Ableitungen der Datenbankeinträge O_{db} verwendet. Diese wurden vorher ebenfalls auf Abweichungen in der Fahrt überprüft und das Ergebnis per Flag gespeichert. Wurde keine Störung in der zu approximierenden 3D-Fahrt erkannt, werden, um genauere Ergebnisse zu erhalten, nur

Odometrie-Datenbankeinträge ohne Störungen herangezogen. Es wird immer die minimalste Abweichung (1) von der zu prüfenden Odometriedatei gesucht und der beste Datenbankeintrag i^* derjenigen Odometriedatei gespeichert

$$i^* = \text{argmin}_i \, d(\boldsymbol{O_{\text{app}}}, \boldsymbol{O_{\text{db,i}}}) \tag{1}$$

Eine Funktion $d(\boldsymbol{O_{\text{app}}}, \boldsymbol{O_{\text{db,i}}})$ berechnet hierbei die Odometrieabweichung zwischen der zu approximierenden und der in der Datenbank liegenden Datei mit der Länge N

$$d(\boldsymbol{O_{\text{app}}}, \boldsymbol{O_{\text{db,i}}}) = \begin{cases} d_{\text{corr}}, & \text{wenn } \boldsymbol{O_{\text{app}}} = \text{störungsfrei} \\ d_{\text{dist}}, & \text{sonst} \end{cases} \tag{2}$$

Je nachdem ob das Abweichungsflag gesetzt ist oder nicht, wird die zugehörige Funktion aufgerufen (Korrekte Fahrt: d_{corr} (3) – gestörte Fahrt: d_{dist} (4)). w_1 bzw. w_2 sind Gewichtungsfaktoren, die die Genauigkeit der Approximation bei Störfahrten erhöhen. w_1 wird daher für korrekte Fahrten auf 1 gesetzt. Bei störbehafteten Fahrten werden $w_1 = 2$ und $w_2 = 4$ gewählt. Die Funktion D_{Reg} berechnet die Regressionsgerade der n vor und nach dem Punkt i liegenden Ableitungen. Diese Maßnahme soll die Genauigkeit hinsichtlich des Nachschwingens bei einer Hindernisüberwindung verbessern

$$d_{\text{corr}} = \sum_{l=0}^{N-1} \sqrt{\begin{aligned} &\sum_{k=0}^{2}(D_F(O_{\text{app,l,k}}) - D_F(O_{\text{db,i,l,k}}))^2 \\ &+w_1 \cdot \sum_{k=0}^{2}(D_A(O_{\text{app,l,k}}) - D_A(O_{\text{db,i,l,k}}))^2 \end{aligned}} \tag{3}$$

$$d_{\text{dist}} = \sum_{l=0}^{N-1} \sqrt{d_{\text{corr}}^2 + w_2 \cdot \sum_{n=1}^{3}(D_{\text{Reg}}(\boldsymbol{O_{\text{app,l,n}}}) - D_{\text{Reg}}(\boldsymbol{O_{\text{db,i,l,n}}}))^2} \tag{4}$$

i^* enthält dann den Datenbankeintrag derjenigen Matrix, die die niedrigste Abweichung von der Originalodometriedatei aufweist. Dies wird für jeden Winkel λ durchgeführt. Danach werden diejenigen korrespondierenden Projektionsmatrizen der Odometrie-Datenbankeinträge mit der kleinsten Abweichung am Projektionswinkel λ gesetzt (5)

$$P_\lambda^* = P_\lambda^{i^*} \tag{5}$$

Um die approximierten Projektionsmatrizen mit den Originalmatrizen zu vergleichen, werden schlussendlich die k Projektionsmatrizen voneinander subtrahiert und aus dem Ergebnis die k Frobeniusnormen [4] der erhaltenen Matrix berechnet. Der erhaltene Wert wird dann wiederum durch k dividiert. Umso näher der Wert sich gegen 0 bewegt, desto höher ist die Genauigkeit der Approximation. Daraus ergibt sich der Fehler der Approximation (6). Damit dieser

Tabelle 1. Abweichungen der approximierten Projektionsmatrizen für 3D-Fahrten sortiert nach dem Schweregrad der provozierten Störung. Im Durchschnitt kann der Fehler um 30.7% gesenkt werden.

Fahrt	Störungsgrad	Fehler ohne Korrektur	Fehler mit Korrektur
1	kein	0.25280	0.22427
2	kein	0.25280	0.26117
3	kein	0.08384	0.07120
4	kein	0.09277	0.06927
5	kein	0.08329	0.20166
6	schwach	1.59156	1.37683
7	schwach	2.40949	1.48036
8	schwach	2.04357	1.13684
9	schwach	2.45058	1.36779
10	schwach	1.98897	1.29668
11	mittel	1.40547	1.27338
12	mittel	2.09694	1.43490
13	mittel	2.13575	1.36560
14	mittel	2.36305	1.80143
15	mittel	2.69442	1.62313
16	stark	2.12311	1.48685
17	stark	1.69686	1.57231
18	stark	1.60749	1.27707
19	stark	1.71238	1.60487
20	stark	2.55049	1.29744
Aus allen Störungen		2.05801	1.42637

Fehler als aussagekräftig angesehen werden kann wurden alle Projektionsmatrizen gleich normiert. Bei allen Matrizen war das zwölfte Element auf 1 normiert

$$\text{Fehler} = \frac{1}{k} \sum_{\lambda=0}^{k-1} ||P_\lambda - P_\lambda^*||_F \qquad (6)$$

3   Ergebnisse

Tab. 1 zeigt den Fehler der Projektionsmatrizen ohne bzw. mit Korrektur durch den Approximationsalgorithmus. Fahrt ist hierbei die jeweilige 3D-Fahrt, deren Projektionsmatrix im leave-one-out-Verfahren berechnet wurde. Störungsgrad gibt das benutzte Latexband an. Hierbei ist zu beachten, dass der Abrisszeitpunkt nicht genau festgelegt werden kann, was Auswirkungen auf die Gesamtabweichung hat. Umso früher der Abriss geschieht, umso höher ist die Gesamtabweichung, was zur Folge hat, dass bei frühem Abriß des schwächsten Bandes die Gesamtabweichung höher sein kann, als bei einem starken Band das spät reißt. Fehler ohne Korrektur listet den Fehler nach (6) auf, wenn einfach die Projektionsmatrizen der Fahrt 1 herangezogen werden (bzw. Fahrt 2 bei Fahrt 1) und Fehler nach Korrektur gibt den Fehler der approximierten Projektionsmatrizen an. Ist der Fehler kleiner als 0.3 kann von einer reproduzierbaren Fahrt ausgegangen werden. Es wird ersichtlich, dass ausser bei Fahrt 5 und Fahrt 2, die Abweichungen durch den Algorithmus signifikant verringert wurden. Alle Ergebnisse der Fahrten 1-5 können als reproduzierbar angesehen werden. Ebenso ist erkennbar, dass je stärker der Abriss zu sein schien desto weniger genau die Approximation wird. Nun wurde mit den ursprünglichen Projektionsmatrizen von Fahrt 13 (Abb. 1(b)) nach altem Schema eine Rekonstruktion durchgeführt, die ebenfalls nur geringe Störungen aufzeigt. Ist eine korrekte Kalibrierung vorhanden, kann also trotz Störung korrekt rekonstruiert werden.

Abb. 2 zeigt die Vergrößerung einer Rekonstruktion von Störfahrt 13 auf eine Metallkugel mit den originalen Projektionsmatrizen (Abb. 3(a)) und ohne (Abb. 3(b)) bzw. mit Korrektur (Abb. 3(c)). Hier wird eine deutliche Verbesserung durch Anwenden des Algorithmus ersichtlich. Das Verfahren verbessert die Ergebnisse bei Hochkontrast (z.B. Metall oder Knochen) für störbehaftete 3D-Fahrten. Eine Auswertung für Niedrig-Kontrast-Anwendungen war nicht möglich, da dass verwendete $5s$-Protkoll nur für Hochkontrast-Anwendungen zugelassen ist. Wir vermuten, dass durch die geringe Anzahl der Datenbankeinträge zu wenig Störfalldateien in der Datenbank sind, um wirklich Abweichungen jeder Art für eine Niederkontrast-Anwendung abdecken zu können. Der Abrisszeitpunkt des Klebebandes liess sich zudem nur schlecht reproduzieren. Eine Datenbankvergrößerung könnte eine ausreichende Approximation auch für störbehaftete Fahrten in diesem Bereich ermöglichen.

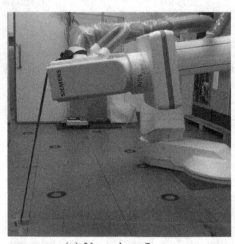 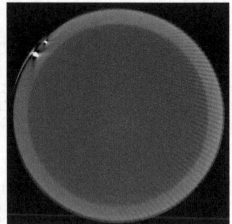

(a) Versuchsaufbau   (b) Rekonstruktion

Abb. 1. Versuchsaufbau zum Generieren der Störfahrten und Rekonstruktion der Fahrt 13 mit originalen Projektionsmatrizen.

Abb. 2. Hochkontrastrekonstruktionen von störbehafteter 3D-Fahrt mit verschiedenen Projektionsmatritzen.

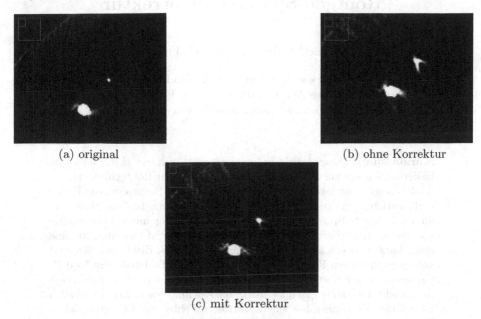

(a) original   (b) ohne Korrektur

(c) mit Korrektur

4   Diskussion

In Zukunft kann darüber nachgedacht werden, bei den Geometriekalibrierungen synchron die Odometriekurven aufzunehmen und in einer Datenbank abzulegen. Treten bei 3D-Fahrten dann Abweichungen auf, die die Rekonstruktion verfälschen, können die Projektionsmatrizen automatisch angepasst werden. Dadurch würde sich eine erhebliche Verbesserung der Genauigkeit beim letztendlichen Einsatzort des Röntgengerätes ergeben. Die Fehlerreduktion von 30.7% ist trotz der geringen Datenbankgröße vielversprechend. Bei den gezeigten Ergebnissen handelt es sich um einen Forschungsprototypen und kein klinisches Produkt.

Literaturverzeichnis

1. Siemens. Sinumerik 840d sl: Funktionsbeschreibung. Erlangen: Siemens AG Industry; 2006.
2. Hoppe S. Accurate Cone-Beam Image Reconstruction in C-Arm Computed Tomography. Dissertation Universität Erlangen-Nürnberg; 2009.
3. Maier A, Choi JH, Keil A, et al. Analysis of vertical and horizontal circular C-arm trajectories. Proc SPIE. 2011; p. 7961231–38.
4. Schwarz HR, Köckler N. Numerische Mathematik. Wiesbaden: Vieweg Teubner; 2011.

Schätzung von Faltungskernen zur Röntgen-Streusignalkorrektur

Christoph Luckner[1,2], Andreas Maier[1], Frank Dennerlein[2]

[1]Lehrstuhl für Mustererkennung, Friedrich-Alexander Universität Erlangen
[2]Siemens AG, Healthcare Sector, Erlangen
christoph.luckner@medtech.stud.uni-erlangen.de

Kurzfassung. Diese Arbeit präsentiert und evaluiert einen faltungs-basierten Ansatz zur Schätzung des Streusignals in Röntgenbildern. Es wird gezeigt, dass aus zwei Aufnahmen derselben Szene ein Abbild des real existierenden Streusignals generiert werden kann. Im Anschluss daran wird eine faltungsbasierte Streusignalschätzung unter Verwendung von parametrisierbaren Streustrahlkernen, bestehend aus einer Summe eines kurz- und eines langreichweitigen Gaußkerns, diskutiert. Anhand von exemplarischen Phantomaufnahmen wird die Stabilität der Modellparameter dieser Kerne und deren Abhängigkeit von der Objektrotation untersucht. Es konnte gezeigt werden, dass es mit diesem Ansatz möglich ist, robuste Ergebnisse mit einem mittleren Fehler von 13% zu erzielen. Weiterhin wurde festgestellt, dass von den Modellparametern lediglich der kurzreichweitige Gaußkern von der Rotation abhängig ist.

1 Einleitung

Die Reduktion der Streustrahlung in medizinischen Röntgenaufnahmen ist nach wie vor ein aktuelles Forschungsthema mit hoher Relevanz für klinische Röntgensysteme. Die von der Streustrahlung verursachten Probleme sind vielfältig und reichen von einem Kontrastverlust im Bild, über eine Erhöhung des Rauschanteils, bis hin zu schwerwiegenden Artefakten bei tomographischen 3D-Rekonstruktionen, die die Aufnahmen im schlimmsten Fall unbrauchbar werden lassen.

Eine etablierte Möglichkeit, um das Streusignal in Röntgenaufnahmen zu unterdrücken, ist der Einsatz eines Streustrahlrasters. Da dieses jedoch sowohl teilweise das diagnostisch wichtige Primärsignal schwächt [1] als auch in manchen Situationen (bspw. bei freien Röntgenaufnahmen) nicht optimal positionierbar ist, ist es nicht immer das Mittel der Wahl.

Die softwarebasierte Korrektur der Streustrahlung ist daher noch immer ein hochaktuelles Forschungsthema. Ein sehr verbreiteter Ansatz zur Streusignalschätzung ist die Faltung des Primärsignals des aufgenommenen Bildes mit einem geschätzten oder gemessenen Streustrahlkern [2]. Weitere Optionen stellen die Interpolation des Kollimatorschattens [3] oder die Nutzung von Beam-Stop-Arrays [4] dar. Die Möglichkeit der Bestimmung per Faltung bietet den Vorteil, dass keine zusätzliche Hardware benötigt wird und sehr gute Schätzungen des Streusignals an jedem Bildpunkt bei kurzer Rechenzeit erreicht werden können.

Eine Variante dieses Ansatzes wird als Superposition der Streustrahlkerne (SKS) bezeichnet und kann sowohl als Fixpunkt-Iterationsverfahren als auch als einfaches Subtraktionsverfahren zur Streustrahlkorrektur eingesetzt werden [5, 6, 7].

2 Material und Methoden

2.1 Theoretischer Hintergund

Jedes, über ein konventionelles Röntgensystem mit potenziellem Einsatz eines Streustrahlrasters, erzeugte Röntgenbild I kann allgemein als Addition des Primärsignals P und Streusignals S betrachtet werden. Werden die Variablen ohne Angabe von Koordinaten verwendet (bspw. I statt $I(x, y)$), so handelt es sich dabei stets um die gesamte Bildmatrix

$$I = T_\mathrm{P} \cdot (P + P^\epsilon) + T_\mathrm{S} \cdot (S + S^\epsilon) \tag{1}$$

wobei P^ϵ und S^ϵ die durch das jeweilige Signal induzierten Rauschterme und T_P bzw. T_S die Transmissionskoeffizienten für Primär- und Streustrahlung sind. Für Aufnahmen ohne Raster gilt $T_\mathrm{P} = T_\mathrm{S} = 1$. Wird ein Beam-Stop-Array (BSA) in den Strahlengang eingebracht, so ergibt sich an diesen Stellen $T_\mathrm{P} = 0$ und $T_\mathrm{S} = 1$. Ein ideales Raster hätte $T_\mathrm{P} = 1$ und $T_\mathrm{S} = 0$. In der Realität liegen diese Werte für ein häufig in der Radiographie verwendetes Raster (Pb15/80) bei $T_\mathrm{P} = 0.745$ und $T_\mathrm{S} = 0.122$. Da hierbei $T_\mathrm{P} < 1$ gilt, wird beim Einsatz eines Streustrahlrasters ein Teil des Primärsignals blockiert, was eine Verschlechterung des Primärsignal-zu-Rauschverhältnisses zur Folge haben kann. Der Rastereinsatz bietet daher insbesondere bei Szenen mit hohem Streustrahlunteil, z.B. für Objekte größer als 10 cm, Vorteile [8].

Da das Streusignal einen niederfrequenten, mit P korrelierten Bildbeitrag darstellt, ist es möglich mittels Tiefpassfilterung des Primärsignals P eine Schätzung des Streusignals $\widehat{S}$ zu erhalten. Der zunächst unbekannte Tiefpassfilter wird in Abschnitt 2.3 diskutiert. Die Rauschterme P^ϵ und S^ϵ werden durch die Tiefpassfilterung weitestgehend eliminiert und daher bei der weiteren Betrachtung nicht weiter berücksichtigt [5, 7].

2.2 Berechnung von Streustrahlbildern

Wird ein Röntgenbild bei gleicher Szene sowohl mit als auch ohne Raster aufgenommen, führt dies zu folgendem Gleichungssystem

$$\begin{pmatrix} I_\mathrm{m} \\ I_\mathrm{o} \end{pmatrix} = \underbrace{\begin{pmatrix} T_\mathrm{P} & T_\mathrm{S} \\ 1 & 1 \end{pmatrix}}_{\mathbf{A}} \cdot \begin{pmatrix} P \\ S \end{pmatrix} \tag{2}$$

wobei I_m hier die Aufnahme mit und I_o die ohne Raster bezeichnet. Da die Matrix $\mathbf{A}$ für $T_\mathrm{P} \neq T_\mathrm{S}$ regulär ist, kann sie invertiert werden

$$\mathbf{A}^{-1} = \frac{1}{T_\mathrm{P} - T_\mathrm{S}} \begin{pmatrix} 1 & -T_\mathrm{S} \\ -1 & T_\mathrm{P} \end{pmatrix} \tag{3}$$

Somit wird eine Zerlegung in Streu- und Primärsignal möglich (Abb. 1) und S bzw. P berechnet sich als

$$S = \frac{T_{\mathrm{P}}}{T_{\mathrm{P}} - T_{\mathrm{S}}} \left(I_{\mathrm{o}} - \frac{I_{\mathrm{m}}}{T_{\mathrm{P}}} \right) \text{ bzw. } P = I_{\mathrm{o}} - S = \frac{1}{T_{\mathrm{P}} - T_{\mathrm{S}}} \left(I_{\mathrm{m}} - T_{\mathrm{S}} \cdot I_{\mathrm{o}} \right) \quad (4)$$

Nachdem bei Phantommessungen Aufnahmen mit prinzipiell beliebig hoher bildwirksamer Dosis durchgeführt werden können, ist es möglich die Rauschterme P^{ϵ} und S^{ϵ} zu vernachlässigen. Dieses so bestimme Streusignal wird im Folgenden zur Anpassung eines modellbasierten Ansatzes zur Streusignalschätzung verwendet. Durch Imperfektionen des realen Rasters und des Messvorgangs kann es passieren, dass in den berechneten Streusignalbildern S Reste des Primärsignals P zu erkennen sind.

Abb. 1. Beispielhafte Zerlegung eines Projektionsbildes I_{o} in Primärsignal P und Streusignal S mittels des Verfahrens der gewichteten Differenzen.

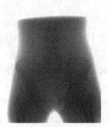 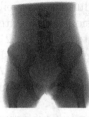 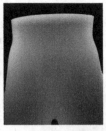

(a) Projektionsbild I_o (b) Primärsignal P (c) Streusignal S

2.3   Schätzung der Streustrahlkerne

Zur modellbasierten Schätzung des Streusignals $\widehat{S}$ innerhalb einer Aufnahme ohne Raster wird ein Verfahren ähnlich dem in [7] vorgestellten Ansatzes verwendet. Dieses setzt sich aus einer Gewichtung der Aufnahme I_{o} und einer anschließenden Faltung zusammen

$$\widehat{S}_{\pi}(x,y) = \iint\limits_{G} \underbrace{I_{\mathrm{o}}(x',y')c_{\alpha,\beta,A}(x',y')}_{\text{Gewichtung des Bildes}} \cdot \underbrace{g_{\sigma_1,\sigma_2,B}(x-x',y-y')}_{\text{Streustrahlkern}} \, \mathrm{d}x'\mathrm{d}y' \quad (5)$$

mit Integrationsgebiet G, das an die Größe m des Faltungskerns angepasst ist und $\pi = \{A, B, \alpha, \beta, \sigma_1, \sigma_2\}$ als Modellparameter der Schätzung. $c_{\alpha,\beta,A}(x,y)$ stellt einen Gewichtungsfaktor dar und berechnet sich mit

$$c_{\alpha,\beta,A}(x,y) = A \cdot \left(\frac{I(x,y)}{I_0} \right)^{\alpha} \cdot \left(-\ln\left(\frac{I(x,y)}{I_0} \right) \right)^{\beta} \quad (6)$$

wobei I_0 den maximalen Intensitätswert der ungeschwächten Strahlung im gesamten Bild beschreibt sowie α und β als Exponenten, die den Gewichtungsfaktor intensitätsbasiert beeinflussen. $g_{\sigma_1,\sigma_2,B}(x,y)$ besteht aus einer gewichteten

Summe aus einem kurz- und einem langreichweitigen Gauß-Kern

$$g_{\sigma_1,\sigma_2,B}(x,y) = \exp\left(-\frac{x^2+y^2}{2\sigma_1^2}\right) + B \cdot \exp\left(-\frac{x^2+y^2}{2\sigma_2^2}\right) \tag{7}$$

2.4 Schätzung der Modellparameter

Zur Bestimmung der Modellparameter π und deren der Variabilität bezüglich der Objektrotation γ wurden Aufnahmen eines Schädelphantoms mit einem Siemens Ysio Radiographiegerät (Siemens AG, Healthcare Sector, Germany) erzeugt. Für die Schätzung der Parameter wurde jeweils eine Aufnahme mit (I_m) und ohne (I_o) Raster sowie ohne Raster mit eingesetztem Beam-Stop-Array (I_{BS}) gemacht. Die Aufnahmen wurden mit Formel 4 in Primär- und Streusignalanteil zerlegt. Ziel war es die Modellparameter π für Gleichung 5 so zu schätzen, dass der Fehler zwischen geschätztem Streusignalbild $\widehat{S}_\pi$ und mittels der Methode der gewichteten Differenzen berechnetem Streusignalbild S minimal wird

$$\pi_\mathrm{opt} = \underset{\pi}{\mathrm{argmin}}\left\{\sqrt{\frac{1}{N}\cdot\sum_{n=1}^{N}\left(\widehat{S}_\pi(x_\mathrm{n},y_\mathrm{n}) - S(x_\mathrm{n},y_\mathrm{n})\right)^2}\right\}, \text{ mit } N\text{: \# der Pixel} \tag{8}$$

Die Bestimmung der Parameter π wurde mittels Rastersuche durchgeführt. Danach ist es möglich, den Streusignalanteil in Aufnahmen ähnlicher Szene mit diesem Parametersatz zunächst zu bestimmen und anschließend zu eliminieren.

3 Ergebnisse

Abb. 2 zeigt das Ausgangsbild I_o für $\gamma = 0°$, das Ergebnis der modellbasierten Schätzung $\widehat{S}_{\pi,\mathrm{opt}}$ sowie als Referenz die nach der Methode der gewichteten Differenz berechnete Version des Streusignals S. Der Plot der gelben Linie aus Abb. 2(a) wird für einen Vergleich der Werte innerhalb der Beam-Stop-Positionen vor und nach der Korrektur verwendet und ist in Abb. 3 dargestellt. Außerdem wurden die Aufnahmen bezüglich der Stabilität der Modellparameter im Hinblick auf die Rotation γ des Phantoms ausgewertet. Die ermittelten optimalen Anpassungsparameter π_opt sowie der nach Gleichung 9 bestimmte Fehler Υ sind in

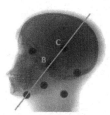

(a) BSA-Aufnahme I_{BS}

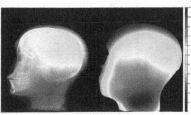

(b) Referenz S und modellb. Schätzung $\widehat{S}_{\pi,opt}$

Abb. 2. Farbcodierte (rot = hoch, blau = niedrig) Version des geschätzten und gemessenen Streusignals sowie die als Referenz verwendete BSA-Aufnahme.

Tabelle 1. Auswertung der Aufnahmen (109 kV, 2.0 mAs) des Schädelphantoms bei $0°$, $90°$ und $135°$ mit $P_{\pi,\mathrm{opt}} = I_\mathrm{o} - \widehat{S}_{\pi,\mathrm{opt}}$.

γ	A	B	α	β	σ_1	σ_2	$\Upsilon(P, I_\mathrm{o})$ / $\Upsilon(P, P_{\pi,\mathrm{opt}})$
$0°$	0.75	0.7	0.29	0.13	20 cm	0.82 cm	0.87 / 0.12
$90°$	0.75	0.7	0.22	0.12	20 cm	2.19 cm	0.43 / 0.14
$135°$	0.75	0.7	0.29	0.11	20 cm	1.48 cm	0.68 / 0.14

Tab. 1 aufgeführt

$$\Upsilon(I_{\mathrm{ref}}, \widehat{I}) = \frac{1}{N} \cdot \sum_{n=1}^{N} \frac{|I_{\mathrm{ref}}(x_\mathrm{n}, y_\mathrm{n}) - \widehat{I}(x_\mathrm{n}, y_\mathrm{n})|}{I_{\mathrm{ref}}(x_\mathrm{n}, y_\mathrm{n})}, \quad \text{mit } N: \# \text{ der Pixel} \qquad (9)$$

4 Diskussion

In dieser Arbeit wurde ein neuartiger Ansatz zur Berechnung des Streusignals aus zwei Röntgenbildern gleicher Szene vorgestellt. Dieser wurde zur Ermittelung eines Streusignalkerns zur Schätzung der Streustrahlung aus einer Röntgenaufnahme benutzt. Es konnte gezeigt werden, dass sich damit Ergebnisse mit einem mittleren Fehler von 13% erzielen lassen. Außerdem wurde die Stabilität der Modellparameter dieser Kerne untersucht, insbesondere deren Abhängigkeit von der Objektrotation. Es wurde festgestellt, dass die Parameter A, B, α, β und σ_1 für das verwendete Kopfphantom weitestgehend rotationsunabhängig sind, während σ_2 zwischen 0.82 und 2.19 variiert.

Die Bestimmung des physikalisch vorhandenen Streusignals aus einem Röntgenbild ohne Raster mit der Methode der gewichteten Differenzen liefert robuste Ergebnisse. Sie eignet sich weiterhin als Referenz für die Optimierungsmethode. Die Objektkanten der in Abb. 2(c) gezeigten Referenz werden durch die enge Fensterung sichtbar. Es konnte gezeigt werden, dass das Ergebnis der modellbasierten Streusignalschätzung um nur $\Upsilon(S, \widehat{S}_{\pi,\mathrm{opt}}) = 16\%$ von der Referenz abweicht, was auch durch den Plot in Abb. 3 bestätigt wird. Zudem sind die bestimmten

Abb. 3. Vorher(I_{BS}: schwarz)-Nachher($I_{\mathrm{BS}} - \widehat{S}_\pi$: blau) Vergleich der Intensitätswerte entlang der gelben Linie in Abb. 2(a); die in rot eingetragenen Zahlen sind die mittleren Intensitätswerte innerhalb der BSAs (A:[120,220], B:[630,730], C:[900,1000]).

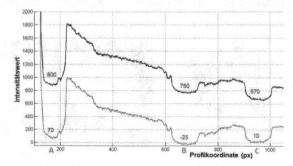

Optimierungsparameter π weitestgehend invariant bezüglich der Rotation γ. Lediglich der Parameter σ_2, der den kurzreichweitigen Gaußkern bestimmt, variiert zwischen $\sigma_{2,\min} = 0.82$ und $\sigma_{2,\max} = 2.19$. Der mittlere Fehler der Schätzungen $\overline{T}(S, \widehat{S}_{\pi,\mathrm{opt}})$ beträgt 13%.

Danksagung. The concepts and information presented in this paper are based on research and are not commercially available. Der Autor dankt Andreas Fieselmann für die interessanten und hilfreichen Diskussionen.

Literaturverzeichnis

1. Kyriakou Y, Kalender W. Efficiency of antiscatter grids for flat-detector CT. Med Phys Biol. 2007;52(20):6275.
2. Seibert J, Boone J. X-ray scatter removal by deconvolution. Med Phys. 1988;15:567.
3. Siewerdsen J, et al. A simple, direct method for x-ray scatter estimation and correction in digital radiography and cone-beam CT. Med Phys. 2006;33:187.
4. Maltz JS, et al. Focused beam-stop array for the measurement of scatter in megavoltage portal and cone beam CT imaging. Med Phys. 2008;35:2452.
5. Ohnesorge B, et al. Efficient object scatter correction algorithm for third and fourth generation CT scanners. Eur Radiol. 1999;9(3):563–9.
6. Rührnschopf E, Klingenbeck K. A general framework and review of scatter correction methods in x-ray cone-beam computerized tomography. Part 1: Scatter compensation approaches. Med Phys. 2011;38:4296.
7. Sun M, Star-Lack J. Improved scatter correction using adaptive scatter kernel superposition. Phys Med Biol. 2010;55(22):6695.
8. Fritz S, Jones A. TU-A-218-07: Quantifying patient thickness for which an antiscatter grid is unnecessary for digital radiographic abdomen exams. Med Phys. 2012;39(6):3895.

Modellierung und Optimierung eines Biosensors zur Detektion viraler Strukturen

Dominic Siedhoff[1], Pascal Libuschewski[2], Frank Weichert[1], Alexander Zybin[3], Peter Marwedel[2], Heinrich Müller[1]

[1]Lehrstuhl für Graphische Systeme, Technische Universität Dortmund
[2]Lehrstuhl für Eingebettete Systeme, Technische Universität Dortmund
[3]Leibniz-Institut für Analytische Wissenschaften – ISAS
siedhoff@ls7.cs.tu-dortmund.de

Kurzfassung. Die echtzeitfähige Detektion mannigfaltiger viraler Strukturen gewinnt zunehmend an Bedeutung. Hier setzt die vorliegende Arbeit an, welche die adaptive Modellierung und Optimierung eines Biosensors vorstellt und zur automatischen Synthese von segmentierten Trainingsdaten nutzt, was den manuellen Aufwand zur Adaption an unterschiedliche Virustypen nachhaltig reduziert. Im vorliegenden Anwendungsfall des PAMONO-Sensors werden über diesen Ansatz die Parameter eines GPGPU-basierten Objekt-Detektors genetisch optimiert. Die Güte des Ansatzes zeigt sich bei der Übertragung der optimierten Parameter auf reale Eingabedaten: Die Qualitätsmaße Precision und Recall erreichen Werte größer als 0.92.

1 Einleitung

Vor dem Hintergrund zunehmender viraler Infektionen und deren Verbreitung ist die Detektion viraler Strukturen und anderer Nano-Partikel von hoher Bedeutung [1]. Der PAMONO-Biosensor (engl. 'Plasmon-Assisted Microscopy of Nanosize Objects') [2] erlaubt beides: Er ermöglicht eine markierungsfreie Detektion intakter Viren in Flüssigkeit durch optische Mikroskopie. Er ist schneller und kostengünstiger als Verfahren wie ELISA und PCR und liefert den indirekten Nachweis einzelner Virusanhaftungen, sowie anderer Nano-Partikel.

Im Hinblick auf die automatische Adaptierung des PAMONO-Biosensors an unterschiedliche Virustypen wird in dieser Arbeit ein Verfahren zur Parameteroptimierung eines Virus-Detektors (allg. Objekt-Detektors) vorgestellt. Da entsprechende Anpassungsvorgänge prinzipiell mit umfangreichen manuellen Segmentierungen verbunden wären, was aber aufgrund des hohen Datenaufkommens hier nicht praktikabel ist, wurde eine Methodik mit minimalem manuellen Segmentierungsaufwand entworfen. Die Kernkomponente ist ein Sensormodell durch das annotierte Trainingsdaten automatisch synthetisiert werden – eine Optimierung auf diesen Trainingsdaten passt die Parameter des Detektors dann vollautomatisch an.

Verwandte Arbeiten lassen sich in die zwei Bereiche unterteilen. Das Problem sehr kleine Objekte bei niedrigem Signal-Rausch-Verhältnis (SNR) zu erkennen wird überblicksartig von Smal et al. [3] behandelt. Es ergibt sich häufig im Zusammenhang mit computergestützter Zellbiologie. Der zum Training gängiger Methoden erforderliche manuelle Segmentierungsaufwand ist hier typischerweise hoch [4, 5]. Der zweite Problembereich ist die Optimierung der Parameter eines Verfahrens, wie von Bartz et al. [6] exemplarisch diskutiert. In der vorliegenden Arbeit liegt der Fokus auf genetischen Algorithmen [7] zur Optimierung der Parameter eines Objekt-Detektors [8]. Zudem ist aufgrund der vorgestellten Synthese keine aufwändige Segmentierung von Trainingsdaten erforderlich.

Ausgehend von dieser einleitenden Darstellung thematisiert Abschnitt 2.1 ein empirisches Modell des PAMONO-Sensors zur Synthese von segmentierten Trainingsdaten. Es kommt innerhalb der Parameteroptimierung des Objekt-Detektors für Nano-Partikel in PAMONO-Daten zum Einsatz (2.2). Abschnitt 2.3 beschreibt den Aufbau der Experimente, deren Ergebnisse in Abschnitt 3 dargestellt und in Abschnitt 4 diskutiert werden.

2 Material und Methoden

Da der PAMONO-Sensor als Ausgangsbasis der weiteren Ausführungen dient, sei dieser hier kurz beschrieben – weitere Details finden sich in der Literatur [2]. Zudem sei angemerkt, dass der Sensor und das vorgestellte Verfahren neben der Detektion viraler Strukturen auch zur Prüfung der Funktionsfähigkeit von Antikörpern und zum Nachweis anderer Nano-Partikel genutzt werden können.

Abbildung 1(a) zeigt den Aufbau des PAMONO Sensors: Eine Diode bestrahlt durch ein Prisma eine mit Antikörpern präparierte Goldschicht. Haftet ein Virus dort an, ändern sekundäre Plasmonenwellen die lokalen Reflektionseigenschaften, sodass ein mikrometergroßer Bereich um das Virus mehr Licht auf einen schräg zur Goldschicht angebrachten CCD Kamerachip reflektiert. Dieser Intensitätsanstieg kann in der Zeitreihe an Bildern, die der CCD aufnimmt, gemessen werden und dient als indirekter Nachweis einer Virusanhaftung. Der Anstieg ist im Vergleich zum näherungsweise konstanten Hintergrundsignal sehr klein. Abbildung 1(b) und (c) zeigen Hintergrundsignal und (bereinigtes und verstärktes) Virussignal.

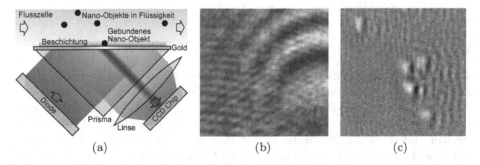

(a)   (b)   (c)

Abb. 1. (a) Aufbau des PAMONO-Biosensors sowie exemplarisches (b) Hintergrundsignal und (c) (zur besseren Sichtbarkeit kontrastverstärktes) Nutzsignal.

2.1 Sensormodell

Die empirische Modellierung des Sensors zur Synthese von Trainingsdaten erfolgt als Zeitreihe der durch den PAMONO Sensor akquirierten Bilddaten

$$I(x,y,t) = (H \cdot P)(x,y,t) + R(x,y,t) \tag{1}$$

Dabei bezeichnet $I(x,y,t)$ die an Ortskoordinate x,y zum Zeitpunkt t gemessene Intensität. Diese setzt sich zusammen aus der Hintergrundkomponente H, multiplikativ moduliert mit dem Nano-Partikelsignal P und additiv überlagert durch das Sensorrauschen R. Der Hintergrund H wiederum wird modelliert als

$$H(x,y,t) = \hat{H}(x,y) \cdot A(x,y,t) \tag{2}$$

wobei $\hat{H}(x,y)$ ein zeitlich konstantes Bild der Sensoroberfläche ist, das allein für die hohen Intensitäten in I verantwortlich ist (Abb. 1(b)). $A(x,y,t)$ ist ein Modulationsterm der störende Artefakte der Messungen modelliert. Die Werte in A streuen geringfügig um 1, ebenso wie die Werte des Partikelsignals

$$P(x,y,t) = (\hat{P}(\circ,\circ,t) ** K_y)(x,y) \tag{3}$$

Das Partikelsignal P, siehe kontrastverstärkte Abbildung 1(c), ist das Nutzsignal der Messung, da es durch die Nano-Partikel verursacht wird und deren indirekten Nachweis ermöglicht. $\hat{P}(\circ,\circ,t)$ bezeichnet das ideale Partikelsignal-Einzelbild des Zeitpunkts t. Im Gegensatz zu P ist es noch nicht durch die geringe Schärfentiefe des optischen Systems degradiert worden. Die geringe Schärfentiefe manifestiert sich deutlich aufgrund der Anordnung des CCD-Chips, der zwar parallel zur seitlichen Prismafläche und zur Linse, aber schräg zur abzubildenden Goldschicht steht (Abb. 1(a)). Die Fokusebene schneidet die Goldschicht in einer Geraden. Partikel die auf Höhe dieser Geraden anhaften sind fokussiert, während die Partikel oberhalb und unterhalb unscharf abgebildet werden. Dieser Effekt wird in (3) durch Faltung mit einer von y abhängigen Punktspreizfunktion (PSF) modelliert. Als Approximation der PSF wird das kreisförmige Kernel K_y verwendet [9] – dies entspricht der kreisförmigen, vollständig geöffneten Apertur der Linse im Sensoraufbau. Der Radius des kreisförmigen Kernels wächst linear mit dem Abstand von y zur Fokusgeraden.

2.2 Optimierung

Abbildung 2 zeigt schematisch das übergeordnete Konzept der Daten-Synthese und der genetischen Parameteroptimierung des Objekt-Detektors für virale Strukturen und andere Nano-Partikel. Ausgangsbasis sind reale Bilddaten des Sensors, mit denen (1) bis (3) gemäß Abschnitt 2.3 berechnet werden. Für die synthetischen Daten ist das Partikelsignal P und damit eine ideale Segmentierung bekannt. Letztere wird im Rahmen einer genetischen Optimierung [7] mit der Ausgabe eines Objekt-Detektors [8] verglichen, um dessen Parameter als Optimierungsvariablen zu verbessern. Als Zielfunktion der Optimierung dient das

Gütemaß Recall [10], welches die Sensitivität des Detektors misst und ermittelt, welcher Anteil der tatsächlich positiven Exemplare gefunden wurde. Das Qualitätsmaß Precision [10] wird verwendet, um in der genetischen Optimierung Parameter zu verwerfen, die zu einer hohen Zahl falsch positiver Erkennungen führen. Precision gibt dabei den positiven Vorhersagewert des Detektors an. Mit den optimierten Parametern werden die realen Eingabedaten des Sensors analysiert. Die so detektierten Objekte sind die Ausgabe des Verfahrens.

2.3 Aufbau der Experimente

Im Folgenden werden vier Ansätze/Experimente zur Berechnung von (1) bis (3) beschrieben, die zum einen der Untersuchung dienen, welche Qualität die auf synthetischen Daten optimierten Parameter des Objekt-Detektors auf realen Sensordaten liefern, und zum anderen bestimmen sollen, welche Daten minimal noch vom Nutzer zur Verfügung gestellt werden müssen – der Fokus liegt auf der Minimierung des manuellen Aufwands.

Als exemplarische Ausgangsbasis dient ein realer Sensor-Datensatz mit 200 nm Polystyren Partikeln in phosphatgepufferter Salzlösung (PBS). Es wurden 20 Bilder pro Sekunde mit einer Auflösung von 1080 × 145 Pixeln mit einer 12 bit CCD Kamera Prosilica GC 2450 aufgenommen. Im Vorfeld erfolgte die Aufnahme von 4000 Bildern ohne die Einleitung von Partikeln. Aus den Aufnahmen wurden vier Datensätze synthetisiert, die sich durch Kombination von zwei Ansätzen zur Generierung des Hintergrundsignals H mit je zwei Ansätzen zur Generierung des Partikelsignals P ergeben.

Der erste Ansatz zur Generierung von H ist die Verwendung des vorab gemessenen realen Signals ohne Partikel. Dieses enthält neben H sowohl die Aufnahme-Artefakte A als auch das Rauschen R. Es wird mit P gemäß (1) moduliert, wobei ignoriert wird, dass so auch R mit P moduliert wird, weil R nicht von H separiert werden kann. Dies ist vernachlässigbar aufgrund der geringen Amplitude von P und der Rausch-Natur von R. Der zweite Ansatz ist die Verwendung eines einzelnen Bildes als $\hat{H}$, sowie $A(\circ, \circ, \circ) = 1$ und die Addition von synthetischem

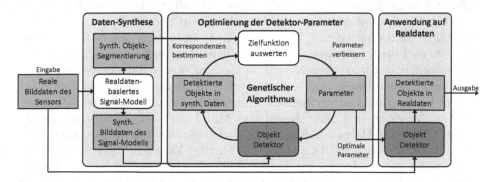

Abb. 2. Schema des Zusammenspiels aus Synthese segmentierter Daten, genetischer Optimierung der Parameter des Detektors und deren Anwendung auf Realdaten.

Tabelle 1. Ergebnisse der Parameter-Optimierung.

| Hintergrund | | Real | | Synthetisch | |
Vorlagen		Real	Synthetisch	Real	Synthetisch
Training	Precision	1.0000	1.0000	1.0000	0.9983
	Recall	0.9484	0.9533	0.9800	0.8983
Test	Precision	1.0000	1.0000	1.0000	0.9983
	Recall	0.9434	0.9266	0.9867	0.8550
Real	Precision	0.9667	0.9476	0.9527	0.9489
	Recall	0.9286	0.9539	0.9286	0.8341

Gaußschen Rauschen R. Mittelwert und Standardabweichung von R orientieren sich an den Eingabedaten. Die beiden Ansätze zur Generierung von P ergeben sich wie folgt: Es können reale Vorlagen für die Partikel-Instanzen verwendet werden, was zur Folge hat, dass der Nutzer vor der Synthese viele Instanzen manuell aus den Eingabedaten segmentieren muss, um die y-abhängigen Variationen aufgrund der geringen Schärfentiefe abzubilden. Eine Faltung wie in (3) entfällt deswegen. Alternativ kann eine einzige Vorlage segmentiert werden, die gemäß (3) bei der Synthese gefaltet wird. Für jede der vier Kombinationen werden die Partikel-Vorlagen an uniform verteilten Koordinaten in P eingefügt und (1) berechnet. Nach diesem Prinzip werden ein Trainingsdatensatz für die Optimierung und ein Testdatensatz zur Qualitätsabschätzung generiert. Ferner wurde zur Validierung der Übertragbarkeit der Parameter auf reale Eingabedaten der reale Datensatz manuell segmentiert. Dies dient ausschließlich der Bewertung der Resultate, nicht der Optimierung. Die erhaltenen Parameter wurden auf Trainings-, Test- und Realdaten angewandt und lieferten die in Abschnitt 3 dargestellten Ergebnisse.

3 Ergebnisse

Tabelle 1 zeigt die Gütemaße Precision und Recall des Detektors nach Optimierung. Die Spalten geben an, wie H und die Vorlagen für P erzeugt wurden. Die Zeilen unterscheiden nach Trainings-, Test- und realen Daten. Für alle Datensätze sind die Schwankungen zwischen Trainings- und Testdatensatz gering; beide wurden nach demselben Modell erzeugt. Im Vergleich dieser Werte mit denen für die realen Daten zeigt sich, dass sie zwar sinken (Ausnahme: Recall bei realem Hintergrund und synthetischen Vorlagen), jedoch nicht stark: Precision sinkt im Vergleich zum Testdatensatz im Mittel um 4.56%, Recall um 1.66%. Alle für die realen Daten erzielten Werte sind größer als 0.92 mit Ausnahme von Recall bei synthetischem Hintergrund und Partikel-Vorlagen. Reale Vorlagen liefern unabhängig von der Art des Hintergrunds sehr ähnliche Ergebnisse, während synthetische Vorlagen auf realem Hintergrund etwas schlechter in Precision und besser in Recall abschneiden.

4   Diskussion

Ausgehend von der Motivation, eine adaptive Detektion viraler Strukturen mittels des PAMONO-Sensors zu ermöglichen, wurden ein Modell dieses Sensors und eine Methodik zur Synthese segmentierter Trainingsdaten entwickelt, welche die automatische, genetische Parameter-Optimierung eines Objekt-Detektors für unterschiedliche Nano-Partikel erlaubt. Als Zielfunktion der Optimierung diente das Gütemaß Recall auf segmentierten, durch das Sensormodell erzeugten Trainingsdaten. Es wurde gezeigt, dass sich die so gefundenen Parameter sehr gut auf reale Sensordaten übertragen lassen und dass durch das Modell die manuelle Segmentierung einer einzigen Partikel-Vorlage zur Generierung geeigneter Trainingsdaten ausreicht – dies reduziert den Aufwand zur Anpassung an verschiedene Arten von Viren/Nano-Partikeln maßgeblich. Insgesamt zeigen die auf realen Sensordaten erzielten hohen Werte für Precision und Recall, dass der Ansatz der Optimierung auf synthetischen Trainingsdaten in Kombination mit dem vorgestellten Sensormodell tragbar ist und praxisrelevante Ergebnisse erzielt.

Zukünftig erfolgt eine weitere Verfeinerung der Methoden des Objekt-Detektors zum Nachweis kleinerer Partikel. Ferner ist mit Blick auf einen mobilen Einsatz des PAMONO-Sensors die Verwendung einer mehrkriteriellen Optimierung geplant, sodass neben der Detektions-Qualität auch die benötigte Energie unter Erhaltung der Echtzeitfähigkeit berücksichtigt werden kann [11].

Danksagung Teile dieser Arbeit wurden von der Deutschen Forschungsgemeinschaft (DFG) im Sonderforschungsbereich 876 „Verfügbarkeit von Information durch Analyse unter Ressourcenbeschränkung", Projekt B2, unterstützt.

Literaturverzeichnis

1. Mairhofer J, Roppert K, Ertl P. Microfluidic systems for pathogen sensing: a review. Sensors. 2009;9:4804–23.
2. Zybin A, et al. Real-time detection of single immobilized nanoparticles by surface plasmon resonance imaging. Plasmonics. 2010;5:31–5.
3. Smal I, et al. Quantitative comparison of spot detection methods in live-cell fluorescence microscopy imaging. Proc ISBI. 2009.
4. Han JW, et al. Radicular cysts and odontogenic keratocysts epithelia classification using cascaded haar classifiers. Proc MIUA; 2008.
5. Pan J, Kanade T, Chen M. Learning to detect different types of cells under phase contrast microscopy. Proc MIAAB. 2009; p. 1–8.
6. Bartz-Beielstein T, et al. The sequential parameter optimization toolbox. Experimental methods for the analysis of optimization algorithms; 2010.
7. Man KF, et al. Genetic Algorithms: Concepts and Designs. Springer; 2001.
8. Libuschewski P, et al. Fuzzy-enhanced, real-time capable detection of biological viruses using a portable biosensor. Proc BIOSTEC. 2013.
9. Sezan MI, Pavlovic G, Tekalp AM, et al. On modeling the focus blur in image restoration. Proc ICASSP. 1991; p. 2485–8.
10. He H, Garcia EA. Learning from imbalanced data. IEEE Trans Knowl Data Eng. 2009;21:1263–84.
11. Libuschewski P, Siedhoff D, Weichert F. Energy-aware design space exploration for GPGPUs. Comput Sci Res Dev. 2013.

Automatic Fovea Localization in Fundus Images

Attila Budai[1], Katja Mogalle[1], Alexander Brost[1], Joachim Hornegger[1],
Georg Michelson[2]

[1]Pattern Recognition Lab, Friedrich-Alexander-Universtität Erlangen-Nürnberg,
Erlangen
[2]Department of Ophthalmology, Friedrich-Alexander-Universtität
Erlangen-Nürnberg, Erlangen
attila.budai@informatik.uni-erlangen.de

Abstract. One of the most common modalities to examine the eye-background is the fundus image. These images are photographs taken through the pupil by a fundus camera. The evaluation of these images is usually carried out by ophthalmologists or experts during visual inspection. The aim of our work is to accelerate this process by a fully-automatic screening. To enable the automatic disease and tissue specific feature extraction, it is necessary to segment the different visible structures in the images. Our group already published methods to extract the vessel tree and estimate the position and diameter of the optic nerve head. In this paper, we present our methods to localize the fovea and the macula region, and compare it to other approaches using the High Resolution Fundus database. Our evaluation showed, that our proposed method is capable of localizing the macula region with an average distance error of 0.1 times optic disk diameter.

1 Introduction

One of the most common modalities to examine the eye-background is the fundus image. These images are photographs of the interior surface of the eye taken through the pupil by a fundus camera. In this section, we describe the standard examination process, image acquisition, and the state of the art methods to localize the macula region.

1.1 Fundus imaging

Fundus cameras in general are low power light microscopes with an attached digital camera. During examination the patient has to look into the device and focus onto a light source acting as a guide. If the focus and all other parameters are set correctly by the technician, the eye-background is illuminated by a strong flash, and a photograph is acquired through the pupil. An example for a fundus camera and an image are shown in Fig. 1. In these images four important structures are visible:

1. Optic nerve head (ONH, or optic disk): A usually circular and bright spot in the retina, where all the nerve fibers and blood vessels enter and leave the eye.
2. Macula: This is a dark spot in fundus images where the density of receptor cells reaches its maximum. The central region of the macula is called fovea, and it is responsible for the sharp vision.
3. Blood vessels: Retinal vessels spreading from the ONH in elliptical paths supplying the retinal tissues with oxygen. In healthy eyes no vessels are visible around the macula, which is called macular avascular zone [1].
4. Background (retina): In the rest of the image the retina is visble, where additional receptor cells can be found for the peripherial vision.

These images are usually evaluated by ophthalmologists or experts through visual inspection. The observer has to look at each of the mentioned structures and analyze them in detail to find signs of irregularities or diseases. This is a long and tiresome process with a high variance between human observers. Our group is working on computer aided and fully automatic screening systems to speed up this process, to unburden the physicians, and to reduce the inter-observer variability.

To facilitate automatic disease and tissue specific feature extraction, it is necessary to segment the different visible structures in the images. Members of our lab already published methods to extract the vessel tree and estimate the position and diameter of the optic nerve head. In this paper, we compare the state of the art methods and present our proposed method to localize the macula region using the results of the above mentioned algorithms.

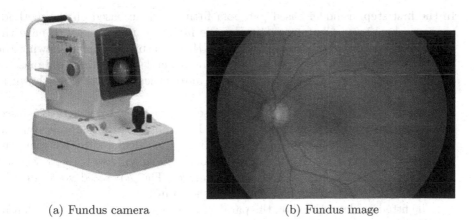

      (a) Fundus camera   (b) Fundus image

Fig. 1. Fundus camera (CANON CF-60UVi) and fundus image showing a glaucomatous eye.

1.2   State of the art

Localization of the fovea is a challenging task due to its low contrast compared to other structures. The only feature which was used for localization is its slightly lower intensity compared to the background [2]. This can easily be mistaken for an illumination artifact or other irregularities. Thus, most of the localization methods use the fact that the macula is in a specific distance and direction from the ONH [3].

For this reason Li and Chutatape [4] proposed a model based method to fit a parabola to landmark points on the main vessels to estimate the location of the fovea. For this approach, two vessels need to be chosen, one below and one above the ONH.

2   Materials and methods

In this paper, we propose a method which combines the main ideas of different localization methods to improve the localization accuracy and robustness. In this section, we introduce our proposed framework for a 2-step localization method. In the first step, an improved model based parabola fitting is used to extract a small region of interest (ROI) at the estimated macula region.

The result is refined in the second step. For this refinement, we propose a distance map based method calculated from the binary vessel image. In the last section, we will describe the evaluation we used to compare our method to other approaches.

2.1   Model based localization

In the first step, a model based parabola fitting is done based on the methods proposed by Li and Chutatape [4]. For the fitting, it is necessary to have the estimated location and diameter of the ONH, and a binary image showing the vessels in the image. These informations are available in the HRF database as a gold standard, or they can be generated automatically as they are shown in Fig. 2.

Instead of fitting a parabola to the vessels themselves, we generate a vessel density image from the binary vessel tree. This simplifies the preprocessing, as no vessels have to be chosen. The density image is calculated by counting the number of pixels segmented as vessels in a local sliding window with a given size depending on the resolution of the input image. The generated vessel density image belonging to the images of Fig. 2 is shown in Fig. 3.

The fitted model is based on the parabola fitting proposed by Li and Chutatape [4], but instead of fitting a single parabola, we use a symmetric double parabola, where the vertex of the parabolas is set to the center of the localized ONH. The localization result of this step will be the point in 2.5 optic disk diameter distance from the ONH position along the symmetry axis of the parabolas, as it is shown in Fig. 3.

Fig. 2. Fundus image and result of the vessel segmentation (white) and ONH localization (red) serving as additional inputs for the fovea localization.

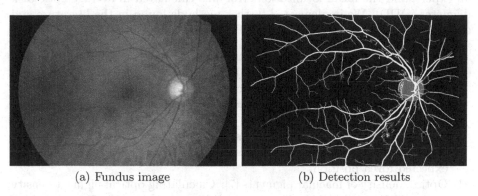

        (a) Fundus image   (b) Detection results

2.2   Refinement step

In a second step, the initial estimation is refined by applying a different method. Therefore, a region of interest is extracted from the images with one optic disk diameter radius around the estimated fovea location. In this ROI a vessel distance map is calculated from the binary vessel image. An example distance map is shown in Fig. 4.

We are searching for a local maximum in this ROI to estimate the position of the fovea. The motivation behind this is the avascular zone around it. Since the shape of the macula is circular, and the fovea is in the center of it, the expected maximum in the distance map should be the fovea.

2.3   Evaluation

We applied our methods on the segmentation dataset of the High Resolution Fundus database [5] to evaluate its accuracy. This database contains 15 images of healthy eyes, 15 images of glaucomatous eyes, and 15 images of eyes with diabetic

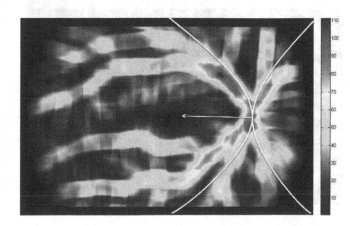

Fig. 3. A model fitted onto the ONH and the density map to estimate the fovea location in 2.5 optic disk diameter distance from the ONH.

retinopathy. The results were compared to a gold standard data measured by an expert, and the mean localization error was calculated in average optic disk diameter (ODD). We implemented further methods found in the literature and combination of some other methods and ideas for comparison:

1. Fast radial symmetry transform (FRST) [6]: A transformation used in computer vision for detecting circular objects is used to detect the center of dark circular objects with different expected radii on each color channel in the ROI. The median of the expected center coordinates are used as expected fovea position.
2. Template matching: the coordinates of maximum response for a Gaussian kernel template matching in L-channel of LAB-color space image is used as expected fovea position
3. Optical density of macular pigments [7]: Calculating optical pigment density in the ROI and calculate the centroid in a density image. The position of the centroid is the estimated fovea location.
4. Morphological operators [2]: Morphological opening is used before finding the minimum of the ROI to estimate fovea position.
5. Mixture of distance transform and FRST: Pixelwise combination of the calculated distance and FRST maps is calculated. In this joint map the maximum position is located and used as the estimated fovea position.

All the methods mentioned above, and further variations of these methods were implemented in Matlab to test their accuracy. The source code of this application is available at [8], and it is free to use for research purposes only.

3   Results

All implemented methods were tested using the High Resolution Fundus database, and the average localization results were compared to a gold standard generated by experts. Tab. 1 shows the measured average localization errors

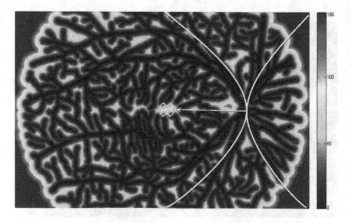

Fig. 4. Distance map generated in the region of interest.

Table 1. Measured average localization error of the tested methods. The proposed distance map based localization outperforms each of the tested methods.

Method	Localization Error (in pixel)	Localization Error (in ODD)
Model based method	145.42 ± 49.98	0.387 ± 0.133
Distance map	$\mathbf{42.54 \pm 23.75}$	$\mathbf{0.113 \pm 0.063}$
FRST	54.31 ± 26.56	0.144 ± 0.070
Template matching	61.69 ± 47.87	0.164 ± 0.127
ODMP	66.29 ± 41.04	0.176 ± 0.109
Morphological operators	51.33 ± 53.82	0.136 ± 0.143
Distance map and FRST	47.12 ± 23.16	0.125 ± 0.061

for each of these methods. Based on these results the model fitting method gives a valuable initial guess, but it needs a refinement step as it is proposed in this paper. The best results are provided by the proposed distance map based method, which was in average about 15% better than the usually used intensity based results.

4 Discussion

We presented a 2-step fovea localization method. We evaluated and compared its results to other state of the art methods using the HRF database. Our evaluation showed, that the proposed method has a localization error of 0.113 ODD, which is better than the state of the art methods. Thus, the method is robust and accurate enough to be applied as preprocessing in computer aided diagnosis systems.

References

1. Bird AC, Weale RA. On the retinal vasculature of the human fovea. Exp Eye Res. 1974;19(5):409–17.
2. Rajaput GG, Reshmi BM, Sidramappa C. Automatic localization of fovea center using mathemathical morphology in fundus images. Int J Mach Intell. 2011;3:172–9.
3. Fleming AD, Goatman KA, Philip S, et al. Automatic detection of retinal antomy to assist diabetic retinopathy screening. Phys Med Biol. 2007;52:331–45.
4. Li H, Chutatape O. Automated feature extraction in color retinal images by a model based approach. IEEE Trans Biomed Eng. 2004;51(2):246–54.
5. Budai A, Odstrcilik J. High resolution fundus image database; 2013. Available from: http://www5.cs.fau.de/research/data/fundus-images/.
6. Loy G, Zelinsky E. A fast radial symmetry transform for detecting points of interest. Eur Conf Comput Vis. 2002; p. 358.
7. Tornow RP, Kopp O. ARVO online abstract: time course and frequency spectrum (0 to 12,5 Hz) of fundus reflection. ARVO Meet Abstr. 2006.
8. Test algorithm for fovea localization; 2013. Available from: http://www5.cs.fau.de/fileadmin/Persons/BudaiAttila/MaculaLocalization.zip.

Geometry-Based Optic Disk Tracking in Retinal Fundus Videos

Anja Kürten[1], Thomas Köhler[1,2], Attila Budai[1,2], Ralf-Peter Tornow[3], Georg Michelson[2,3], Joachim Hornegger[1,2]

[1]Pattern Recognition Lab, FAU Erlangen-Nürnberg
[2]Erlangen Graduate School in Advanced Optical Technologies (SAOT)
[3]Department of Ophthalmology, FAU Erlangen-Nürnberg
anja-kuerten@web.de

Abstract. Fundus video cameras enable the acquisition of image sequences to analyze fast temporal changes on the human retina in a non-invasive manner. In this work, we propose a tracking-by-detection scheme for the optic disk to capture the human eye motion on-line during examination. Our approach exploits the elliptical shape of the optic disk. Therefore, we employ the fast radial symmetry transform for an efficient estimation of the disk center point in successive frames. Large eye movements due to saccades, motion of the head or blinking are detected automatically by a correlation analysis to guide the tracking procedure. In our experiments on real video data acquired by a low-cost video camera, the proposed method yields a hit rate of 98% with a normalized median accuracy of 4% of the disk diameter. The achieved frame rate of 28 frames per second enables a real-time application of our approach.

1 Introduction

Fundus photography is a widely used modality to diagnose diseases such as diabetic retinopathy or glaucoma by detection of anomalies in single 2-D images. Novel fundus video cameras enable the observation of fast temporal changes on the retina for new applications such as the measurement of the time course of the fundus reflection to analyze the cardiac cycle [1]. During examination, the human eye undergoes natural as well as guided movements. For applications such as patient guidance or the fixation of a certain position on the fundus by a stimulus, eye motion must be captured on-line as feedback in a control system. Tracking algorithms determine the position of an object in successive frames and can be used to capture eye motion. Therefore, the optic disk (OD) visible as bright elliptical spot, represents a robust feature for tracking.

While there are numerous approaches for OD localization, OD tracking remains challenging and has been less considered in literature. Difficulties arise due to the decreased image quality in terms of resolution and illumination conditions of common fundus video cameras compared to conventional fundus cameras [2]. Furthermore, tracking has to deal with large eye movements due to saccades, head motion or blinking during examination. In an early work, Koozekanani et al. [3] have proposed a method to track the OD using a tiered detection scheme containing Hough transform, eigenimage analysis and geometric analysis. However, this approach is computationally demanding which makes a real-time application cumbersome. In terms of object detection methods, Loy and Zelinsky [4] have introduced the fast radial symmetry transform (FRST) as a point of interest detector to highlight points of high radial symmetry. Compared to the circular Hough transform, this method has a low computational complexity and thus it is well suited for real-time applications. Recently, the FRST has been proposed by Budai et al. [5] for OD localization in high-resolution fundus photographs.

In this paper, we propose a tracking algorithm that exploits the geometry of the OD to capture its radius and position in successive frames of a fundus image sequence. Therefore, our method employs the FRST in a tracking-by-detection scheme. Large eye motion due to saccades or head movements are detected automatically by a correlation analysis to guide the tracking procedure. The proposed method enables real-time OD tracking during examination.

2   Materials and methods

2.1   Fast radial symmetry transform

For every pixel p in the input image I, the position of the center point candidate $c(p)$ is given by $c(p) = p + \left\lceil \frac{\nabla I(p)}{\|\nabla I(p)\|_2} \cdot r \right\rceil$, where $\nabla I(p)$ is the gradient of the input image and r is the radius. An orientation projection image O_r and a magnitude projection image M_r of the same size as I are initialized with zeros. Then, the values are incremented for every center point candidate according to

$$O_r(c(p)) := \begin{cases} O_r(c(p)) + 1 & \text{if } \gamma \geq \nabla I(p) \geq \beta \\ O_r(c(p)) & \text{otherwise} \end{cases} \tag{1}$$

$$M_r(c(p)) := \begin{cases} M_r(c(p)) + \|\nabla I(p)\|_2 & \text{if } \gamma \geq \nabla I(p) \geq \beta \\ M_r(c(p)) & \text{otherwise} \end{cases} \tag{2}$$

where $O_r(c(p))$ and $M_r(c(p))$ denote the orientation projection and magnitude projection image for center point candidate $c(p)$, β is a gradient threshold parameter to exclude small gradients caused by noise and γ is a gradient threshold parameter to exclude high gradients that are likely to be caused by blood vessels [5]. The projection images are combined to a single map $F_r(p)$ according to

$$F_r(p) = \frac{M_r(p)}{k_r} \left(\frac{|\tilde{O}_r(p)|}{k_r} \right)^\alpha, \text{ where } \tilde{O}_r(p) = \begin{cases} O_r(p) & \text{if } O_r(p) < k_r \\ k_r & \text{otherwise} \end{cases} \tag{3}$$

where α is the radial strictness parameter and k_r is a normalization factor. Finally, the radial symmetry contribution map S_r is computed as $S_r = F_r * A_r$, where A_r is a two-dimensional Gaussian with standard deviation $\sigma = 0.25n$. Local maximums in S_r indicate bright regions of high radial symmetry and are detected for OD localization.

2.2 Tracking algorithm

The proposed algorithm is divided into two steps: (i) During the initialization, the OD is localized and its radius is estimated. (ii) For tracking, the position of the OD is updated for every frame. In a preprocessing step for each frame, we apply a Gaussian filter for noise reduction and a dilation with subsequent erosion to suppress blood vessels that influence the detection of circular objects.

Radius estimation. The radial symmetry contribution map $S_r(I)$ is calculated for a set of radii $R = \{r_1, r_2, ...\}$ in image I. We search for the maximum in all maps $S_r(I)$ and estimate the OD radius $\hat{r}$ as

$$\hat{r}(I) = \arg \max_{r \in R}(\max(S_r(I))) \tag{4}$$

where $\max(S_r(I)))$ is the maximum in the radial symmetry contribution map $S_r(I)$. As the radius estimation in a single image may be affected by noise, we estimate the radius in a number of successive frames during initialization and compute the median radius $\tilde{r}$ over all estimates $\hat{r}$. In order to improve efficiency and since the OD size is fixed over time, this radius is used for tracking based on the FRST in all subsequent frames.

Position update. The OD position is detected by computing the FRST map $S_{\tilde{r}}(I)$ for the current frame based on the radius estimate $\tilde{r}$. Then, the center point is updated by detecting the position of the maximum value $\max(S_{\tilde{r}}(I))$. The efficiency of the position update is improved by computing $S_{\tilde{r}}(I)$ only in a quadratic window centered on the OD position of the previous frame with an edge length of l times the OD diameter. In case of large eye movements due to saccades, the OD leaves the window and its new position cannot be detected relative to the previous frame. Therefore, we compute the normalized cross-correlation ρ between optic disk windows in successive frames. For $\rho < \rho_0$, we detect a saccade and update the OD position using the FRST in the whole image. Additionally, frames affected by blinking are excluded from tracking. We compute the Bhattacharyya coefficient [6] b between the histogram of the first image and the histogram of the current frame to exclude frames with $b < b_0$.

2.3 Experiments

We evaluated our algorithm on a set of fundus image sequences acquired with a low-cost video camera that was constructed by Dr. Ralf-Peter Tornow. The camera uses LED illumination and a CCD camera (640 x 480 pixels) to acquire video sequences with up to 50 frames per second (fps) and a field of view of 15° without dilating the pupil. We captured image sequences from the left eye of six healthy subjects under two scenarios: (i) The subject fixated on a bright spot, so that the fixation position was stable. (ii) The subject fixated on different points in order to produce saccades. After three seconds of fixating on the starting

Table 1. Hit rate and accuracy measured in OD diameter (ODD) of the proposed tracking-by-detection algorithm (TbD) and mean shift tracking (MST). We also evaluated the inter-observer variance between expert A and expert B.

	Hit rate [%]		Mean error [ODD]		Median error [ODD]	
	A	B	A	B	A	B
TbD (proposed)	98.0	98.9	0.13 ± 0.21	0.12 ± 0.18	0.03	0.04
MST	86.9	88.9	0.35 ± 0.43	0.32 ± 0.41	0.20	0.19
Expert A				0.03 ± 0.02		0.03
Expert B			0.03 ± 0.02		0.03	

point, the subject alternated between looking to the right, fixating on the starting point and looking to the left. Each sequence has a duration of 15 seconds and was taken with two different frame rates: 25 and 50 fps. Two ophthalmic imaging experts created ground truth data by labeling the OD center in every 15th frame and measuring the vertical OD diameter in the first frame. The data from one subject was used for parameter adjustment and was excluded from the results. The range of the radii was set to $R = \{90, 95, \ldots, 120\}$. Six frames were used for initialization. The edge length of the OD window was chosen as 1.25 times the OD diameter. The saccade threshold was set to $\rho_0 = 0.25$ and the blink threshold was set to $b_0 = 0.7$. For the FRST, the radial strictness parameter was selected to be $\alpha = 2$ and the gradient thresholds were set to $\beta = 10$ and $\gamma = 80$.

Our method was compared to intensity-based mean shift tracking (MST) [6]. All algorithms were implemented in C++ and runtimes were evaluated on an Intel i3 CPU with 2.4 GHz and 4 GB RAM. Robustness was assessed by computing the hit rate for each algorithm. A hit is detected if the estimated OD center is inside the labeled OD. The accuracy of tracking was evaluated by computing the euclidean distance between the detected and the labeled center.

3   Results

The accuracy achieved by mean shift tracking and the proposed method itemized for the examined subjects is shown as boxplot in Fig. 1. The measuring unit is OD diameter (ODD), which is the euclidean error of the center point detection normalized with the corresponding ground truth OD diameter. For both algorithms, tracking was more reliable for video data acquired with a lower frame rate (25 fps) and thus improved conditions in terms of illumination and contrast. Mean shift tracking showed higher errors for saccade sequences. Tab. 1 summarizes the hit rates as well as mean, standard deviation and median of the accuracy over all test sequences. Our algorithm achieved a mean hit rate of 98.0%, a mean accuracy of 0.13 ± 0.21 ODD and a median accuracy of 0.04 ODD which is in the range of the median inter-observer variance of 0.03 ODD. Mean shift tracking achieved a mean hit rate of 86.9% with a mean accuracy of 0.35 ± 0.43 ODD and a median accuracy of 0.20 ODD. A qualitative comparison between both methods for two different subjects is presented in Fig. 2. In particular, the proposed method was able to detect the OD even in case of saccades whereas mean shift resulted in erroneous center point detections. In terms of run-time, we achieved a mean frame rate of 28 fps. The mean shift approach achieved a frame rate of 200 fps. We used the same initialization to estimate the OD radius for all methods, which had a mean runtime of 1.9 seconds.

4   Discussion

We proposed a tracking-by-detection framework to capture the position and the radius of the OD in successive frames of retinal fundus image sequences. The FRST is employed for tracking and exploits the circular shape of the OD. Compared to intensity-based mean shift tracking, the proposed method shows improved robustness with respect to large eye movements due to saccades. Our

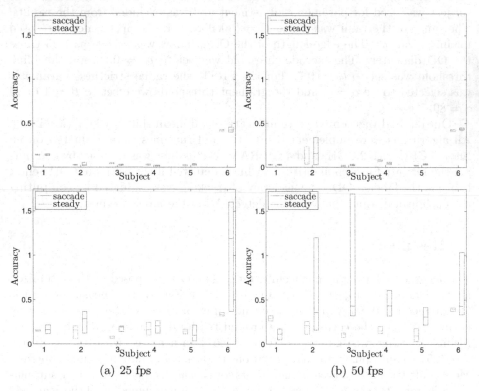

(a) 25 fps   (b) 50 fps

Fig. 1. Boxplots of the tracking accuracy for the proposed method (top row) and mean shift tracking (bottom row) normalized by the OD diameter (ODD) for 25 fps (a) and 50 fps (b). We evaluated the euclidean distance between the estimated OD center point and the mean of two experts used as ground truth.

Fig. 2. Tracking results for different frames obtained by mean shift tracking (dotted blue line) and the proposed method (magenta line).

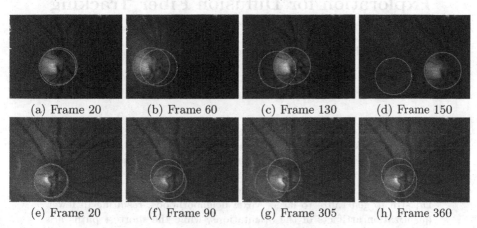

| (a) Frame 20 | (b) Frame 60 | (c) Frame 130 | (d) Frame 150 |
| (e) Frame 20 | (f) Frame 90 | (g) Frame 305 | (h) Frame 360 |

proof-of-concept implementation enables a real-time application for 25 fps video data. A GPU implementation holds great potential to speed-up our algorithm.

In our approach, the OD detection and position update may be affected by blood vessels which have a shape and gradient similar to the OD boundary as shown in Fig. 3(g). In this case, the inclusion of vascular information as proposed by [3] could improve the robustness. Future work will focus on a hybrid approach to integrate color and texture information to the proposed algorithm in order to improve tracking reliability.

Acknowledgement. The authors gratefully acknowledge funding of the Erlangen Graduate School in Advanced Optical Technologies (SAOT) by the German National Science Foundation (DFG) in the framework of the excellence initiative.

References

1. Tornow RP, Kopp O, Schultheiss B. Time course of fundus reflection changes according to the cardiac cycle. Invest Ophthalmol Vis Sci. 2003;44:Abstract 1296.
2. Köhler T, Hornegger J, Mayer M, et al. Quality-guided denoising for low-cost fundus imaging. Proc BVM. 2012; p. 292–7.
3. Koozekanani D, Boyer KL, Roberts C. Tracking the optic nervehead in oct video using dual eigenspaces and an adaptive vascular distribution model. IEEE Trans Med Imaging. 2003;22(12):1519–36.
4. Loy G, Zelinsky A. Fast radial symmetry for detecting points of interest. IEEE Trans Pattern Anal Mach Intell. 2003;25(8):959–73.
5. Budai A, Aichert A, Vymazal B, et al. Optic disk localization using fast radial symmetry transform. Proc CBMS. 2013; p. 59–64.
6. Comaniciu D, Ramesh V, Meer P. Kernel-based object tracking. IEEE Trans Pattern Anal Mach Intell. 2003;25(5):564–77.

Interactive Volume-Based Visualization and Exploration for Diffusion Fiber Tracking

Dominik Sibbing, Henrik Zimmer, Robin Tomcin, Leif Kobbelt

Computer Graphics and Multimedia, RWTH Aachen University
sibbing@cs.rwth-aachen.de

Abstract. We present a new method to interactively compute and visualize fiber bundles extracted from a diffusion magnetic resonance image. It uses Dijkstra's shortest path algorithm to find globally optimal pathways from a given seed to all other voxels. Our distance function enables Dijkstra to generalize to larger voxel neighborhoods, resulting in fewer quantization artifacts of the orientations, while the shortest paths are still efficiently computable. Our volumetric fiber representation enables the usage of volume rendering techniques. No complicated pruning or analysis of the resulting fiber tree is needed in order to visualize important fibers. In fact, this can efficiently be done by changing a transfer function. The interactive application allows the user to focus on data exploration.

1 Introduction

Diffusion Magnetic Resonance Imaging (dMRI) is a non invasive imaging method, that measures the diffusion of water within living tissue. Fibers, membranes and other molecular structures are pipelines or obstacles for the water molecules and thus influence their movements into certain directions, i.e. water majorly flows along fibers. Diffusion MRI measures this flow and translates these measurements to oriented distribution function (ODFs), which locally characterize the probability of water flowing into a certain direction. We use Diffusion Tensor Imaging (DTI) to demonstrate the effectiveness of the suggested pipeline, but a generalization to High Angular Resolution Diffusion Imaging (HARDI) such as Q-Ball Imaging [1] is just a matter of adapting a distance function.

To better understand the connectivity within the human brain, the ultimate goal is to reconstruct the "true" fiber pathways from these ODFs. We present an efficient method to compute and visualize such globally connected fiber tracts based on Dijkstra's shortest path algorithm and represent the resulting pathways in a volumetric fashion. Related approaches typically use 26 neighbors defining the edge relation of Dijkstra's graph, leading to discretization artifacts, especially problematic for HARDI data.

Classical tractography traces possible nerve tracts starting from a seed position. Early deterministic approaches are the streamline tracking technique (STT) and tensor deflection (TEND) [2]. A number of probabilistic tractography techniques have been presented based on modeling and sampling an ODF in each voxel [3, 4]. Difficulties in probabilistic tractography mainly involve the reported running times [5], which can range to 24h using Monte Carlo-based sampling [3] or need to be implemented on modern GPUs to reduce the computation time [6]. Some recently proposed tracking algorithms are based on a weighted graph-structure [5, 7]. Using shortest path algorithms enables globally optimal, deterministic results and allows to bridge tract connections otherwise lost in other approaches. As noted in [5] more than 26 neighboring voxels may be required to correctly capture fiber tract orientations, which leads to a computationally more involved tracing approach, but no practical details on implementational aspects or analysis of different neighborhoods are given. The most related work to our approach is [7]. The main difference is that we use physically motivated weights and allow for arbitrarily sized neighborhoods, which are efficiently integrated in Dijkstra's algorithm. Additionally we do not require any heuristics for pruning the shortest path tree. Simultaneously visualizing all pathways in 3D, often affects the clarity of the illustration. To enhance explorability, some approaches filter the computed tracts [8, 7] in a pre-processing step. Additionally visualizing scalar properties such as uncertainties, densities or distances from a seed is often limited to separate 2D opaque images [5, 7]. 3D volume rendering has been used to render local scalar quantities, such as uncertainty of probabilistic tractography pathways [9], or local tensor orientations [10]. Our visualization is also based on volume rendering. Since, highlighting important fibers requires only the adaption of a transfer function, which can be done in real time. The visualized information is purely based on the shortest path tree and thereby follows up on the future work posed in [7] to further exploit the Dijkstra information for a better visualization.

In this paper, we explore the usage of larger neighborhoods and thereby reduce such artifacts. Our approach efficiently integrates the ODF along a path between neighboring voxels and controls the directional sensitivity of the propagated front by a single parameter.

2   Materials and methods

The idea of our volumetric fiber representation is to count the number of pathways (computed during Dijkstra) that run through a given voxel. We adapt a transfer function, commonly used in volume visualization, to continuously blend in and out fibers instead of tediously trace and prune the obtained tree structure.

2.1   Fiber extraction pipeline

Our approach to transform the information given as local diffusion tensors into globally connected pathways representing the fibers is based on Dijkstra's shortest path algorithm. This algorithm takes an edge weighted graph $G = (V, E)$ as input, starts from a given (set of) seed node(s) and sequentially conquers the remaining nodes of the graph in the order of increasing distances to the seed (Fig. 1). Since a predecessor map $pre[v]$ is stored for each node v, it is always possible to trace back a unique path to the seed. In our setting the nodes of the graph are a subset of the DT image voxels and the weight between two neighboring nodes shall be small if the ODF indicates a large flow between them. To represent the fibers we use the resulting predecessor map to trace all possible pathways back to the seed and thereby count for every voxel the number of pathways that run through it. We use volume rendering techniques to highlight regions with a high count value, i.e. regions containing many fibers.

2.2　Tracing the DTI volume

The simultaneous motion of water molecules in different directions (Brownian motion) can be described by a tensor $T \in \mathbb{R}^{3 \times 3} = U \cdot D \cdot U^T$, where U is an orthogonal matrix storing the main diffusion axes column-wise and $D = \mathrm{diag}(\lambda_1, \lambda_2, \lambda_3)$ is the diagonal matrix of eigenvalues of T. Given a direction $\mathbf{r}$ this tensor can be used to compute the flow of water into this direction $f(\mathbf{r}) = \mathbf{r}^T \cdot T \cdot \mathbf{r}$.

To restrict our computations to the white matter of the human brain we define the nodes V of G to be those voxels with a fractional anisotropy (FA) > 0.1 [8]. This filters out voxels with no pronounced fiber directions.

When defining the connectivity of G and thereby the set E of edges, one typically uses the 26 neighbors of the 1-ring of a voxel for simplicity. To more accurately capture the tensor directions in strongly anisotropic regions, we present an efficient way to also handle arbitrary n-ring neighborhoods. Since the goal of using larger voxel neighborhoods is to increase the number of directions, we can save memory and compute time by discarding redundant edges whose orientations are already covered by shorter edges (top left image of Fig. 1). When using n-ring neighborhoods with $n \geq 2$ some care has to be taken during Dijkstra when conquering a voxel v. To avoid back and forth motion of the front we need to conquer all voxels between v and $pre[v]$. In a preprocessing step we intersect each possible edge with a smaller grid defining the neighborhood stencil and store a list of visited voxels $\{v_i\}$ and a corresponding list of line segments of length $\{l_i\}$ (bottom left image of Fig. 1). During Dijkstra all voxels between v and $pre[v]$ can then simply be tagged by traversing the respective list $\{v_i\}$.

Imagine the edge e is embedded in a continuous tensor field $T_{\mathbf{x}}$, with $\mathbf{x} \in \mathbb{R}^3$. Intuitively spoken the contribution to the edge distance $d[e]$ of one infinitesimal line segment dt at position $\mathbf{x}$ should be low if the local tensor indicates a strong flow into the edge direction $\mathbf{r}$ ($\|\mathbf{r}\| = 1$). We base the edge distance on the inverse metric tensor and define $d[e] = \int_e \left(\mathbf{b}^T \cdot \mathrm{diag}\left(\frac{1}{\lambda_1^\alpha}, \frac{1}{\lambda_2^\alpha}, \frac{1}{\lambda_3^\alpha}\right) \cdot \mathbf{b} \right) dt$, where $\mathbf{b} = U^T \cdot \mathbf{r}$. The introduced parameter α controls the sensitivity to the anisotropy of this flow metric. When increasing α, the front rapidly moves along significant fibers first (Col. 2 of Fig. 3). This integral over an edge is discretized by a Riemann sum with nearest neighbor sampled tensors $\{T_i\}$ of the voxels $\{v_i\}$ intersected along the edge and weighted by the length of the respective segments $\{l_i\}$ (Fig. 1) such that $d[e] \approx \sum_i \left(\mathbf{r}^T \cdot T_i^{-\alpha} \cdot \mathbf{r} \right) l_i$.

2.3 Representing fibers

The unique predecessor relation $pre[v]$ (Fig. 1) defines a tree of globally optimal shortest paths along nerve fibers starting from a seed node. Instead of extracting an explicit tree topology, we represent the structure of this tree in a volumetric fashion by tracing back all end points to the seed (end points are defined as tree nodes having a predecessor but no successors and are found by building a successor map from the predecessor information). Whenever we traverse a voxel during this process we increase a value stored at that voxel by the respective partial edge length l_i. The result is a volumetric image where voxels have high intensity values if intersected by many pathways.

3 Results

We used a DT image with 128x120x75 voxels, from which we extracted 171041 nodes with FA > 0.1. We simultaneously visualize an anatomical image and the volumetric fiber representation (Sec. 2.3) using direct volume rendering. By designing a transfer function that maps intensities I smaller than a user defined value I_a to blue and opacity 0 and intensities larger I_b to red and opacity 1, we can continuously prune fibers by interactively adapting I_a and I_b. Within the interval we linearly interpolate opacity and hue values. Defining a narrow interval at the right spectrum of intensities only visualizes the main fibers, while a wide interval also reveals fine structures (Col. 4 of Fig. 3). Exploring the volume and simultaneous seed placement using a 3D mouse is possible at high frame rates of about 50 fps on an Intel(R) Core(TM) i7 CPU with 2.67 GHz. Since all computations (Sec. 2.1) run in a separate thread and updates are displayed immediately after computation, the application is highly interactive.

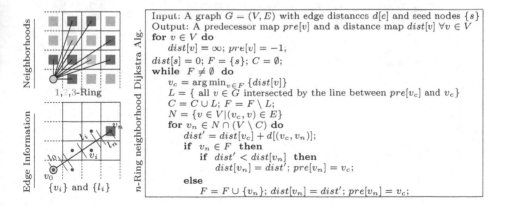

Fig. 1. On the top left a quadrant of a 2D visualization of different neighborhood sizes is shown. Omitted, linear dependent directions are color-coded in gray. The information (intersected voxels and lengths) stored for each $e \in E$ is shown on the bottom left.

Table 1. Timings (in ms) for different portions (25% to 100%) and neighborhood sizes (the 0-ring has 6 neighbors).

Cells (%)	0-Ring	1-Ring	2-Ring	3-Ring
100	160/160	240/160	420/160	660/155
75	135/110	190/120	350/140	600/155
50	90/80	140/75	255/105	450/118
25	35/28	100/50	105/40	300/70

Since voxels with a high flow rate are conquered first, the last conquered nodes of G usually do not contain many paths. This allows us to speed up the computation by only conquering a certain portion of the graph. Our experiments indicate that all important pathways have been extracted, when aborting the computation after conquering 50% of the nodes (Col. 1 of Fig. 3). While timings for Dijkstra are mainly affected by the neighborhood size (first numbers in Tab. 1), the timings for tracing back endpoints (second numbers) are mainly influenced by the amount of endpoints, which depends on the portion of nodes to be conquered. Col. 2 of Fig. 3 shows how the parameter α can be used to influence the anisotropic movement of the front. Keeping α small results in a more spherical expansion pattern while high values for α force the front to quickly follow important paths. In this example we place the seed near the left eye and major pathways end near the visual cortex. Using the 1-ring results in pathways similar to using larger neighborhoods (Col. 3 of Fig. 3). This is good, since such neighborhoods were often used in previous works. Nevertheless, including voxels from the 2-ring reveals more, finer structures. When using larger neighborhoods we only gain a bit more information, so we use the 2-ring by default.

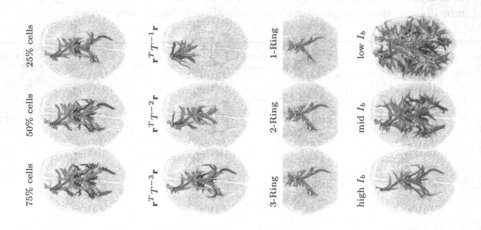

Fig. 2. Connection between the eyes and the visual cortex. Col. 1: Effect of conquering different portions of the graph. Col. 2: Influence of α. Col. 3: Different neighborhood sizes. Col. 4: Visual pruning of the tree by changing the transfer function.

4 Discussion

We presented an efficient method based on Dijkstra's algorithms to compute and visualize globally connected pathways. Since our visualization approach is based on volume rendering, highlighting important fibers is just a matter of adapting a transfer function. Enhancing the anisotropic movement of the front (parameter α in Sec. 2.2) and using larger voxel neighborhoods yield plausible and smooth pathways.

To visualize specific nerve bundles, we plan to interactively define a target region besides the seed, which requires the user to have some anatomical knowledge. After computing Dijkstra one can automatically select those endpoints, whose paths to the seed intersect the user defined target region. We expect that tracing back (Sec. 2.3) those paths would restrict the visualization to specific connections. In our current system we represent the ODF by a single elliptically shaped tensor. In future work we would like to use arbitrary ODFs to compute the edge distances. Then, this approach also works for HARDI data like Q-Ball Images, which would lead to even more reliable representations of the fibers.

Acknowledgement. This work was partially supported by the DFG (IRTG 1328).

References

1. Tuch DS. Q-ball imaging. Magn Reson Med. 2004;52(6):1358–72.
2. Crettenand S, Meredith SD, Hoptman MJ, et al. Quantitative analysis and comparison of diffusion tensor imaging tractography algorithms. Ir Signals Syst Conf. 2006; p. 105–10.
3. Behrens TE, Woolrich MW, Jenkinson M, et al. Characterization and propagation of uncertainty in diffusion-weighted MR imaging. Magn Reson Med. 2003;50(5):1077–88.
4. Friman O, Farneback G, Westin CF. A bayesian approach for stochastic white matter tractography. IEEE Trans Med Imaging. 2006;25(8):965–78.
5. Zalesky A. DT-MRI fiber tracking: a shortest paths approach. IEEE Trans Med Imaging. 2008;27(10):1458–71.
6. McGraw T, Nadar MS. Stochastic DT-MRI connectivity mapping on the GPU. IEEE Trans Vis Comput Graph. 2007;13(6):1504–11.
7. Everts MH, Bekker H, Roerdink JBTM. Visualizing white matter structure of the brain using Dijkstra's algorithm. Proc ISPA. 2009; p. 569–74.
8. Sherbondy A, Akers D, Mackenzie R, et al. Exploring connectivity of the brain's white matter with dynamic queries. IEEE TVCG. 2005;11(4):419–30.
9. Rick T, von Kapri A, Caspers S, et al. Visualization of probabilistic fiber tracts in virtual reality. Stud Health Technol Inform. 2011;163:486–92.
10. Kindlmann G, , Westin CF. Diffusion tensor visualization with glyph packing. IEEE TVCG. 2006;12(5):1329–36.

On Feature Tracking in X-Ray Images

Moritz Klüppel[1], Jian Wang[1], David Bernecker[1], Peter Fischer[1,2],
Joachim Hornegger[1,2]

[1] Pattern Recognition Lab, FAU Erlangen-Nürnberg
[2] Erlangen Graduate School in Advanced Optical Technologies (SAOT)
moritz.klueppel@medtech.stud.uni-erlangen.de

Abstract. Feature point tracking and detection of X-ray images is challenging due to overlapping anatomical structures of different depths, which lead to low-contrast images. Tracking of motion in X-ray sequences can support many clinical applications like motion compensation or two- or three-dimensional registration algorithms. This paper is the first to evaluate the performance of several feature tracking and detection algorithms on artificial and real X-ray image sequences, which involve rigid motion as well as external disturbances. A stand-alone application has been developed to provide an overall test bench for all algorithms, realized by OpenCV implementations. Experiments show that the Karhunen Loeve Transform-based Tracker is the most consistent and effective tracking algorithm. Considering external disturbances, template matching provides the most sufficient results. Furthermore, the influence of feature point detection methods on tracking results is shown.

1 Introduction

In interventional radiology, fluoroscopy provides real-time two-dimensional (2D) X-ray images. To enhance the 2D X-ray images with additional planning information, the images can be overlaid with pre-operative 3D CT or MRI images. The registration of three-dimensional (3D) volume and real-time 2D fluoroscopic images is one of the key challenges for image-guided interventional radiology [1]. However, motion of the patient or distinct organs can occur, which needs to be compensated for an accurate 2D/3D overlay. Therefore, motion has to be detected and characterized first. One way to achieve this step is to apply feature point tracking algorithms, which find 2D correspondences between neighboring frames.

Previous work on patient motion compensation mostly falls into two categories, namely model-driven [2] and data-driven [3]. An example for the methods used in the latter category is the optical flow-based Karhunen Loeve Transform (KLT)-Tracker [4], which is the starting point of our evaluation.

In computer vision, most of the feature tracking methods were designed for natural images. Tracking in X-ray images is a more challenging task due to the lower contrast. Furthermore, overlapping structures of different depths lead to a low distinction. To authors' knowledge, no previous work has been published so far, which assesses the standard behavior of tracking algorithms on X-ray images. This work presents an evaluation of state of the art feature tracking approaches for estimating the patient motion from 2D X-ray images. The tracking methods are evaluated on both digitally reconstructed radiography (DRR) image sequences and clinical X-ray images.

2   Materials and methods

Feature tracking relies on the robust detection of salient points or regions, which appear over several frames. For this task, several methods are evaluated in the following section. An implementation of all methods can be found in the open-source computer vision library OpenCV. Although no direct comparison between the OpenCV algorithms and the reference implementations has been performed, this library is widely used in the field of computer vision and is permanently enhanced. The next section then describes how the detected feature points are tracked over time.

2.1   Feature detection and description

In this evaluation, the following feature point detection methods are considered.

- Good Features To Track (GFTT) [4]
- Features from Accelerated Segment Test (FAST) [5]
- Scale Invariant Feature Transform (SIFT) [6]
- Speeded Up Robust Features (SURF) [7]
- Binary Robust Invariant Scalable Keypoints (BRISK) [8]

Out of the five methods, GFTT was developed for the use in conjunction with a specific tracking algorithm, the KLT-Tracker. GFTT aims at finding feature points which exhibit optimal characteristics for this tracking method. Since the KLT-Tracker uses patches around the feature points for tracking, GFTT is a pure feature point detector. In contrary, FAST, SIFT, SURF and BRISK do not only detect feature points, but also encode information about the surrounding region of the feature point. These descriptor values, which are usually invariant to scaling and rotation, can be used to establish correspondences between feature points in successive frames.

2.2   Feature tracking

For the actual tracking of the detected feature points over the neighboring frames, three different methods are considered.

The Kanade-Lucas-Tomasi tracker (KLT-Tracker) uses small image patches around the detected feature points to compute the sparse optical flow between two neighboring frames. One drawback of this method is that it can only cope with small displacements of the individual feature points. As comparison, the descriptor values obtained from the each feature points can be used for descriptor matching between the two successive frames. For computing the correspondences between the feature points, we either use a brute-force nearest neighbor algorithm, or the Fast Library for Approximate Nearest Neighbors (FLANN) [9]. As a third tracking method, we have used template matching, where relative larger patches surrounding the feature points are used. Each patch is compared to its surrounding in the next frame using normalized sum of squared differences (SQD), normalized correlation coefficient (COEF) or normalized cross correlation (NCC). The displacement for the feature point is then given by the displacement which exhibits the smallest difference or highest correlation measure of the image patch.

2.3 Experiments

With the application of interventional imaging in mind, the feature tracking algorithms need to be evaluated under the aspect of real-time capability and the actual quality and accuracy of the tracking results. Following performance metrics and experimental results are based on these two evaluation points.

Performance metrics The computational efficiency is affected by operations performed on the whole image (e.g. detecting feature points) and operations performed for each detected point (e.g. descriptor calculation). The rate between the number of tracked feature points and the costs for tracking each of these points can be described by the relative computational efficiency

$$t_{\mathrm{rel}} = \frac{T}{\# \text{ of detected/tracked features}} \tag{1}$$

where T is the overall execution time for one frame.

The consistency of tracking results is a decisive factor for a successful tracking method. The proposed modified tracking rate (mTR) computes the ratio of feature points in I_0 and the number of actually tracked feature points in I_t

$$\mathrm{mTR} = \frac{\# \text{ of tracked features in } I_t}{\# \text{ of features in } I_0} \tag{2}$$

For the case of known ground-truth movement $\boldsymbol{u}_i^*$ of a set of points, the Object tracking error (OTE) is used for measuring tracking accuracy. Based on

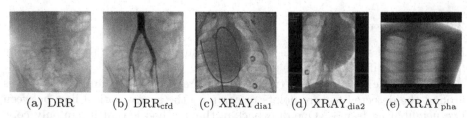

    (a) DRR   (b) DRR$_{\mathrm{cfd}}$ (c) XRAY$_{\mathrm{dia1}}$ (d) XRAY$_{\mathrm{dia2}}$ (e) XRAY$_{\mathrm{pha}}$

Fig. 1. The different datasets which are used for experimental evaluation. Each set provides a sequence of images, acquired under motion.

Table 1. Computational efficiency of feature detection and tracking procedures. Mean computation time as well as corresponding standard deviation are presented in milliseconds (ms).

Detection	GFTT	FAST	SIFT	SURF	BRISK		
t_{rel}[ms]	1.095	0.009	5.573	0.433	0.181		
$\sigma(t_{rel})$[ms]	0.11	0.001	5.515	0.106	0.019		
Tracking	KLT	tmSQD	tmNCC	tmCOEF	dmSIFT	dmSURF	dmBRISK
t_{rel}[ms]	0.068	1.728	1.733	1.749	61.636	7.866	4.381
$\sigma(t_{rel})$[ms]	0.027	2.863	2.857	2.837	69.712	4.689	4.238

the tracked feature points, the error of the estimated motion $\hat{u}_i$ of all the N frames is combined in the modified tracking error

$$\text{mTE} = \frac{1}{N} \sum_{i=1}^{N} \|u_i^* - \hat{u}_i\|^2 \tag{3}$$

This measure describes tracking accuracy and the consistency of the tracking result at the same time.

Experimental materials The evaluation is performed on artificial and real-world data. An illustrative overview of the used image sequences is given in Fig. 1. For the simulated digitally reconstructed radiography (DRR) images the ground truth motion is known. The motion consists of translations and rotations in 3D which were projected to 2D motion in the images. For both kind of motions, one dataset was evaluated respectively. For tracking algorithms in a clinical background, external disturbances in image sequences are common. Interventional devices or contrast agent can suddenly appear in the image and cause sustainable changes of the image data. Therefore, the behavior of the feature point tracking algorithms is also evaluated for such sequences in one dataset (DRR$_{cfd}$), where blood flow was simulated by Computational Fluid Dynamics (CFD). The real image sequences are acquired using a C-arm CT and have unknown ground truth data. For these datasets, only the computational efficiency and the mTR can be calculated. Two datasets (XRAY$_{dia1}$, XRAY$_{dia2}$) provide X-ray images of real patients, and one sequence (XRAY$_{pha}$) consists of images of a phantom model. In this dataset patient motion was simulated by moving the phantom during image acquisition.

3   Results

Tab. 1 presents the results of different feature detection methods in milliseconds (ms). As expected, SIFT is much more time-consuming than BRISK and FAST. The high variance of SIFT performance leads to a wide gap in efficiency while detecting a small and large number of features. Despite its scale-space approach, SURF provides higher computational efficiency. Except for SIFT, all methods are in an acceptable range, also for large numbers of feature points. Similarly, Tab. 1 shows the timing results of tracking procedures. BRISK gives the best result, while the descriptor matching algorithms are very slow. The brute-force method is applied for SIFT (dmSIFT) and SURF (dmSURF), while FLANN is applied for BRISK (dmBRISK). Compared to the other algorithms, the KLT-Tracker has the highest computational efficiency. Meanwhile, all three comparison methods (tmSQD, tmNCC, tmCOEF) of template matching also provide high efficiency.

The experimental results of $\overline{mTR}$ for the KLT-Tracker are not substantially different from the template matching algorithms good results. All are in the range of more than 97%. In contrast, the descriptor matching approaches provide bad tracking rates of 5-80%. Furthermore, the respective standard deviations are high, which means no consistency is established. A reason for this behavior could be the qualitative ranking of the matches by the respective algorithms, so the matches are admittedly computed correctly, but are not followed constantly over each frame.

The tracking error mTE is shown in Fig. 2. It shows that the descriptor matching procedures fail while following the feature points. In comparison, the KLT-Tracker provides the best results as illustrated by the first five bar sets. However, the error is increased when combined with the highly efficient FAST detector. In contrast, the features detected by SIFT are well tracked, but the low efficiency of this detector (Tab. 1) has to be considered. For the CFD dataset, the template matching algorithms provide the best results. For the KLT-Tracker, the feature points get 'washed' away if the blood flow appears, but the templates can be tracked again when the disturbance is gone.

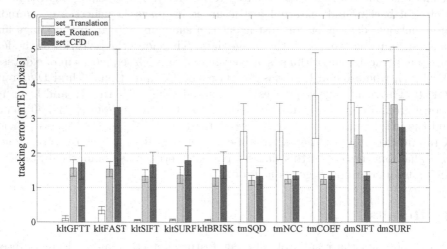

Fig. 2. The tracking error mTE for each DRR dataset is illustrated in this figure. Each tracking procedure has been evaluated. The deficient results of the descriptor matching algorithm in combination with BRISK had been skipped for illustrative purpose.

4 Discussion

In this paper, different popular feature tracking algorithms are evaluated on X-ray images. The evaluation is performed in a single framework that provides an identical test environment and I/O parameters. Experiments are designed to investigate the behaviors of anatomical feature detection and tracking in both simulated (DRR) and real X-ray images. Different 3D motion patterns are considered in the experiments. In general, the computational efficiency decreases with increasing detection accuracy of the feature detection algorithms. The KLT-Tracker is highlighted as an efficient, accurate and consistent tracking approach. Furthermore, template matching provides sufficient results during external disturbances in the image sequences. As the mTR and mTE metrics showed, the descriptor matching algorithms generally failed, which means extensions are needed in further investigations.

As the presented results showed the success and efficiency of optical flow, realized by the KLT-Tracker, future work will have to focus on further implementations of optical flow algorithms. Baker et al. present a benchmark of multiple optical flow implementations [10]. To counter the tradeoff between high quality features and low computational efficiency, further SIFT implementations could be improved by parallelization. In addition, future experimental evaluation procedures should be able to use real ground truth 2D motion of the X-ray image to provide more precise test results.

References

1. Markelj P, Tomažević D, Likar B, et al. A review of 3D/2D registration methods for image-guided interventions. Med Image Anal. 2012;16(3):642–61.
2. Cao Y, Wang P. An adaptive method of tracking anatomical curves in X-ray sequences. Proc MICCAI. 2012; p. 173–80.
3. Wang J, Borsdorf A, Hornegger J. Depth-layer-based patient motion compensation for the overlay of 3D volumes onto X-ray sequences. Proc BVM. 2013; p. 128–33.
4. Tomasi C, Kanade T. Detection and Tracking of Point Features. School of Computer Science, Carnegie Mellon University; 1991.
5. Rosten E, Reitmayr G, Drummond T. Real-time video annotations for augmented reality. Adv Vis Comput. 2005; p. 294–302.
6. Lowe DG. Distinctive image features from scale-invariant keypoints. Int J Comput Vis. 2004;60(2):91–110.
7. Bay H, Tuytelaars T, Van Gool L. Surf: speeded up robust features. Eur Conf Comput Vis. 2006; p. 404–17.
8. Leutenegger S, Chli M, Siegwart RY. BRISK: binary robust invariant scalable keypoints. Proc IEEE ICCV. 2011; p. 2548–55.
9. Muja M, Lowe DG. Fast approximate nearest neighbors with automatic algorithm configuration. Proc VISIGRAPP. 2009; p. 331–40.
10. Baker S, Scharstein D, Lewis J, et al. A database and evaluation methodology for optical flow. Int J Comput Vis. 2011;92(1):1–31.

Detektion chirurgischer Schrauben in 3D C-Bogen Daten

Joseph Görres[1], Michael Brehler[1], Jochen Franke[2], Ivo Wolf[3], Sven Y. Vetter[2], Paul A. Grützner[2], Hans-Peter Meinzer[1], Diana Nabers[1]

[1]Abteilung für Medizinische und Biologische Informatik, DKFZ Heidelberg
[2]Berufsgenossenschaftliche Unfallklinik, Ludwigshafen
[3]Institut für Medizinische Informatik, Hochschule Mannheim
j.goerres@dkfz-heidelberg.de

Kurzfassung. Frakturen am Fersenbein werden mit Hilfe offener Reduktion und interner Fixation korrigiert. Eine anatomisch korrekte Rekonstruktion beteiligter Gelenke ist notwendig, um Knorpelschäden und verfrühte Arthrose vorzubeugen. Um intraartikuläre Schraubenplatzierungen zu vermeiden wird der mobile 3D C-Bogen eingesetzt. Die detaillierte Analyse der Schraubenlage anhand des erzeugten 3D Bildes ist jedoch auf eine zeitaufwändige Mensch-Computer-Interaktion angewiesen. Etablierte Interaktionsprozeduren basieren auf wiederholtem Positionieren und Rotieren von Schnittebenen, wodurch die intraoperative Kontrolle der Schraubenplatzierung die Dauer der Operation wesentlich verlängert. Um die Interaktion mit 3D C-Bogen Daten zu erleichtern schlagen wir eine automatische Schraubendetektion vor, mit der eine direkte Anwahl relevanter Schnittebenen möglich wird. Unser Ansatz setzt sich aus zwei Schritten zusammen. Im ersten Schritt werden zylindrische Charakteristiken anhand lokaler Gradientstrukturen mit Hilfe von RANSAC ermittelt. Diese Charakteristiken werden dann durch die Anwendung des DBScan Clustering Algorithmus im zweiten Schritt gruppiert. Jedes detektierte Cluster repräsentiert abschließend eine Schraube. Unsere Evaluation mit 309 Schrauben in 50 Bildern zeigt robuste Ergebnisse. Der Algorithmus detektierte 97.4% der Schrauben korrekt.

1 Einleitung

Interartikuläre Frakturen am Fersenbein werden mit Hilfe von offener Reduktion und interner Fixation korrigiert. Dazu werden die Knochenfragmente mit einer Kalkaneusplatte und mehreren Schrauben fixiert. Um Arthrose vorzubeugen dürfen keine Schrauben in benachbarte Gelenke ragen [1]. Diese Voraussetzung lässt sich mit Hilfe des mobilen 3D C-Bogens intraoperativ sicherstellen. Im Gegensatz zu einzelnen 2D Röntgen-Aufnahmen, kann die Kontrolle der Schraubenlage mit Hilfe des 3D C-Bogen Daten unter einer höheren Genauigkeit erfolgen. Somit senkt der Einsatz von mobilen 3D C-Bogen die Rezidivrate für Osteosynthesen am Fersenbein und verringert außerdem die Notwendigkeit eines postoperativen CT Scans [2].

Um die relevanten Schrauben in dem dreidimensionalen Datensatz präzise kontrollieren zu können, muss der Chirurg die Orientierung der Schnittebenen manuell auf die Längsausrichtung der Schraube anpassen. Dies ist ein zeitaufwändiger Prozess, der für jede Schraube durchgeführt werden muss. Um diesen manuellen Prozess zu automatisieren, stellen wir ein Detektionsverfahren vor, dass Schrauben in den Bilddaten findet, womit sich die Schnittebenen bestimmen lassen. Die Detektion von Schrauben in 3D C-Bogen Daten ist dabei herausfordernd, da Metallimplantate und Schrauben stark die Bildqualitiät beeinflussen. Außerdem sind Schrauben und die Kalkaneusplatte miteinander verbunden und liegen im gleichen Bildintensitätsbereich von Metall. Aus diesen Gründen ist es nicht möglich das Problem mit einer einfachen Intensitätsklassifikation zu lösen.

Die Detektion von chirurgischen Schrauben ist ein weitgehend unerforschtes Gebiet. Unser Verfahren weist die größte Ähnlichkeit mit Ansätzen zur Zylinderdetektion auf. Die eindeutige Gradientenstruktur am Zylinderrand kann ausgenutzt werden um Zylinderrichtungen zu ermitteln. Zu diesem Zweck haben Chaperon et al. [3] RANSAC und Rabbani et al. [4] eine Hough Transformation angewandt. Beide Ansätze beruhen jedoch auf der Annahme, dass ein Großteil der untersuchten Gradienten am Zylinderrand befindlich sind. Diese Annahme mag für synthetische oder industrielle Bilddaten mit wohlgeformten Zylindern ausreichend sein, aber in unserem Fall bilden Gradienten an der Schraubengrenze eine Minderheit innerhalb des gesamten Bildes und stechen daher nicht statistisch heraus. Aus diesem Grund untersuchen wir Gradienten lediglich lokal in kleinen Bildregionen. Bezüglich der medizinischen Anwendung gibt es eine verwandte Arbeit von Zhou et al. [5] zur Segmentierung von Nadeln in 3D Ultraschall Bildern mit einer 3D Hough Transformation. Eine Geradendetektion ist jedoch nicht ausreichend diskriminativ bei unseren Bilddaten, da Knochengrenzen und Kalkaneusplatten ebenfalls zahlreiche Geraden mit hoher Bildintensität präsentieren.

Mit diesem Beitrag stellen wir eine automatische Schraubendetektion vor, die als Grundlage für eine vereinfachte Interaktion mit 3D Bilddaten dient. Eine Bestimmung von lokalen zylindrischen Charakteristiken wird angewandt, um Schrauben von Knochengrenzen und Kalkaneusplatten zu separieren.

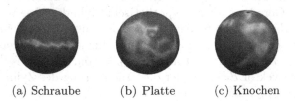

(a) Schraube   (b) Platte   (c) Knochen

Abb. 1. Orientierungshistogramme für verschiedene Bildregionen: (a) eine Schraube, (b) ein Teil einer Kalkaneusplatte und (c) ein Teil einer Knochengrenze. Die Farben beschreiben die normalisierte Summe der Gradientenbeträge für die jeweilige Richtung. Rot steht für die niedrigsten Werte und blau für die höchsten.

2   Material und Methoden

Chirurgische Schrauben haben eine zylindrische Form, die im Bild eine eindeutige Gradientenstruktur am Zylinderrand aufweist. Allgemein betrachtet zeigen alle Gradientenrichtungen an der Mantelfläche in Richtung der zentralen Zylinderachse. Werden dort befindliche Gradienten unabhängig von ihren Positionen untersucht, dann liegen diese alle in der selben zweidimensionalen Ebene. Diese Charakteristik lässt sich in unseren Bilddaten feststellen und kann mit Hilfe von Orientierungshistogrammen visualisiert werden. Abb. 1 zeigt ein Beispiel für eine Bildregion, die nur eine Schraube enthält und stellt dies zwei Bildregionen, die eine Kalkaneusplatte, bzw. eine Knochengrenze zeigen, gegenüber.

Wir nutzen die beschriebene Gradientenstruktur aus, indem wir den Random Sample Consensus (RANSAC) Algorithmus [6] anwenden. Hierzu müssen das notwendige Modell und die Fehlerfunktion definiert werden, um unsere gewünschte Gradientenstruktur zu ermitteln. Wir definieren das Modell als eine Ebene durch den Ursprung, die durch zwei randomisiert gewählte Gradienten $a_1 = \nabla i(x_1)$ und $a_2 = \nabla i(x_2)$ aufgespannt wird. Diese Gradienten befinden sich an den Positionen $x_1, x_2 \in \mathbb{R}^3$ aus der Bildregion R im Bild i. Wir stellen sicher, dass der Betrag eines randomisiert gewählten Gradienten mindestens halb so groß ist wie der maximale Betrag aller Gradienten in Region R. Die Ebenennormale n ist dann definiert durch $n = (\hat{a}_1 \times \hat{a}_2)$. Unsere Fehlerfunktion f bewertet die Distanzen aller Gradientenrichtungen zur gewählten Ebene und wird beschrieben mit Hilfe der Notationen $\hat{x} = \frac{x}{||x||}$, $||x||^2 = \langle x, x \rangle$

$$f(R) = \frac{\sum_{r \in R} ||\nabla i(r)|| \cdot m(\hat{n}, \widehat{\nabla i(r)})}{\sum_{r \in R} ||\nabla i(r)|| + \epsilon}, \quad \text{mit } m(x, y) = \left(\frac{\langle x, y \rangle}{0.1} \right)^2 \quad (1)$$

Wir generieren zahlreiche Regionen für das gesamte Bild indem wir eine Schrittweite von $w \in \mathbb{N}$ Pixeln entlang aller Dimensionen wählen. Die Regionen haben eine feste Größe von $\lfloor \frac{m}{v} \rfloor \times \lfloor \frac{m}{v} \rfloor \times \lfloor \frac{m}{v} \rfloor$ Voxeln mit dem geschätzten Schraubendurchmesser $m = 4$ mm und dem Schichtabstand v, der bei allen Dimensionen gleich ist. Auf jeder gewählten Bildregion wenden wir RANSAC an. Liefert $f(R)$ einen kleinen Wert, dann haben wir die Präsenz einer zylindrischen Charakteristik in der Bildregion R ermittelt. Diese Charakteristik beschreiben wir durch eine Gerade, die eine hypothetische Zylinderachse repräsentiert und bezeichnen sie als Zylinderkandidat. Wir wählen entsprechend einen Schwellwert $\tau \in \mathbb{R}^{>0}$ und erzeugen einen Zylinderkandidat für jede Bildregion R, die die Bedingung $f(R) < \tau$ erfüllt. Jeder Kandidat $c_k = (p_k, d_k)$, $k \in \mathbb{N}^{\geq 0}$ setzt sich aus einem Richtungsvektor $d_k \in \mathbb{R}^3$, der die Orientierung des Zylinders beschreibt, und einem Punkt $p_k \in \mathbb{R}^3$, der die Position des Zylinders beschreibt, zusammen. Der Kandidatenpunkt p_k auf der hypothetischen Zylinderachse wird durch die Berechnung des Mittelpunkts der kürzesten Strecke zwischen zwei windschiefen Geraden geschätzt. Die windschiefen Geraden setzen sich zusammen aus den Richtungen a_1, a_2 und ihrer Positionen im Bild. Die Kandidatenrichtung d_k ist bestimmt durch die Normale der Kandidatenebene, die durch RANSAC ermittelt wird. In wenigen Fällen können alle betrachteten Gradienten einer Bildregion in die gleiche Richtung zeigen und liegen somit in der gleichen Ebene, z.B. an ebenen Objektgrenzen. Um solche Kandidaten zu entfernen überprüfen wir, dass verschiedene Gradientenrichtungen in der Bildregion vorhanden sind.

Für jede chirurgische Schraube erhält man viele Kandidaten. Diese sind dicht besiedelt und zeigen in gleiche Richtungen, die ungefähr parallel zur zentralen Schraubenachse liegen. In Abb. 2 werden alle Kandidaten für ein Bildbeispiel gezeigt, woran sich diese Eigenschaft gut erkennen lässt. Um diese Kandidatenansammlungen zu ermitteln wenden wir den DBScan Algorithmus [7] an. Dieser ist ein dichtebasierter Ansatz zur Clusteranalyse, der durch alle Kandidaten iteriert und rekursiv ein Cluster aufbaut, wenn die Zahl der Nachbarn innerhalb eines vorgegebenen Radius $r \in \mathbb{R}^{>0}$ größer als $n \in \mathbb{N}$ ist. Die Distanz d zwischen zwei Kandidaten c_1, c_2 ist definiert durch $d^2(c_1, c_2) = (\cos^{-1}\langle \hat{d}_1, \hat{d}_2 \rangle)^2 + (s(c_1, c_2)/\lfloor \frac{m}{v} \rfloor)^2$. Wir definieren s als das Maximum der zwei kürzesten Distanzen von Punkt p_1 zur Geraden (p_2, d_2) und p_2 zu (p_1, d_1).

Für jedes ermittelte Cluster berechnen wir abschließend einen mittleren Kandidaten und die räumliche Ausdehnung entlang seiner Richtung. Jedes Cluster repräsentiert somit eine detektierte Schraube.

3 Ergebnisse

Unser Evaluationsdatensatz besteht aus 50 Bildvolumen, die während einer chirurgischen Operation direkt nach dem Einsetzen von Schrauben aufgenommen wurden. Die Bildquelle ist ein Arcadis® Orbic von Siemens, ein isozentrischer mobiler C-Bogen Scanner für Cone-Beam CT. In unserer Konfiguration erstellt das Gerät Bilder mit einer Auflösung von $256 \times 256 \times 256$ Voxeln bei einer Voxelgröße von 0.485 mm. Jedes Bild zeigt das vollständige Fersenbein und in der Bildmitte meist das untere Sprunggelenk. Wir haben eine verlässliche Ground-Truth erstellt, indem wir 309 chirurgische Schrauben manuell annotiert haben. Jede

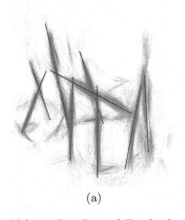

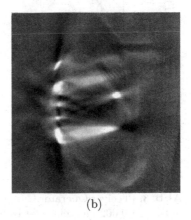

(a)   (b)

Abb. 2. Die Ground-Truth, dargestellt als blaue Linie, wird den Kandidaten in (a) gegenübergestellt. Ein axialer Schnitt des Eingabebildes wird in (b) abgebildet.

Schraube wird durch einen Punkt an seiner Spitze und einen Punkt an seinem Kopf beschrieben. In jedem Bild gibt es zwischen zwei und neun Schrauben (6.2 ± 1.4 pro Bild) mit Dicken zwischen 2 mm und 6 mm. Viele verschiedene Schraubentypen sind präsent und in 48 Bildvolumen ist außerdem eine Kalkaneusplatte vorhanden. Eine Schraube wird als detektiert bezeichnet, wenn der Abstand d zwischen Ergebnis c_r und Ground-Truth c_g die Bedingung $d(c_r, c_g) < 0.5$ erfüllt.

Unser Ansatz wurde auf jedes Bild im Evaluationsdatensatz mit den Parametern $(r, n, w) = (0.04, 12, 4)$ angewandt. Den kritischen Parameter τ haben wir von 0 bis 0.258 bei einer Schrittweite von 0.002 variiert. Die Detektionsleistung für verschiedene τ ist in Abb. 3 dargestellt. Wird akzeptiert, dass im Mittel jede dritte detektierte Schraube falsch positiv ist, erreicht das Verfahren eine True-Positive-Rate (TPR) von 97.4%. Soll im Mittel jedoch nicht mehr als jede zehnte (zwanzigste) detektierte Schraube falsch positiv sein, sinkt die TPR auf 75.4% (50%). Die Berechnungszeit ist dabei etwa 15 Sekunden, wenn nur ein Prozessorkern verwendet wird. Die Berechnung wurde mit C++ Programmcode auf einem einzelnen Prozessorkern eines Intel®Core™i7 CPU X990 mit 3.47GHz durchgeführt. Die Entwicklung und Evaluation wurde mit dem Medical Imaging Interaction Toolkit (MITK, http://www.mitk.org [8]) umgesetzt.

4 Diskussion

Eine vollständig automatische Methode zur Detektion von chirurgischen Schrauben in Bildern mobiler 3D C-Bogen Geräte wurde präsentiert. Durch das Ausnutzen zugrundeliegender Gradientenstrukturen sind wir in der Lage zylindrische und nicht-zylindrische Bildregionen zu separieren. Chirurgische Schrauben

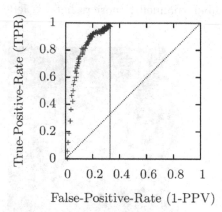
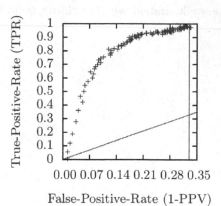

Abb. 3. Receiver Operator Curve (ROC), die bei der Variation von τ bei einer Schrittweite von 0.002 entsteht. Die Daten streuen geringfügig aufgrund der randomisierten Gradientenwahl durch RANSAC. Im rechten Schaubild ist eine Detailansicht der ROC für den Bereich, der durch die rote Linie eingegrenzt ist, dargestellt.

werden verlässlich detektiert, obwohl ihr Intensitätsbereich mit Knochengrenzen und Kalkaneusplatten überlappt. Mit unserem Ansatz lassen sich gewünschte Bildregionen um eine Schraube herum direkt anwählen. Chirurgen können somit schnell relevante Bildregionen betrachten, ohne durch manuelle Interaktion im Arbeitsfluss behindert zu werden.

Die Evaluation zeigt eine hohe Robustheit des Verfahrens bei gleichzeitig akzeptabler Berechnungszeit, wodurch sich das Verfahren für den intraoperativen Einsatz eignet. Die Berechnungszeit lässt sich außerdem drastisch reduzieren, da die teuersten Rechenschritte mit Hilfe massiver Parallelisierung durchgeführt werden können. Für die Zukunft planen wir unser Verfahren auf andere Operationen zur Behandlung von Knochenfrakturen zu übertragen.

Danksagung. Die Autoren möchten sich bei Dr. Karl Barth und Dr. Gerhard Kleinszig für den technischen Support und die bereitgestellten Informationen über das C-Bogen CT System bedanken. Dieses Projekt wurde von Siemens Healthcare (X-ray Products) teilfinanziert.

Literaturverzeichnis

1. Sanders R. Current concepts review: displaced intra-articular fractures of the calcaneus. J Bone Joint Surg. 2000;82(2):225–50.
2. Franke J, Recum J, Wendl K, et al. Intraoperative three-dimensional imaging: beneficial or necessary? Unfallchirurg. 2013;116(2):185–90.
3. Chaperon T, Goulette F. Extracting cylinders in full 3D data using a random sampling method and the gaussian image. Proc VMV. 2001; p. 35–42.
4. Rabbani T, van den Heuvel FA. Efficient hough transform for automatic detection of cylinders in point clouds. Proc ISPRS Workshop Laser Scanning. 2005; p. 60–5.
5. Zhou H, Qiu W, Ding M, et al. Automatic needle segmentation in 3D ultrasound images using 3D improved Hough transform. Proc SPIE. 2008;6918:691821–1 – 691821–9.
6. Fischler MA, Bolles RC. Random sample consensus: a paradigm for model fitting with applications to image analysis and automated cartography. Com ACM. 1981;24(6):381–95.
7. Ester M, Kriegel HP, Sander J, et al. A density-based algorithm for discovering clusters in large spatial databases with noise. Knowl Discov Data Min. 1996; p. 226–31.
8. Nolden M, Zelzer S, Seitel A, et al. The medical imaging interaction toolkit: challenges and advances. Int J Comput Assist Radiol Surg. 2013;8(4):607–20.

3D-Symmetrietransformation zur Gefäßsegmentierung in MRT-TOF-Daten

Regina Pohle-Fröhlich[1], Derik Stalder[2]

[1]iPattern – Institut für Mustererkennung, Hochschule Niederrhein, Krefeld
[2]Gamma Knife Zentrum Krefeld
regina.pohle@hsnr.de

Kurzfassung. Im Beitrag wird ein Verfahren zur Gefäßdetektion in 3D MRT-TOF-Bilddaten vorgeschlagen, das auf der Auswertung von Symmetrieinformation beruht. Die Ergebnisse der entwickelten Symmetrietransformation werden mit denen der Skalenraumfilterung verglichen. Die neue Transformation liefert eine detailreichere Darstellung des Gefäßbaums in den Ergebnissen und erlaubt gleichzeitig eine Separierung der Gefäße nach bestimmten Gefäßdurchmessern.

1 Einleitung

Vor einer Gamma Knife Behandlung von Gefäßmalformationen werden diagnostische 2D-Angiographien mit entsprechenden Markern angefertigt, um die genaue Position des zu bestrahlenden Areals festzulegen. Außerdem werden für die Bestrahlungsplanung 3D MRT-TOF-Bilddaten, die ebenfalls die Marker enthalten, benötigt. Durch eine Registrierung der beiden Bildmaterialien anhand der Markerpunkte lässt sich die Position des zu bestrahlenden Areals in die MRT-Daten übertragen. Da zur Bilderzeugung der Angiographien eine für den Patienten belastende Kontrastmittelgabe notwendig ist, soll untersucht werden, ob zur Registrierung extern angefertigte 2D-Angiographien aus Voruntersuchungen genutzt werden können. In diesen Aufnahmen fehlen jedoch verwertbare Markerpositionen, so dass zur Registrierung natürliche Marker verwendet werden sollen, wie z.B. große Gefäße. In einem ersten Schritt ist es deswegen notwendig, die Gefäße in den 3D Bilddaten zu segmentieren. Gesucht ist ein Verfahren, welches sowohl für 3D- als auch für 2D-Bilddaten funktioniert und zur Verfolgung einer grob-zu-fein Stategie bei der Registrierung gleichzeitig eine Differenzierung zwischen unterschiedlichen Gefäßdurchmessern erlaubt.

Die in der Literatur beschriebenen Ansätze zur Segmentierung von Blutgefäßen in 3D-Aufnahmen unterscheiden sich hinsichtlich des eingesetzten Modellwissens. So werden häufig wahrnehmungsbasierte Modelle, die davon ausgehen, dass die Gefäße in den Aufnahmen heller als die Umgebung sind, mit geometrischen Modellen kombiniert. Diese legen eine zylinderförmige Gestalt der Blutgefäße zugrunde [1].

Bei den in der Praxis eingesetzten Segmentierungsverfahren müssen bei der Detektion minimaler Pfade [2] und dem Einsatz deformierbarer Modelle [3] Startpunktinitialisierungen bzw. Gewichtungsfaktoren vorgegeben werden, so dass sie immer Benutzerinteraktion benötigen. Eine Differenzierung zwischen unterschiedlichen Gefäßgrößen ist bei beiden Methoden nur über einen Nachverarbeitungsschritt möglich.

Bei den statistischen Ansätzen [4] hängt die Genauigkeit der Segmentierung von dem zugrunde gelegten Modell ab. Ein Problem ist hier, dass sich das Kontrastmittel nicht gleichmäßig in den Gefäßen verteilt und dadurch Intensitätsschwankungen auftreten. Verfahren, die den Gradientenfluss auswerten [5] haben ihre Beschränkungen bei der Segmentierung schmaler, gekrümmter Gefäße sowie an Verzweigungspunkten. Auch bei diesen Segmentierungsmethoden muss die Gefäßstärke anschließend separat berechnet werden.

Der am häufigsten eingesetzte Segmentierungsansatz basiert auf einer Skalenraumfilterung [6]. Hierbei wird durch die Faltung des Bildes mit Gaußfiltern unterschiedlicher Größe und die anschließende Auswertung der Eigenwerte der Hesse-Matrix an jedem Voxel eine Verstärkung der Blutgefäße erreicht. Das Ergebnis kann dann entweder direkt visualisiert werden oder es schließen sich andere Segmentierungsverfahren, wie z.B. ein Schwellwertverfahren, an. Die Qualität des Ergebnisses wird bei dem Verfahren durch Strukturen in der Umgebung der Gefäße beeinflusst, da diese ebenfalls vom Gaußfilterkern überdeckt werden. Durch die Verwendung verschiedener Auflösungsstufen ist außerdem eine Differenzierung zwischen verschiedenen Gefäßdurchmessern sehr einfach zu realisieren. Aus diesem Grund soll dieses Verfahren auch als Vergleichsmethode für den von uns entwickelten Algorithmus dienen.

2 Material und Methoden

Bei unserem Ansatz wird die Tatsache ausgenutzt, dass sich die Blutgefäße in den MRT-TOF-Bilddaten im Grauwert von der Umgebung unterscheiden und eine annähernd zylindersymmetrische Gestalt besitzen. Deshalb schlagen wir zur Gefäßdetektion eine Symmetrietransformation vor. In der Literatur sind zahlreiche Verfahren zur Symmetrieerkennung beschrieben. Einen guten Überblick über existierende Verfahren gibt [7]. Analog zum allgemeinen Ansatz zur Symmetriedetektion wird bei dem entwickelten Verfahren im ersten Schritt ein Kennwert für die Symmetrie für jeden Voxel berechnet. Zur Registrierung mit den 2D Angiographien verwenden wir im Moment eine Maximumintensitätsprojektion (MIP) dieser Daten. Ein Problem bei der Berechnung des Symmetriekennwertes ist, dass dafür idealerweise nur solche Voxel herangezogen werden sollten, die auch zum Objekt gehören. Die Größe eines symmetrischen Objekts ist aber im Vorfeld nicht bekannt. Einige Verfahren benötigen die Größe der symmetrischen Objekte deshalb als Eingabeparameter, bei anderen Verfahren werden alle möglichen Radien durchgetestet, was sehr rechenintensiv ist. Bei dem verwendeten Ansatz von Dalitz et. al. [8] wird hingegen die Größe des Objekts während der Berechnung geschätzt. Es muss lediglich ein maximaler Radius für die Objekte vorgegeben werden. Dieses für 2D-Daten entwickelte Verfahren haben wir im Rahmen der Untersuchung für die Segmentierung der Blutgefäße in den MRT-TOF-Aufnahmen auf 3D erweitert.

Bei der Spiegelung einer 3D-Struktur an einem Punkt verlaufen die Gradientenvektoren $G(x + \Delta)$ und $G(x - \Delta)$ parallel und genau in entgegengesetzter Richtung (Abb. 1), so dass das Skalarprodukt ($\langle.,.\rangle$) negativ wird. Daher wird folgende Größe an Symmetriezentren maximal

$$S(x, r) = - \sum_{(\Delta_x, \Delta_y, \Delta_z) \leqq r} \langle G(x - \Delta), G(x + \Delta) \rangle \tag{1}$$

In der Gleichung wird eine Invertierung des Symmetriewertes vorgenommen, damit im Ergebnis höhere Symmetriewerte eine höhere Wahrscheinlichkeit für eine Symmetrieachse wiedergeben. ähnlich wie bei der Berechnung der 2D-Symmetrie-Transformation nach [8] können durch Anwendung einer rekursiven Berechnungsvorschrift die Symmetriekennzahlen für alle Radien $r = 1, .., r_{max}$ ohne zusätzlichen Rechenaufwand bestimmt werden.

Um sicherzustellen, dass in der späteren MIP sowohl kleinere als auch größere Gefäße die gleiche Intensität aufweisen, ist eine Normierung der berechneten Symmetriekennzahlen erforderlich. Bei der rekursiven Symmetrieberechnung in 2D erfolgt in jedem Rekursionsschritt die Berechnung der Symmetrie für eine quadratische Region, so dass sich für jeden Pixel r_{max} unterschiedliche Symmetriekennzahlen ergeben. Bei der Erweiterung der Rekursion um eine weitere Dimension werden nun in den Zwischenschritten solange Regionen in Form quadratischer Säulen mit einer Kantenlänge r_{xy} der Grundfläche und einer Seitenlänge r_z betrachtet, bis ein Würfel mit der Kantenlänge r_{max} erreicht ist. Bei Zugrundelegung einer zylinderförmigen Gestalt wächst der Symmetriescore S proportional zu $r_{xy} \cdot r_z$. Um dies zu kompensieren normieren wir S mittels

$$S_n(x, r_{xy}, r_z) = S(x, r_{xy}, r_z) / (r_{xy} \cdot r_z) \tag{2}$$

Zur Bestimmung der Kombination von Gefäßradius und Gefäßlänge R_{xy} und R_z für einen Voxel x wird die Position (R_{xy}, R_z) des Maximums bei den normierten Symmetriekennzahlen erfasst

$$(R_{xy}, R_z) = \arg\max\{S_n(x, r_{xy}, r_z) \,|\, r_{xy}, r_z = 1, .., r_{max}\} \tag{3}$$

Der normierte Symmetriewert kann dann an der entsprechenden Position ausgelesen werden

$$S_n(x) = S_n(x, R_{xy}, R_z) \tag{4}$$

Abb. 1. Die Spiegelung des Punktes $x + \Delta$ an der Symmetrieachse führt zu einem parallelen und genau entgegengesetzten Gradientenverlauf.

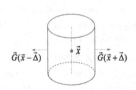

Anhand des Gradienten im geglätteten Symmetriebild kann anschließend entschieden werden, welcher der beiden Werte (R_{xy} oder R_z) dem Gefäßradius entspricht.

3 Ergebnisse

Das entwickelte Verfahren haben wir anhand von drei verschiedenen Datensammlungen evaluiert und mit den Ergebnissen der Skalenraumfilterung verglichen. Im ersten Evaluationsschritt sollte festgestellt werden, wie gut das Verfahren unter optimalen Bedingungen funktioniert. Dazu wurde ein künstliches Testbild mit einem sich verzweigenden Zylinder verwendet. Das Ergebnis in Abb. 2 zeigt, dass die Symmetrieachsen in diesem Fall fast ohne Störungen gefunden wurden. Zur Erzeugung des 3D-Plots mit dem Ergebnis der Symmetrietransformation wurden die ermittelten Radien verwendet, die zu den zwei höchsten Symmetriewerten in einer Schicht gehörten. Ein visueller Vergleich mit der 3D Darstellung des Originaldatensatzes zeigt, dass die Radienschätzung zumeist korrekte Ergebnisse liefert. Nur im Bereich der Verzweigung ist, wie zu erwarten war, ein falscher Radius geschätzt worden. Auch bei dem Ergebnis des Vergleichsverfahrens ist im Bereich der Verzweigung und an den jeweiligen Enden eine leichte Veränderung des Objektes gegenüber dem Original zu erkennen.

Für den zweiten Evaluationsschritt wurden die Bilddaten eines simulierten T_1-Datensatzes vom Gehirn mit Shading [9] mit den Bilddaten von 10 verschiedenen simulierten Gefäßbäumen [10] additiv verknüpft. Für die Evaluation haben wir sowohl die simulierten Gefäßbäume als auch die Ergebnisse der Symmetrietransformation und des Vergleichsverfahrens der zehn verschiedenen Datensätze in die drei Hauptebenen projiziert und die Gefäßsegmente, die in dieser Darstellung eine Grauwertdifferenz von mindestens 20 Grauwerten zu ihren Nachbarpixeln aufwiesen gezählt. Ein Beispiel für die genutzte Darstellung ist in Abb. 3 zu sehen. Von den 788 in den simulierten Bilddaten vorhandenen Gefäßsegmenten wurden 35 in den Ergebnissen der Symmetrietransformation nicht detektiert, was einer Fehlerrate von 4.4% entspricht. Hierbei handelt es sich ausschließlich um schmale Segmente von 1 Pixel Breite und weniger als 5 Pixeln Länge in der Projektion. Mit dem Vergleichsverfahren wurden 6.2% der Gefäßsegmente nicht

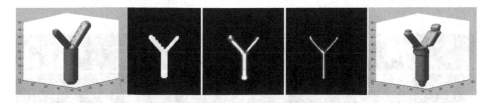

Abb. 2. von links nach rechts: 3D-Darstellung des künstlichen Testdatensatzes, Maximumintensitätsprojektionen des unbearbeiteten Datensatzes, des Ergebnisses der Skalenraumfilterung, des Ergebnisses der Symmetrietransformation und 3D-Darstellung anhand der Radienschätzung.

Abb. 3. von oben nach unten: MIP des Originaldatensatzes, MIP der Symmetrietransformation und MIP der Skalenraumfilterung.

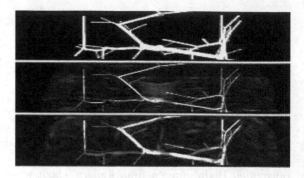

detektiert. An diesen Testdatensätzen wurde weiterhin untersucht, wie gut die geschätzten Gefäßradien mit den realen Radien übereinstimmten. Hierzu wurde in jedem Schnittbild der Radius des Voxels mit dem höchsten Symmetriewert betrachtet. Bei den untersuchten 560 Schichten wurde in 89,4% der Fälle der korrekte Radius ermittelt. Fehler traten verstärkt dann auf, wenn das Gefäß in 45° zu allen drei Achsen verlief. In diesem Fall lag der gesuchte Radius zwischen den ermittelten Radien R_{xy} und R_z. Weiterhin konnte gezeigt werden, dass anhand der geschätzten Radien eine Differenzierung zwischen großen und kleinen Gefäßen vorgenommen werden kann (Abb. 4).

Im dritten Evaluationsschritt haben wir reale TOF-Datensätze verwendet. Das Ergebnis der Gefäßdetektion für einen Beispieldatensatz ist in Abb. 5 im Vergleich zur Skalenraumfilterung zu sehen. Hier ist zu erkennen, dass durch die Symmetrietransformation mehr Details im Bild erhalten bleiben. Dies liegt darin begründet, dass bei der Skalenraumfilterung durch die Anwendung der Gaußfilterung kleine, schwach kontrastierte Gefäße entfernt werden.

4   Diskussion

Das vorgestellte Verfahren zur Gefäßdetektion basierend auf einer 3D Symmetrietransformation liefert eine hohe Erkennungsrate und eine detailreiche Gefäßdarstellung. Vorteilhaft ist im Vergleich zu anderen Verfahren die Möglichkeit der Differenzierung zwischen Gefäßen unterschiedlicher Stärke. Im nächsten Schritt soll eine Weiterverarbeitung der Daten durch Nutzung einer 3D-Skelettierung auf

Abb. 4. MIP des simulierten Gefäßbaums (links oben) und Ergebnisse der Symmetrietransformation für Gefäße mit einem Radius kleiner als 2 Voxel (links unten), mit einem Radius gleich 2 Voxel (rechts oben) und größer als 2 Voxel (rechts unten).

Abb. 5. Die MIP der Skalenraumfilterung (oben) zeigt im Vergleich zur MIP der Symmetrietransformation (unten) für einen Beispiel TOF-Datensatz weniger Gefäße und stellt diese auch unscharf und vergrößert dar.

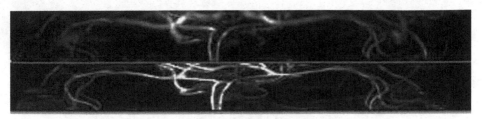

Grauwertbildern unter Berücksichtigung der Radieninformation erfolgen, um eine Segmentierung der Gefäße zu erreichen. Dies ist notwendig, um Aussagen zur Genauigkeit der Methode treffen zu können. Weiterhin soll die Radienschätzung für schräg verlaufende Gefäße verbessert werden. Hier ist zu untersuchen, ob dies durch eine Erweiterung der Symmetrietransformation auf rechteckige statt wie bisher quadratische Bereiche in der einen Ebene erreicht werden kann.

Literaturverzeichnis

1. Lesage D, Angelini E, Bloch I, et al. A review of 3D vessel lumen segmentation techniques: models, features and extraction schemes. Med Image Anal. 2009;13(6):819–45.
2. Lin Q. Enhancement, detection, and visualization of 3D volume data. PhD Thesis No 824, Linköping University. 2003.
3. de Bruijne M, van Ginneken B, Viergever M, et al. Adapting active shape models for 3D segmentation of tubular structures in medical images. Proc IPMI. 2003; p. 136–47.
4. El-Baz A, Elnakib A, Khalifa F, et al. Precise segmentation of 3-D magnetic resonance angiography. Biomed Eng. 2012;59(7):2019–29.
5. Law M, Chung A. Efficient implementation for spherical flux computation and its application to vascular segmentation. IEEE Trans Image Process. 2009;18(3):596–612.
6. AF Frangi KVea WJ Niessen. Multiscale vessel enhancement filtering. Lect Notes Comput Sci. 1998;1496:130–7.
7. Liu Y, Hel-Or H, Kaplan C, et al. Computational symmetry in computer vision and computer graphics. Now Publishers; 2010.
8. Dalitz C, Pohle-Fröhlich R, Bolten T. Detection of symmetry points in images. Proc VISAPP. 2013; p. 577–85.
9. BrainWeb: simulated brain database; 1997. Online; accessed 17-July-2013. http://www.bic.mni.mcgill.ca/brainweb/.
10. Hamarneh G, Jassi P. VascuSynth: simulating vascular trees for generating volumetric image data with ground truth segmentation and tree analysis. Comput Med Imaging Graph. 2010;34(8):605–16.

Segmentierung intrahepatischer Gefäße mit Vesselness-Verfahren

Peter A. Behringer[1], Andre Mastmeyer[1], Dirk Fortmeier[12],
Constantin Biermann[3], Heinz Handels[1]

[1]Institut für Medizinische Informatik, Universität zu Lübeck
[2]Graduiertenschule für Informatik in Medizin und Lebenswissenschaften
[3]Klinik für Radiologie und Nuklearmedizin, Universitätsklinikum Schleswig-Holstein
Campus Lübeck
behringe@miw.uni-luebeck.de

Kurzfassung. Segmentierungsverfahren spielen bei der Operationsplanung von Lebereingriffen eine tragende Rolle. Die Identifikation der Gefäße aus den Intensitätsdaten zu interpretierbaren Objekten bringt insbesondere bei der risikominimierenden Planung chirurgischer Eingriffe bedeutende Vorteile. In diesem Beitrag wird ein semi-automatisches Verfahren zur Detektion und Segmentierung der intrahepatischen Strukturen, namentlich der Blut-, sowie der Gallengangsgefäße in 3D CT-Bildern vorgestellt. Die Gefäßverstärkung wurde mittels Vesselness-Verfahren nach Sato et al. [1] und Frangi et al. [2] durchgeführt. Zur Segmentierung wurde schließlich ein Volumenwachstumsverfahren mit anschließender Analyse zusammenhängender Komponenten verwendet. Die Segmentierungsergebnisse von zehn Patientendatensätzen wurden qualitativ durch optischen Vergleich mit einer zuvor erstellen manuellen Segmentierung eines medizinisches Experten, sowie quantitativ unter Zuhilfenahme des DICE-Koeffizienten bewertet.

1 Einleitung

Die Perkutane Transhepatische Cholangiodrainage (PTCD) kann in der Praxis nur unzureichend trainiert werden, da die Übung am Patienten eine große Anzahl an Gefahren und Komplikationen mit sich bringt. Ein Gallengangspunktionssimulator soll dieses Problem durch die realitätsnahe Simulation der Prozedur lösen und so ein risikofreies Training ermöglichen. Um das Punktionstraining so alltagsnah wie möglich zu gestalten, soll das Training patienten-individuell durchführbar sein. Auf diese Weise können real anstehende Punktionseingriffe im Vorfeld vom Operateur trainiert und geplant werden.

Diese Arbeit befasst sich mit der semi-automatischen Verstärkung und Segmentierung der intrahepatischen Gefäßstrukturen in 3D CT-Datensätzen. Zur Gefäßverstärkung wurden die Vesselnessfilter von Sato et al. [1] und Frangi et al. [2] implementiert und getestet. Beide Filter analysieren die Eigenwerte der Ableitungen zweiter Ordnung voxelweise auf verschiedenen Skalen. Auf diese Weise ordnen sie jedem Voxel einen Vesselnesswert zu, welcher als Klassifikationsmerkmal zur eigentlichen Gefäßsegmentierung verwendet wird. Der Algorithmus wurde auf CT-Daten der Leber angepasst und entsprechende Parameter optimiert. Zur Evaluation der vorgestellten Methoden wurden zehn CT-Bilddatensätze des Abdomens unterschiedlicher Patienten verwendet. Bei den aufgenommen Bildern handelt es sich um gefäßkonstastierte Aufnahmen zu diagnostischen Zwecken während der portal-venösen Phase. Bei allen Patienten sind die Gallengänge pathologisch verändert (Cholestase) und treten infolgedessen als erweiterte, dunkle Gefäße im Lebergewebe hervor. Zur Bewertung der Ergebnisse des Verfahrens wurden zuvor manuelle Segmentierungen der Lebergefäße in Kooperation mit einem medizinischen Experten angefertigt. Die Segmentierung wurde im Anschluss sowohl optisch, als auch mit Hilfe des DICE-Koeffizienten verglichen und bewertet.

2   Material und Methoden

Abb. 1 zeigt den Ablauf der Gefäßsegmentierung. Die sechs Kernprozesse lassen sich in die Phasen der Vorverarbeitung (2.1) sowie der Gefäßverstärkung und Segmentierung (2.2) zusammenfassen.

Die Schritte wurden pro CT-Datensatz jeweils für die Blutgefäße und Gallengänge angewandt. Zur Verarbeitung der dunklen Gallengangstrukturen wurden die Bilddaten nach der Maskierung der Leber invertiert. Die Überlagerung der beiden Segmentierungen bildet schließlich das fertige Ergebnis. Anschließend können die beiden Segmentierungen in einem Multi-Label-Bild zum Patientenatlas hinzugefügt werden.

2.1   Vorverarbeitung

Um die intrahepatischen Gefäße lokal zu bearbeiten, wurde die Leber in einem ersten Vorverarbeitungsschritt maskiert. Hierzu wurden Lebermasken verwendet, die zuvor manuell erstellt wurden. Um Gefäße verschiedener Größen zu berücksichtigen, muss die Vesselness auf verschiedenen Skalen σ_s berechnet werden. Zu

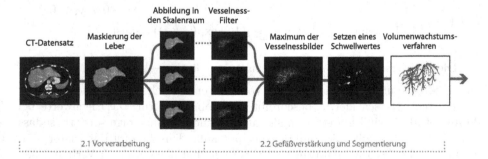

Abb. 1. Visualisierung der sechs Schritte der Segmentierungspipeline, die sich von links nach rechts aus Vorverarbeitung, Gefäßverstärkung und Segmentierung zusammensetzt.

diesem Zweck wird das Bild vor der Bestimmung der Vesselness mit Gauß-Filtern der verschiedenen Standardabweichungen σ_s geglättet. Die Vesselness $V(x)$ entspricht schließlich dem Maximum innerhalb aller Skalen

$$V(x) = \max_{\sigma_{s_{min}} \leq \sigma_s \leq \sigma_{s_{max}}} V(\sigma_s, x) \tag{1}$$

Für intrahepatische Gefäße haben sich die von Drechsler et al. [3] ermittelten Skalen $\sigma_s = 2, 3, 4$ als solide erwiesen.

2.2 Gefäßverstärkung und Segmentierung

Um gefäßartige Strukturen aus den Daten extrahieren zu können, wurde ein Vesselnessfilter angewandt. Dieser zeigte bereits in der Vergangenheit gute Ergebnisse bei der Segmentierung von zerebralen Gefäßstrukturen [4], Lungengefäßen [5], sowie bei Gefäßen des Atmungstraktes [6]. Der Filter interpretiert die zweite Ableitung eines Bildes. Hierbei nutzt er die drei Eigenwerte $\lambda_1, \lambda_2, \lambda_3$ der lokalen Hessematrix. Diese werden bei dreidimensionalen Bilddaten voxelweise berechnet, auf unterschiedliche Arten interpretiert [1, 2] und schließlich in einem Vesselnesswert festgehalten. Dieser nimmt einen hohen Wert an, falls das Voxel zu einem Gefäß gehört und ist nahe 0, falls nicht. Die Vesselnessfunktion nach Sato et al. [1] ist wie folgt gegeben

$$V(x) = \begin{cases} \exp\left(\frac{-\lambda_1^2}{2(\alpha_1\lambda_c)^2}\right)\lambda_c & \lambda_1 \leq 0, \lambda_c \neq 0 \\ \exp\left(\frac{-\lambda_1^2}{2(\alpha_2\lambda_c)^2}\right)\lambda_c & \lambda_1 > 0, \lambda_c \neq 0 \\ 0 & \lambda_c = 0 \end{cases} \tag{2}$$

wobei $\lambda_c = min(-\lambda_2, -\lambda_3)$ und $\alpha_1 < \alpha_2$ einstellbare Parameter sind. Die Eigenwerte sind bei Sato et al. [1] in absteigender Richtung sortiert, sodass $\lambda_1 \geq \lambda_2 \geq \lambda_3$ gilt. Als zweite Funktion zur Gefäßverstärkung wurde die Vesselness von Frangi et al. [2] getestet

$$V(x) = \begin{cases} 0 & \lambda_2 > 0 \vee \lambda_3 > 0 \\ \left(1 - \exp(-\frac{\Re_a^2}{2\alpha^2})\right)\exp(-\frac{\Re_b^2}{2\beta^2})(1 - \exp(-\frac{S^2}{2c^2})) & \text{sonst} \end{cases} \tag{3}$$

Diese unterscheidet durch die Verhältnisse $\Re_a = \frac{|\lambda_1|}{\sqrt{|\lambda_2||\lambda_3|}}$ bzw. $\Re_b = \frac{|\lambda_2|}{|\lambda_3|}$ in wieweit die unterliegende Struktur von platten-ähnlichen bzw. linienförmigen Strukturen unterscheidet. S beschreibt die Frobeniusnorm. Die Eigenwerte bei Frangi et al. [2] sind in betragsmäßig aufsteigender Reihenfolge sortiert, sodass $|\lambda_1| \leq |\lambda_2| \leq |\lambda_3|$ gilt. Die Funktion enthält außerdem die drei Parameter α, β und c, welche die Sensitivität des Filters gegenüber den einzelnen Verhältnissen festlegen. In den Versuchen wurde nach Drechsler et al. [3] $\alpha = \beta = 0,5$ gewählt und c manuell justiert um optimale Ergebnisse zu erhalten. Um das Rauschen im Bild zu entfernen, sowie kleinere, falsch detektierte Gefäße der Segmentierung zu entziehen, wurde ein Schwellwertoperator mit einer experimentell ermittelten Schwelle g angewandt. Im letzten Schritt wurden die Voxel durch ein Volumenwachstumsverfahren zu zusammenhängenden Gefäßstrukturen zusammengefügt. Hierzu wurde das MeVisLab-Modul [1] „Connected Components" mit den Grundeinstellungen benutzt.

3 Ergebnisse

Abb. 2 zeigt die Ergebnisse der Segmentierung als 3D-Modelle. Die Vesselness wurde nach der Methode von Sato et al. [1] berechnet. In der linken Spalte sind die manuellen Segmentierungen zu erkennen, in der Mitte das Ergebnis der Pipeline und rechts eine gemeinsame Darstellung. Die obere Zeile zeigt einen Blutgefäßbaum, die untere ein Gallengangsystem. Der Ductus hepaticus communis befindet sich außerhalb des Lebergewebes und ist infolgedessen nicht dargestellt. Folgende Beobachtungen können festgehalten werden: Erstens ist erkennbar, dass das automatisch erzeugte Ergebnis der Segmentierungs-Pipeline, insbesondere bei Gefäßenden, einen höheren Detailgrad aufweist. Zweitens sind die Gefäßzüge seltener unterbrochen. Zum Teil sind die Gefäße des Ergebnisses etwas dünner als in der Referenz. Die Vesselnessfunktion nach Sato et al. [1] zeigte im Vergleich zur Bestimmung nach Frangi et al. [2] bei Segmentierungen der Blutgefäße, sowie bei Gallengängen besondere Vorteile bei den Gefäßabzweigungen. Es wurden DICE-Koeffizienten bis zu 0,65 ermittelt. Der Durchschnittswert des DICE-Koeffizienten liegt für Blutgefäße bei $0,52 \pm 0,09$ und für Gallengänge bei $0,46 \pm 0,12$. Die besten Ergebnisse wurden mit Satos Funktion aus Gl. (2) mit $\alpha_1 = 0,5$ und $\alpha_2 = 2$ erzielt. Der Schwellwert zeigte sowohl bei den Blutgefäßen, als auch bei den Gallengängen die besten Ergebnisse bei $g = 1,2$. Die Laufzeit des kompletten Verfahrens beträgt im Schnitt etwa 10 Minuten.

4 Diskussion

In dieser Arbeit wurde eine Pipeline zur Gefäßsegmentierung intrahepatischer Gefäße aus CT-Daten vorgestellt. Blutgefäße sowie Gallengänge können mit dieser Methode erfolgreich extrahiert und dargestellt werden. Die entwickelte Pipeline ermöglicht ein patienten-individuelles Training im Gallengangspunktionssimulator und legt alle verwendeten Parameter offen. Eine Trennung der arteriellen und venösen Strukturen war aufgrund der niedrigen Bildqualität nicht möglich. Die Pipeline greift auf Masken der Leber zurück, die zuvor segmentiert wurden. Für einen vollständig automatisierbaren Algorithmus müssten diese im Vorfeld durch geeignete Level-Set-Ansätze oder Volumenwachstumsverfahren aus dem CT-Datensatz extrahiert werden. Die ermittelten Parameter für die Vesselnessfunktion von Sato et al. [1] sind fix, und bedürfen keiner weiteren Einstellungen. Frangis Vesselnessfunktion hingegen bedarf pro Datensatz einer

---

[1] www.mevislab.de

manuellen Einstellung des Parameters c und ist somit für einen vollständigen Automatismus aus Sicht des Autors schlechter geeignet. Die Schwellwertoperation ist für den Anspruch eines vollautomatischen Algorithmus zwar eher ungeeignet, jedoch in Anbetracht der hohen Sensitivität des Filters unabdingbar. Sofern keine geeignete Referenzsegmentierung vorliegt, muss die Wahl des Schwellwertes für das gefäßverstärkte Bild als einziger Parameter datensatzabhängig durch eine optische Bewertung erfolgen. In den Versuchen zeigte sich, dass der Suchraum

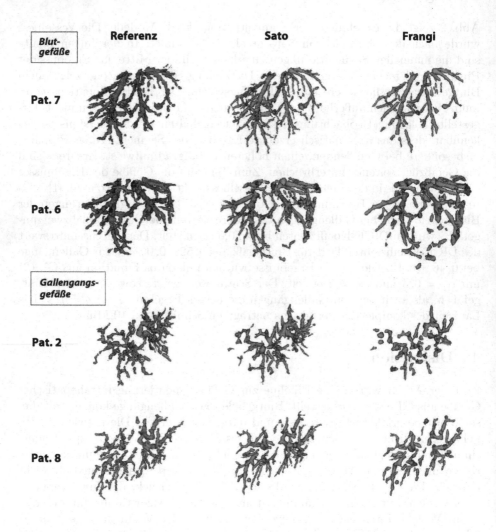

Abb. 2. Automatisch erzeugte Ergebnisse der Segmentierungspipeline mit Vesselness nach Sato und Frangi (hellblau), sowie manuelle Referenz (grün: Gallengänge; rot: Blutgefäße). Die oberen sechs Objekte sind extrahierte Blutgefäßbäume aus den CT-Datensätzen von Patient 7 und 6. Die unteren dagegen sind extrahierte Gallengangsysteme der Patienten 2 und 8.

auf das Intervall [0,8; 1,4] in 0,2-er Schritten beschränkt werden kann. Dies kann in einer klinischen Applikation durch einen Slider im GUI abgebildet werden. Eine automatische Bestimmung eines Schwellwertes ist schwierig, da eine manuelle Referenzsegmentierung zur Anpassung des Wertes notwendig ist. Für eine Verbesserung der DICE-Koeffizienten und der Laufzeit des Algorithmus könnte zukünftig das Vesselness-Verfahren nach Erdt et al. [7] in den Vergleich miteinbezogen werden. Dieses kommt nach Angaben der Autoren komplett ohne Parameter aus und ist durch Nutzung von Grafik-Hardware wesentlich schneller. Ebenso könnten neuere Verfahren wie das von Quian et al. [8] als Alternative zur Vesselnessfunktion untersucht werden.

Danksagung. Diese Arbeit wird von der DFG gefördert (DFG-HA 2355/10-1).

Literaturverzeichnis

1. Sato Y, Nakajima S, et al NS. Three-dimensional multi-scale line filter for segmentation and visualization of curvilinear structures in medical images. Med Image Anal. 1998;2:143–68.
2. Frangi AF, Niessen WJ, et al KLV. Multiscale vessel enhancement filtering. Med Image Comput Comput Assist Interv. 1998; p. 130–7.
3. Drechsler K, Oyarzun CL. Comparison of vesselness functions for multiscale analysis of the liver vasculature. Proc ITAB. 2010; p. 1–5.
4. Forkert ND, Säring D, Wenzel K, et al. Fuzzy-based extraction of vascular structures from time-of-flight MR images. IOS Press; 2009.
5. Staring M, Xiao C, et al DPS. Pulmonary vessel segmentation using vessel enhancement filters. Proc ISBI. 2012; p. 1–8.
6. Rudzki M. Vessel detection method based on eigenvalues of the hessian matrix and its applicability to airway tree Segmentation. Proc Int PhD Workshop. 2009; p. 100–5.
7. Erdt M, Raspe M, Suehling M. Automatic hepatic vessel segmentation using graphics hardware. Med Imaging Augmented Real Lect Notes Computer Sci. 2008;5128:403–12.
8. Qian X, Brennan MP, et al DPD. A non-parametric vessel detection method for complex vascular structures. Med Image Anal. 2009;13:49–61.

Segmentierung von ischämischen Schlaganfall-Läsionen in multispektralen MR-Bildern mit Random Decision Forests

Oskar Maier[1,2], Matthias Wilms[1], Janina von der Gablentz[3], Ulrike Krämer[3], Heinz Handels[1]

[1]Institut für Medizinische Informatik, Universität zu Lübeck
[2]Graduate School for Computing in Medicine and Live Science, Universität zu Lübeck
[3]Klinik für Neurologie, Universität zu Lübeck
maier@imi.uni-luebeck.de

Kurzfassung. Die vorliegende Arbeit beschäftigt sich mit der automatischen Segmentierung von ischämischen Schlaganfall-Läsionen in Magnetresonanztomographie (MR) Bildern. Eine geeignete Methode muss inhomogene Regionen verschiedener Größen und Formen im Gehirn lokalisieren. Wir stellen einen neuen Segmentierungsansatz vor, der auf lokalen Merkmalen basiert, welche aus multispektralen MR Daten extrahiert werden und so gewählt sind, dass sie menschliche Entscheidungskriterien modellieren. Ein Random Decision Forest Klassifizierer wird mit Expertensegmentierungen trainiert und dann auf unbekannte Datensätze angewendet. Der Ansatz wird an acht Fällen mittels Leave-One-Out-Kreuzvalidierungsverfahren evaluiert und die relative Eignung jedes Merkmales und jeder MR-Sequenz untersucht. Ein Vergleich zeigt höhere Dice-Koeffizienten als andere Methoden aus der Literatur.

1 Einleitung

In der Global Burden of Disease Studie von 2010 wird Schlaganfall als die zweithäufigste Todesursache weltweit aufgeführt. Ischämische Schlaganfälle werden durch eine Unterbrechung der Blutversorgung ausgelöst und führen zum Absterben des Gewebes. Die betroffenen Bereiche, Läsionen genannt, können mit Hilfe der Magnetresonanztomographie (MR) dargestellt werden [1].

Genaue Information über die Lage und Größe der Läsionen kann wertvolle Hinweise für die Diagnose und Behandlungsentscheidungen liefern [2]. Auch im wissenschaftlichen Kontext werden zeitaufwendige Segmentierungen der Läsionen in MR Bildern benötigt, so z. B. in den kognitiven Neurowissenschaften, um einen Zusammenhang zwischen anatomischen Regionen und funktionellen Arealen herzustellen. Eine automatische Segmentierung von Schlaganfall-Läsionen wird dadurch erschwert, dass sie in unterschiedlichen Bereichen des Gehirns auftreten, von verschiedener Form und Größe sind, alle gesunden Gehirngewebe betreffen können und kein einheitliches Erscheinungsbild oder Intensitätsprofil aufweisen [1].

Die meisten veröffentlichten Ansätze zur Segmentierung von Schlaganfall-Läsionen verwenden nur eine Sequenz [3, 4]. Um die große Varianz der Läsionen zu besser zu erfassen, kombinieren wir verschiedene MR-Sequenzen zu multispektralen Datensätzen. In [5] berichten die Autoren von guten Ergebnissen, die sie mit Support Vector Machines (SVM) auf multispektralen Bilddaten erzielten.

In diesem Beitrag stellen wir eine neue Methode vor, die auf Random Decision Forests (RDF) [6] basiert und sich an dem Multiple Sklerose (MS) Segmentierungsframework von [7] orientiert. Für unseren Ansatz extrahieren wir verschiedene lokale Merkmale für jeden Bildpunkt, die versuchen menschliche Entscheidungskriterien zu modellieren. Ein RDF wird mit den Merkmalsvektoren trainiert und auf unbekannte Datensätze angewendet. Weiterhin bestimmen wir die relative Wichtigkeit jedes Merkmales und jeder MR-Sequenz für die Problemlösung. Schließlich vergleichen wir unseren Ansatz mit anderen veröffentlichten Methoden.

2 Material und Methoden

Wir verwenden einen Voxel-Klassifizierungsansatz zur Segmentierung von Schlaganfall-Läsionen. Die MR-Daten werden vorverarbeitet, multispektrale Merkmale für jeden Voxel extrahiert und ein RDF Klassifizierer trainiert. Die resultierenden Segmentierungen werden durch ein Nachverarbeitungsschritt verbessert.

Für diese Studie sind die folgenden MRI-Sequenzen verfügbar: fluid attenuated inversion recovery (FLAIR), T1 turbo field echo (T1-TFE), T2 turbo spin echo (T2-TSE), zwei diffusion weighted (DW) Aufnahmen (b $0, 1000 \, \mathrm{s/mm^2}$), und ein apparent diffusion coefficient (ADC) Bild, berechnet aus den beiden DW-Sequenzen (alle ohne Kontrastmittel). In einem Vorverarbeitungsschritt werden die Gehirne extrahiert, Rauschen mit einem Anisotropic Diffusion Filter gemildert und schließlich die verschiedenen Sequenzen mit einem Mutual Information Ähnlichkeitsmaß rigide co-registriert um Patientenbewegungen zu kompensieren. Jeder Datensatz kann als ein multispektrales Bild mit sechs Kanälen aufgefasst werden.

2.1 Klassifikation mit Random Decision Forests

RDF [6] ist eine häufig eingesetzte (z.B. [7]) Methode für überwachtes Lernen von nicht-linearen Klassifizierungsaufgaben. Eine große Menge unkorrelierter Entscheidungsbäume wird auf wiederholten bootstrap-Stichproben der Trainingsdaten gebildet, wobei die Entscheidung an jedem Knoten über einer zufälligen Untermenge der vorhandenen Prädikate gebildet wird. Sie stellen damit eine robustere Erweiterung der bekannten Methode des bagging dar. Die Klassenzugehörigkeit eines Bildpunktes wird durch einen Mehrheitsbeschluss der Bäume bestimmt. RDFs neigen nicht zu Überanpassung, sind robust gegen die Wahl ihrer Parameter und einfach parallelisierbar.

Die Wahl der Trainingsdaten kann großen Einfluss auf die Klassifizierungsgüte haben. Auch wenn RDFs nicht zu Überanpassung neigen, ist es in Hinblick auf die Trainingszeiten dennoch wünschenswert, nur eine repräsentative Untermenge der verfügbaren Trainingsdaten zu verwenden. Schlaganfall-Läsionen machen meist deutlich unter 50% der Gehirnmasse aus, es besteht also ein Bias zum gesunden Gewebe. Viele Autoren eliminieren dieses Ungleichgewicht während der Auswahl der Stichprobe [8]. Wir haben empirisch festgestellt, dass es vorteilhaft ist das innewohnende Klassenverhältnis beizubehalten. Wir verwenden eine geschichtete Zufallsstrichprobe von 3.000 Elementen aus jedem Trainingsdatensatz und erreichen damit eine durchschnittliche Trainingszeit von 1.5 Minuten.

Unser Verfahren berücksichtigt nicht die räumliche Verbundenheit der Bildpunkte, sodass vereinzelte Fehlklassifizierungen fern der Zielläsion oder in ihrem Innern auftreten. Diese entfernen wir nachträglich, indem wir die größte Zusammenhangskomponente auswählen und morphologisches Schließen anwenden.

2.2 Bildpunktmerkmale

Wir extrahieren insgesamt sieben Merkmale für jeden Bildpunkt, die idealerweise differenzierend und unkorreliert sind. Bei der Auswahl orientieren wir uns an Kriterien, die auch von einem menschlichen Beobachter zur Unterscheidung herangezogen werden.

Eines der wichtigsten Kriterien ist der Vergleich zwischen den Gehirnhälften [3]. Wir teilen die Aufnahme entlang der Fissura longitudinalis, spiegeln die eine erhaltene Hälfte auf die Andere und bilden sie mit einer affinen Registrierung aufeinander ab. Die Hypothese ist, dass die läsionsbedingten Unterschiede ausgeprägter sind als die natürlichen Abweichungen zwischen den Hemisphären. Der normalisierte, absolute Differenzwert zwischen den Hemisphären bildet die hemispheric-difference.

Läsionen zeigen sich häufig als Hypo- oder Hyperintensitäten in MR Bildern. Als intensities-Merkmal wählen wir deshalb die Grauwerte an den Bildpunkten. Die lokale Nachbarschaft berücksichtigen wir, indem wir einen Gaussfilter auf drei Stufen (sigma=3, 7, 11 mm) anwenden und damit drei neighbourhood-Merkmale erhalten. Für das 19-elementige localhistogram-Merkmal wird ein Histogramm mit 19 Bins über eine $5\,\text{mm}^3$ Region um jeden Bildpunkt erstellt und normalisiert. Das letzte Merkmal, centerdistance, wird aus der Distanz der Bildpunkte zum vermuteten räumlichen Gehirnzentrum gebildet und bietet Information zur anatomischen Lage.

Unser Merkmalsvektor setzt sich damit aus hemispheric-difference, intensities, 3×neighbourhood, localhistogram und centerdistance zusammen. Außer der centerdistance und clusterdistance werden alle Merkmale auf jeder MR-Sequenz berechnet.

3 Ergebnisse

Wir evaluieren unsere Methode an acht Patienten mit Schlaganfall-Läsionen im chronischen Stadium, als Goldstandard dienen Expertensegmentierungen in den

Tabelle 1. Ergebnisse für alle acht Patienten und der Mittelwert.

Patient	Recall	Precision	DC	HD [mm]	SD [mm]	Läsionsgröße [ml]
01	0.72	0.90	0.80	17.89	2.14	127
02	0.70	0.99	0.82	12.37	1.84	171
03	0.81	0.70	0.75	09.22	0.96	8
04	0.52	0.96	0.67	43.61	4.19	338
05	0.84	0.79	0.81	13.64	0.99	42
06	0.58	0.96	0.72	26.19	4.02	141
07	0.73	0.92	0.82	21.93	1.95	120
08	0.87	0.72	0.79	22.38	2.18	44
Mittelwert	0.72	0.87	0.77	20.90	2.28	
STD	±0.12	±0.11	±0.05	±10.11	±1.14	

FLAIR Bildern. Aufgrund der geringen Anzahl Datensätze verwenden wir Leave-One-Out-Kreuzvalidierung auf Patientenbasis zur Evaluierung. Zur Bewertung der resultierenden Segmentierung berechnen wir precision und recall. Weiterhin geben wir den Dice-Koeffizient (DC), die Hausdorff-Metrik (HD) und die Mittlere Oberflächen Distanz (SD) an.

Die Evaluationsergebnisse für jeden Datensatz und die Durchschnittswerte sowie Standardabweichungen sind in Tab. 1 gelistet. Der monospektrale Fall mit nur der FLAIR-Sequenz als Eingabe führte zu recall=0.69, precision=0.80, DC 0.71, HD=26 und SD=3.28 im Mittel. Abb. 1 zeigt zusätzlich jeweils eine Schicht des besten und schlechtesten Falles.

3.1 Individueller Beitrag der Merkmale und MR-Sequenzen

RDF bietet die Möglichkeit die relative Wichtigkeit eines Merkmals direkt während der Konstruktion der Entscheidungsbäume durch Permutation der out-of-bag Daten zu berechnen. Abb. 2(a) zeigt die relative Wichtigkeit unserer Merkmale auf. Neben den Merkmalsbewertungen sind auch die relativen Beiträge der einzelnen MR-Sequenzen gegeben (Abb. 2(b)). Die Werte, die zu einer Summe

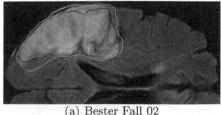
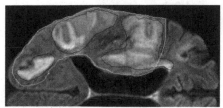

(a) Bester Fall 02   (b) Schlechtester Fall 04

Abb. 1. Segmentierungsbeispiele des besten (a) und schlechtesten (b) DC-Wertes. Segmentierung in schwarz und Goldstandard in hellgelb auf FLAIR Sequenz.

von Eins fehlen, sind die Beiträge von sequenzunabhängigen Merkmalen wie der Distanz zum Hirnzentrum.

4 Diskussion

Wir haben RDF Klassifizierer erfolgreich für eine Segmentierung von Ischämieläsionen im Gehirn eingesetzt und gezeigt, dass dieser Ansatz überdurchschnittlich gute Ergebnisse liefert. Mehrere klinisch motivierte Merkmale wurde vorgestellt und ihre relativen Beiträge evaluiert, mit teilweise überraschendem Ergebnis. Unsere automatische Methode arbeitet auf multispektralen Bilddaten und verbindet somit mehrere Informationsquellen. Eine Überprüfung der Kanäle fand keine MRI-Sequenzen entbehrlich. Der schon zuvor beobachtete Vorteil von multispektralen gegenüber monospektralen Ansätzen [7] konnte damit weiter gefestigt werden.

Im Vergleich zu anderen Ansätzen aus der Literatur erreicht unsere Methode mit einem durchschnittlichen Dice-Koeffizienten von 0.77 ± 0.05 ein deutlich besseres Ergebnis mit sehr geringer Standardabweichung bei einer vergleichbaren Anzahl Datensätze: Wilke et al. [3] berichten von Werten bis zu 0.60 für ihren halbautomatischen und 0.49 für ihren automatischen Ansatz, Hevia-Montiel et al. [9] kommen auf Dice-Koeffizienten bis zu 0.54 ± 0.18 und Seghier et al. [4] veröffentlichten Ergebnisse von 0.64 ± 0.1. Allerdings kommen in den verglichenen Veröffentlichungen andere Daten zum Einsatz.

Das Ranking der MR-Sequenzen wird von FLAIR angeführt, die weiteren Sequenzen unterscheiden sich in ihrer Wichtigkeit kaum. Jede Sequenz trägt ihren Teil zum Ergebnis bei und keine kann verlustlos weggelassen werden, was durch die monospektralen FLAIR Resultate bestätigt wird. Weitere Experimente haben gezeigt, dass schon das Fehlen der ADC Aufnahmen zu einer Absenkung der Ergebniswerte führt. Der starke FLAIR Beitrag kann teilweise dadurch erklärt werden, dass der Goldstandard in dieser Sequenz erstellt wurde und somit ein Bias darstellt.

Bei den Merkmalen heben sich die lokalen Histogramme deutlich ab. Das Mittelfeld bilden die Gauss-gefilterten Sequenzen und die räumliche Position

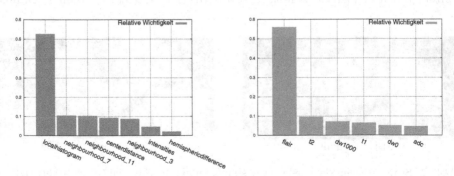

Abb. 2. Relative mittlere Wichtigkeit der (a) Merkmale und (b) MR-Sequenzen.

der Bildpunkte, ausgedrückt durch die Distanz zum Hirnzentrum. Der geringe
Beitrag der Intensitätswerte kann dem Bildrauschen geschuldet sein, dass trotz
Filterung nicht ausreichend entfernt werden konnte. In [7] berichten die Autoren
von Schwierigkeiten zwischen läsionsbedingten und natürlichen Unterschieden
zwischen den Hemisphären zu differenzieren. Dies könnte den geringen Einfluss
des Hemisphärendifferenzmerkmales erklären. Die relativen Wichtigkeiten, die
hier präsentiert werden, müssen mit Vorsicht behandelt werden, da dem berechneten Wert die Annahme von Unabhängigkeit der Merkmale bzw. Sequenzen zu
Grunde liegt, die aber z.B. für die neighourhood-Merkmale nicht gegeben ist.

Während unsere Methode vorteilhaft im Vergleich mit anderen abschneidet,
so besteht noch Raum für Verbesserungen. Für die Zukunft wäre es wünschenswert eine Studie an einer deutlich größeren und frei verfügbaren Datenbank
durchzuführen. Weiterhin sollten neue Merkmale entworfen und eingeführt bzw.
vorhandene optimiert werden. Auch wäre es interessant, verschiedene Kombination von MR-Sequenzen zu vergleichen. Als nächsten Schritt planen wir die
Ergebnisse unseres Ansatzes als Ausgangspunkt für andere Segmentierungsmethoden zu verwenden, die eine anfängliche Schätzung benötigen. Im besonderen
wollen wir zur Verbesserung der Genauigkeit regionen-basierte Graph Cuts [10]
auf multispektrale Daten erweitern.

Literaturverzeichnis

1. Srinivasan A, Goyal M, Azri FA, et al. State-of-the-art imaging of acute stroke.
   Radiographics. 2006;26(suppl 1):75–95.
2. Lövblad KO, Laubach HJ, Baird AE, et al. Clinical experience with diffusion-
   weighted MR in patients with acute stroke. Am J Neurorad. 1998;19(6):1061–6.
3. Wilke M, de Haan B, Juenger H, et al. Manual, semi-automated, and automated delineation of chronic brain lesions: a comparison of methods. Neuroimage.
   2011;56(4):2038–46.
4. Seghier ML, Ramlackhansingh A, Crinion J, et al. Lesion identification using
   unified segmentation-normalisation models and fuzzy clustering. Neuroimage.
   2008;41(4-3):1253–66.
5. Maier O, Wilms M, von der Gablentz J, et al. Ischemic stroke lesion segmentation
   in multi-spectral MR images with support vector machine classifiers. Procs SPIE,
   in press. 2014.
6. Breiman L. Random forests. Mach Learn. 2001;45(1):5–32.
7. Geremia E, Clatz O, Menze BH, et al. Spatial decision forests for MS lesion segmentation in multi-channel magnetic resonance images. Neuroimage. 2011;57(2):378 –
   90.
8. Lao Z, Shen D, Liu D, et al. Computer-assisted segmentation of white matter lesions in 3D MR images using support vector machine. Academic Radiol.
   2008;15(3):300–13.
9. Hevia-Montiel N, Jimenez-Alaniz JR, Medina-Banuelos V, et al. Robust nonpa-
   rametric segmentation of infarct lesion from diffusion-weighted MR images. Proc
   IEEE EMBS. 2007; p. 2102–5.
10. Maier OMO, Jimenez D, Santos A, et al. Segmentation of RV in 4D cardiac MR
    volumes using region-merging graph cuts. Comput Cardiol. 2012; p. 697–700.

Computer-Aided Detection of Lesions in Digital Breast Tomosynthesis Images

Martin Prinzen[1], Florian Wagner[1], Sebastian Nowack[1],
Rüdiger Schulz-Wendtland[2], Dietrich Paulus[3], Thomas Wittenberg[1]

[1]Department of Image Processing and Medical Engineering,
Fraunhofer Institute for Integrated Circuits IIS, Erlangen
[2]Institute of Diagnostic Radiology, Erlangen University Hospital
[3]Institute for Computational Visualistics, University of Koblenz-Landau
martin.prinzen@iis.fraunhofer.de

Abstract. The most common cancer among women in the western world is breast cancer. Early detection of lesions greatly influences the progress and success of its treatment. Digital breast tomosynthesis (DBT) is a new imaging technique that facilitates a three-dimensional reconstruction of the breast. DBT reduces superimposition of breast tissues and provides better insight into the breast compared to the common digital mammography. In order to assist radiologists with the examination and assessment of the large amount of DBT data, a computer aided detection (CADe) of focal lesions can be an essential tool, leading to increased sensitivity and specificity. We present and compare two different approaches for a fully automated detection of lesions in DBT data using voxel-wise classification, one being the state of the art and the other one an enhancement. Multiple difference of Gaussians detect lesions based on their common higher intensity and contrast in relation to surrounding tissue. A gradient orientation analysis detects round and spiculated lesions, even when they are weak in contrast and intensity. By combining these features and using a support vector machine, a classification performance of 88% can be achieved.

1 Introduction

Worldwide, breast cancer is the most common cancer among women and represents the leading cause of mortality for women in their fifties [1]. The early detection and appropriate treatment of lesions considerably increases the chance of survival. The 5-year survival rate for patients with breast cancer in early stage has been reported with up to 97% [2]. In the late stage this rate drastically decreases to about 23% [2]. To date, mammography is the only image based technique for early detection of breast cancer that verifiably decreases the mortality rate [3]. Mammography utilizes low dose X-Rays for the acquisition of high resolution X-Ray images of the breast. Lesions are possible indications for breast cancer. They are most often depicted as conspicuous bright areas on the X-Rays since they commonly have a higher density compared to surrounding

healthy tissue. Unfortunately, 10 to 30% of breast cancer cases remain undetected in conventional mammography due to overlapping tissue and low contrast
lesions that occur especially in dense breasts [2]. Digital breast tomosynthesis
(DBT) is a new imaging technique that resembles computed tomography (CT)
in a way that a series of X-Ray images are acquired by shifting the X-Ray emit-
ter along an partial arc around the breast. A series of X-Ray images are then
used to three-dimensionally reconstruct the breast. The DBT acquisition and
some three-dimensional reconstructed slices are depicted in Fig. 1. This imaging
technique considerably decreases the amount of overlapping tissue and hence
provides better insight into the breast. A survey among radiologists shows that
DBT provides comparable (to 51%) or better image quality (to 37%) in 89% of
all considered cases in comparison to conventional mammography [5].

Manual screening for lesions and signs of breast cancer in DBT or digital
mammograms is a time consuming and complex task which is prone to mistakes
by the examining radiologist [3]. In this process, a computer aided detection
(CADe) system becomes an important tool for supporting the clinical examination and clinical decision making. Studies show that a CADe system may
increase the detection rate of lesions about 20% [6]. It is capable of providing
an objective second opinion of constant quality, reducing the workload of radiologist and saving time and costs. In this work we present a CADe system that
reads available DBT data and highlights all voxels that are likely to belong to a
lesion. The more likely a region in the DBT mammogram belongs to a lesion, the
brighter it gets highlighted in the feature map. The sensitivity and specificity of
the output remains controllable by the radiologist to fit personal preferences.

2   Materials and methods

The overall process of the developed CADe system consists of two parts. The
first part classifies all voxels separately in possible lesions and non-lesions pur-

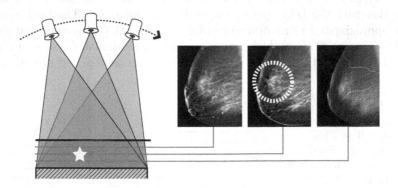

Fig. 1. Scheme of a DBT acquisition of a compressed breast (left) and the output
slices (right). The lesion (white star) in the breast is clearly visible in the center slice
(white circle). After [4].

suing a high sensitivity (true positive rate). In the second part, the number of false positives is reduced to achieve a high specificity (true negative rate) whilst remaining the high sensitivity. Both parts consist of preprocessing, feature extraction, feature selection and classification. In the following, we present, evaluate and compare two approaches for the first part, a gradient orientation analysis and an intensity filter using multiple difference of Gaussians. These approaches are evaluated both separately and combined using a support vector machine (SVM). The area under curve (AUC) is used as an evaluation measure on the basis of a ground truth of 100 DBT data sets from [7], each consisting of 57 slices on average and with a resolution of $0.085 \times 0.085 \times 1\,\mathrm{mm}^3$ per voxel.

First, the DBT data gets rescaled using a tri-linear interpolation in order to reduce the computational effort. The rescaled resolution of $0.4 \times 0.4 \times 1\,\mathrm{mm}^3$ per voxel ensures, that the smallest lesions in the used ground truth is still sufficiently represented by $10 \times 10 \times 5$ voxels. The reduction of image noise has been examined but had no significant influence on the classification performance. The out-of-plane noise caused by the dense skin of the breast (so called skinline noise) causes considerable artifacts in intensity features. Therefore the skinline is masked and the skinline noise is reduced using a novel approach in which each slice of the DBT data is multiplied with its specifically normalized and gamma corrected distance transform. Each slice in the resulting DBT data is then mirrored at the resulting edge of the breast to the background (first in x-, then in y-direction) to avoid border artifacts.

2.1 Difference of Gaussians

Many lesions become visible due to their high density of tissue resulting in bright areas in the DBT mammogram. These areas depict a higher intensity compared to their background. If convoluted with the Laplacian of Gaussian (LoG) operator, these areas get highlighted. In order to compensate for lesions of different sizes, the LoG operator is applied using multiple scales. The scale that most accurately resembles the size of a lesion leads to the maximum output of the convolution with the LoG operator according to this scale. The LoG operator can be approximated using difference of Gaussians (DoG) according to sigmas with $\sigma_i = 1.6\sigma_{i+1}$. This enables the reuse of already calculated gaussian filtered slices for the calculation of DoG of subsequent scales as depicted in Fig. 2. The

Fig. 2. Multiple difference of Gaussians (DoG) of a slice. The output value of a voxel is the maximum intensity found in all DoG.

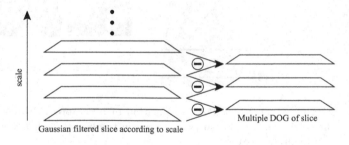

output value of these multiple DoG is given by the maximum intensity found in all DoG (maximum intensity projection). These intensities mark areas in the DBT projection mammogram proportional to their probability of being a true lesion.

2.2 Gradient orientation analysis

Some lesions are not visible due to a higher intensity compared to their background but rather by their margin and geometric form. A gradient orientation analysis (GOA) enables the detection of margins that are likely to belong to a lesion by investigating the gradients and their orientation and searching for convergences. In case of a round (spiculated) lesion, the gradients (edges) point towards the center of the lesion. The gradient orientations are calculated slice-wise using the Scharr operator that provides robust rotational invariance [8]. Additionally, the roughly approximated tissue orientations of the regarded breast is calculated by applying the Scharr operator on the distance transform of each binarized slice of the DBT mammogram. A custom neighborhood, as depicted in Fig. 3, is defined.

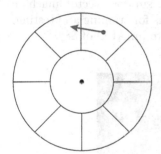

Fig. 3. The neighborhood of a point (center dot) for a GOA. It is defined by the outside of an inner and the inside of an outer circle. This 'hose' is divided into disjoint sectors, eight in this instance. An exemplary gradient orientation which belongs to the neighborhood is shown as a vector. The radii of the outer and inner circle of the neighborhood are calculated from the scale at which the DoG feature (see previous section) returns its maximum value response. If this response is below a threshold, the radii are set to default values.

Two GOA features are calculated for both round lesions (subscript c) on the basis of oriented gradients and for spiculated lesions (subscript s) on the basis of oriented edges inside this neighborhood. The first feature GOA_{c1} (GOA_{s1}) counts the number of gradient (edge) orientations that intersect the inner circle of the neighborhood. Additionally, gradient (edge) orientations that run across the estimated tissue orientation are weighted higher by factor two.

For the second feature GOA_{c2} (GOA_{s2}), the number n^+ of estimated gradient (edge) orientations that are intersecting the inner circle is calculated inside one sector, given uniformly distributed random gradient (edge) orientations. The second feature GOA_{c2} (GOA_{s2}) then counts the number of sectors which have more than n^+-many gradient (edge) orientations that intersect the inner circle. This ensures that not only one or two sectors contribute the gradient (edge) orientations converging towards the center of the neighborhood as is the case with vessels for instance.

3 Results

Fig. 4 shows the output of the two presented DoG and GOA features. They are evaluated using a ground truth of 100 downsized DBT mammograms from [6] which leads to roughly 11 Gigabyte of data. The features are calculated for each voxel of all slices and the area under curve (AUC) of specificity to sensitivity is calculated by stepwise incrementation of a global threshold. The lower the threshold the less voxels are classified as lesions. With increasing threshold, more voxels get classified as lesions. At full threshold, all mammogram data is classified as lesions. The AUC describes the quality of this classification. An AUC of 50% is similar to random classification. An AUC of 100% describes a perfect classificator that classifies all voxels as lesions that are actual lesions and all voxels as non-lesions that are actual non-lesions.

The AUC of the proposed methods are 85% for DoG, 82% for GOA_{c1}, 82% for GOA_{c2}, 80% for GOA_{s1} and 80% for GOA_{s2}. It is feasible that the features responding to round lesions (GOA_{c1} and GOA_{c2}) do not response as good to spiculated lesions as features responding to spiculated lesions (GOA_{s1} and GOA_{s2}) and vice versa. The same takes effect on features designed to response to intensities (DoG) and gradient orientation convergences (GOA). Therefore, we evaluated the combination of all features using a support vector machine (SVM) with equally sized sets of 50 DBT mammograms for training and testing. This improves the classification performance, leading to an AUC of 88%.

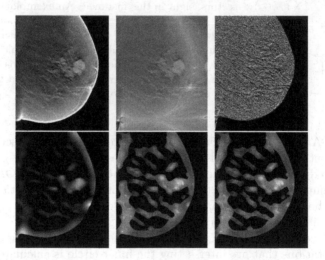

Fig. 4. From left to right: Input slice showing a round lesion, the preprocessed slice with masked skinline, reduced skinline noise and mirrored and the oriented gradients using the Scharr operator (upper row). The DoG, the GOA_{c1} and the GOA_{c2} feature maps (lower row). The round lesion is clearly visible as highlighted area in all feature maps.

4 Discussion

It has been shown that for the purpose of a high sensitivity in the first part of the developed CADe system, the voxel-wise classification of DBT mammograms provides a robust and reliable output giving an AUC of 88%. Two features have been presented and evaluated individually and combined using a SVM.

Some promising new findings and possible improvements can be deduced from the results. An interesting fact lies in the higher classification performance of the DoG feature in comparison to the GOA features. Compared to their application to conventional digital mammograms, the DoG feature not only performs better than the GOA features but DoG performs considerably better than any other single feature seen individually [9]. This shows the better visibility by means of intensity and contrast of lesions in DBT, probably due to the decreased amount of overlapping tissue in DBT mammograms compared to conventional digital mammograms. Furthermore, most of the false positives regarding the DoG feature occur due to the dense pectoral muscle which leads to high intensity artifacts that are falsely regarded as lesions. It is feasible that the classification performance using the DoG feature can further increase if a segmentation of the DBT mammogram into breast and pectoral muscle is applied in a preprocessing step.

It has been shown that a combination of features improves the classification performance. Further improvements are possible in the development of a SVM or the use of a classificator that is able to handle the large amount of DBT data, as well as the continuous extension of the ground truth by new cases, as it would be applicable in clinical use.

References

1. Cancer facts & figures 2012. American Cancer Society; 2012.
2. Singh S, Baydush A, Harrawood B, et al. Mass detection in mammographic ROIs using Watson filters. Procs SPIE. 2006.
3. Wittenberg T, Wagner F, Gryanik A. Towards a computer assisted diagnosis system for digital breast tomosynthesis. Biomed Tech. 2012.
4. Smith A. Fundamentals of Breast Tomosynthesis; 2008. Available from: http://www.hologic.com/de/.
5. Good WF, Abrams GS, Catullo VJ, et al.. Digital breast tomosynthesis: a pilot observer study; 2012.
6. Borsdorf A. Adaptive filtering for noise reduction in X-ray computed tomography; 2009.
7. Universitätsklinik Erlangen. Brust-Tomosynthesedaten der IMoDe (Imaging and Molecular Detection); 2013. Studie der Universitätsklinik Erlangen, März 2013.
8. Prinzen M. Lokalisation von Vegetation in Bildern von Architekturumgebungen. Bachelor-Thesis, Universität Koblenz-Landau; 2009.
9. te Brake GM. Computer aided detection of masses in digital mammograms; 2000.

Fast Interpolation of Dense Motion Fields from Synthetic Phantoms

Andreas Maier[1,2], Oliver Taubmann[1], Jens Wetzl[1], Jakob Wasza[1],
Christoph Forman[1,2], Peter Fischer[1,2], Joachim Hornegger[1,2], Rebecca Fahrig[3]

[1] Pattern Recognition Lab, FAU Erlangen-Nuremberg
[2] Erlangen Graduate School in Advanced Optical Technologies (SAOT)
[3] Radiological Sciences Lab, Stanford University
andreas.maier@fau.de

Abstract. Numerical phantoms are a common tool for the evaluation of
registration and reconstruction algorithms. For applications concerning
motion, dense deformation fields are of particular interest. Phantoms,
however, are often described as surfaces and thus motion vectors can only
be generated at these surfaces. In order to create dense motion fields,
interpolation is required. A frequently used method for this purpose is
the Parzen interpolator. However, with a high number of surface motion
vectors and a high voxel count, its run time increases dramatically. In
this paper, we investigate different methods to accelerate the creation
of these motion fields using hierarchical sampling and the random ball
cover. In the results, we show that a 64^3 volume can be sampled in less
than one second with an error below 0.1 mm. Furthermore, we accelerate
the interpolation of a 256^3 dense deformation field to only $\bar{6}.5$ minutes
using the proposed methods from days with previous methods.

1 Introduction

The systematic evaluation and comparison of non-rigid image registration and
reconstruction methods requires the availability of ground truth data in the form
of dense deformation fields. Ideally, this data should not come from a regularized registration or interpolation methods in order to to prevent bias towards a
certain approach, e.g. ground truth from a thin-plate-spline-based interpolation
will favor other thin-plate-spline based methods although they might be a more
realistic with respect to anatomy [1].

The 4D extended cardio-torso (XCAT) phantom [2] defines per-organ deformations over time and can be used to generate medical image sequences with
somewhat realistic respiratory or cardiac motion and also provides corresponding
sparse displacement vector fields defined on its parametric surfaces.

The main contribution of this article is a graphics processing unit (GPU)
accelerated method to compute dense displacement vector fields estimating the
motion inside and outside of organs from the given surface motion.

2   Materials and methods

In our two-step method (Fig. 1), we first generate accurate point approximations of the parametric B-spline surfaces [3]. The motion sparsely defined at each of these points is then interpolated efficiently on a dense regular grid to obtain full respiratory and/or cardiac motion fields covering the upper body.

2.1   Efficient point approximation of parametric surfaces

In order to find point samples that will serve as nodes for the interpolation, we finely tessellate the parametric surfaces $s(u, v, t)$ defined in terms of control points $c_{\text{l,k,i}}$ and their weights $\beta(u)$ of degree 3

$$s(u, v, t) = \sum_i \sum_k \sum_l c_{\text{l,k,i}} \beta(u - l)\beta(v - k)\beta(t - i) \qquad (1)$$

$$\text{with} \quad \beta(u) = \begin{cases} 0, & |u| \geq 2 \\ \frac{1}{6}(2 - |u|)^3, & 1 \leq |u| < 2 \\ \frac{2}{3} - \frac{1}{2}|u|^2(2 - |u|), & |u| < 1 \end{cases} \qquad (2)$$

Note that this tessellation can be implemented even more efficiently using texture units on the graphics card [3] at the cost of slightly decreased accuracy. For the present work, we used double precision CPU computations, as we wanted to investigate the accuracy of our interpolation approaches.

2.2   Fast interpolation of deformations on a regular grid

We now consider a regular 3D grid with the desired properties, e.g. size, location and spacing. For each grid point x, we aim to find an estimate of its motion $d_\sigma(x)$ from a combination of the displacements defined at the closest surface points. In the following, we only consider the evaluation of a deformation field from time t_0 to t_1, i.e. the n surface points at time t_0 are denoted as $x_i := s(u_i, v_i, t_0)$

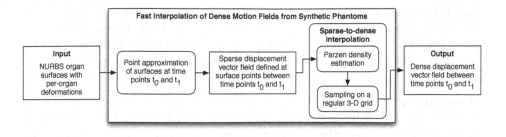

Fig. 1. System overview.

and their deformation as $d_i := s(u_i, v_i, t_1) - s(u_i, v_i, t_0)$. For interpolation, we employ a Parzen density estimation [4] with a Gaussian kernel function

$$\hat{d}_\sigma(x) = \frac{1}{\sum_{i=1}^{n} w(x, x_i \sigma)} \sum_{i=1}^{n} w(x, x_i, \sigma) d_i, \tag{3}$$

$$\text{with} \quad w(x, x_i, \sigma) = \exp\left(-\frac{\|x - x_i\|_2^2}{2\sigma^2} + K\right) \tag{4}$$

The parameter σ is used to control the smoothness of the interpolation and K is a constant that is added to increase numerical stability of the Gaussian kernel. Note that as the weights $w(x, x_i, \sigma)$ appear in the numerator and the denominator, K cancels out. In our experiments, we chose $K = 70$.

The performance bottleneck of this approach is the summation over i, which has to be repeated for each voxel. Given a grid of 256^3 points and sparse vector field with about 700,000 vectors, $1.0 \cdot 10^{13}$ evaluations of (4) have to be performed. Such computations usually take hours to days to finish. However, as the weight decays exponentially with increasing distance, we are able to reduce the number of points that have to be considered at each voxel. In the following, we will describe two hierarchical methods to achieve this reduction, and one randomized method.

Slice selection. For parallelization on the GPU, we chose to run each kernel execution for an individual slice. Thus, it makes sense to preselect only points that are close to the current slice. As the distance threshold T_z, we selected 10 % of the volume size in the z direction plus 6 standard deviations σ of the Gaussian kernel. This leads to a reduced list of motion vector points per slice $x_{i,S}$ for use in (3) instead of x_i.

Gridding. In addition to Slice Selection, we can further reduce the number of points per voxel by a Gridding approach. For each slice, we first create a list of points g_j forming a sub-grid at a lower resolution than the sampling grid with step size p. Next, a list of close points x_{i,g_j} is created for each g_j. Each $x_{i,S}$ that is closer than $T_p := 2p + 6\sigma$ is added to this list. For the evaluation, first the correct sub-list x_{i,g_j} has to be selected by finding the g_j that is closest to x. Next, (3) is applied using x_{i,g_j} instead of x_i which leads to a dramatic reduction of search points. A sub-sampling factor of 16 was used in our experiments.

Random ball cover. The selection process described in the previous section bears striking similarity to the Random Ball Cover (RBC) [5]. Thus, we propose an adaptation of this method. Instead of using a regular grid as in the previous method, we use the structure of the data vectors and select representatives g_r randomly. Again, a list for each representative has to be generated. In order to pick an appropriate distance threshold, we have to determine the maximal minimum distance p^* between all points. Then the threshold T_r is found as

$$T_r = p^* + \min(6\sigma, p^*) \tag{5}$$

which evaluates to $p^* + 6\sigma$ for few representatives and $2p^*$ for many representatives. The list x_{i,g_r} is then built in the same way as in the previous approach and used in (3).

3   Experiments and results

All steps of the proposed methods have been implemented and optimized to run on the GPU using the Open Computing Language (OpenCL) framework. Our implementation will be made available as part of the CONRAD software platform [6] designed for simulating basic processes in X-ray imaging and the evaluation of image reconstruction algorithms [7].

In order to measure the evaluation accuracy, we investigated our methods using the XCAT heart using a 64^3 voxel volume only. The voxel size was 2.5 mm (isotropic). In total, 4,500 vectors have to be interpolated at each grid point. The ground truth motion field obtained without any search point reduction is shown in Fig. 2. We measured total computation time, kernel execution time, number of points used for interpolation, and the root mean square error (RMSE) between each method and the ground truth deformation field computed with CPU double accuracy. The results are given in Tab. 1. With varying σ, we observe that the thresholds we chose yield stable results for all methods. Errors are virtually always below 0.1 mm. With the presented parameters, RBC performs best. However, reduction rates are the highest with the Gridding approach, which comes with a slight increase in computational error.

Next, we evaluated the three methods with a bigger sampling grid using 256^3 voxels with an isotropic size of 1.5 mm and 700,000 motion vectors. With this number of vectors, we are not able to evaluate the plain OpenCL and the Slice Selection approach, as the computation time per slice exceeds 2 s. This causes the graphics driver to terminate the kernel execution. While there are ways to circumvent this, we generally do not want to pursue this direction as execution times are too long. For the Gridding approach, we were able to compute the complete deformation field in 389 s with about 200 vectors used per representative. For the RBC, we were not able to obtain similar results. With 50,000 representatives, the memory required to store the search list exceeded our graphics card memory. With 500,000 representatives, we already need $3.5 \cdot 10^{11}$ distance comparisons just to build the RBC list. This is almost as complex as the original problem. Thus, only the Gridding approach was suitable for the large problem size. Fig. 3 shows the resulting motion vector field.

4   Conclusion

We have developed a fast method to generate dense motion vector fields from phantom data. In the small problem size, all three proposed methods worked

Table 1. Results using a 64^3 deformation field of the XCAT heart phantom.

σ	Algorithm	Kernel time [s]	Total time [s]	Used vectors [%]	RMSE [mm]
1	CPU	-	274.107	100.0	0.0
	OpenCL	4.961	5.241	100.0	$2.66 \cdot 10^{-6}$
	Slice Selection	1.591	1.903	27.5	$2.44 \cdot 10^{-6}$
	Gridding	1.544	1.857	3.9	0.096
	RBC 500	0.951	1.498	13.5	0.012
	RBC 250	0.874	1.435	15.6	0.029
	RBC 50	1.077	1.450	18.7	0.137
5	CPU	-	432.691	100.0	0.0
	OpenCL	4.960	5.289	100.0	$2.66 \cdot 10^{-6}$
	Slice Selection	3.027	3.432	56.4	0.084
	Gridding	3.244	3.619	14.5	0.084
	RBC 500	1.685	2.247	28.3	0.001
	RBC 250	2.013	2.480	38.0	0.001
	RBC 50	2.793	3.198	53.1	$2.72 \cdot 10^{-5}$

well with an error of less than 0.1 mm. For the large problem size, only the Gridding approach could be successfully applied, as it reduced the number of interpolation vectors by the largest factor. In this case, we report a runtime of about 6.5 minutes.

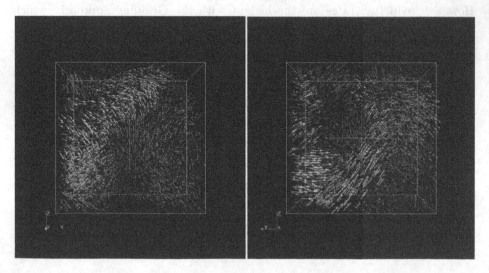

Fig. 2. Two perpendicular views of the cardiac motion field generated with the XCAT heart and the given configuration. The figure nicely shows the complexity of the 3D pumping motion of the heart.

Fig. 3. Two perpendicular views of the breathing motion field representing an inhalation, generated with the XCAT torso and the given configuration. The vectors pointing downward are linked to the downward motion of the diaphragm in the center of the volume. The upward (along the z direction) and outward (against the y direction) motion shows the expanding chest motion.

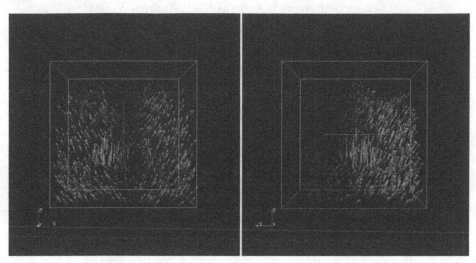

Acknowledgement. The authors gratefully acknowledge funding of the Erlangen Graduate School in Advanced Optical Technologies (SAOT) and the Research Training Group Heterogeneous Imaging Systems by the German Research Foundation (DFG) in the framework of the German excellence initiative.

References

1. von Berg J, Barschdorf H, Blaffert T, et al. Surface based cardiac and respiratory motion extraction for pulmonary structures from multi-phase CT. Proc SPIE;6511:65110Y–1–11.
2. Segars WP, Sturgeon G, Mendonca S, et al. 4D XCAT phantom for multimodality imaging research. Med Phys. 2010;37(9):4902–15.
3. Maier A, Hofmann H, Schwemmer C, et al. Fast simulation of X-ray projections of spline-based surfaces using an append buffer. Phys Med Biol. 2012;57(19):6193–210.
4. Parzen E. On estimation of a probability density function and mode. Ann Math Stat. 1962;33(3):1065–76.
5. Neumann D, Lugauer F, Bauer S, et al. Real-time RGB-D mapping and 3-D modeling on the GPU using the random ball cover data structure. Proc IEEE ICCV. 2011; p. 1161–67.
6. Maier A, Hofmann H, Berger M, et al. CONRAD: a software framework for cone-beam imaging in radiology. Med Phys. 2013;40(11):111914–1–8.
7. Kak AC, Slaney M. Principles of Computerized Tomographic Imaging. Piscataway, NJ, USA: IEEE; 1988.

The Effect of Endoscopic Lens Distortion Correction on Physicians' Diagnosis Performance

Michael Gadermayr[1], Andreas Uhl[1], Andreas Vécsei[2]

[1]Department of Computer Sciences, University of Salzburg, Austria
[2]Department of Pediatrics, St. Anna Children's Hospital, Austria
mgadermayr@cosy.sbg.ac.at

Abstract. In endoscopic images, significant barrel-type distortions are introduced in case of deploying wide-angle lenses. In this work, the effect of lens distortion correction on the human experts' classification performance is investigated. Especially, the discrimination between healthy patients and patients suffering from celiac disease is examined. Furthermore, the classification results of human experts are compared with those achieved with state-of-the-art computer aided decision support systems. This paper considers a two- as well as a four-classes case. Finally we come to the conclusion, that distortion correction does not improve the human experts' classification performance.

1 Introduction

Celiac disease is an autoimmune disorder that affects the small bowel in genetically predisposed individuals after introduction of gluten containing food. Characteristic for this disease is an inflammatory reaction in the mucosa of the small bowel caused by a dysregulated immune response triggered by ingested gluten proteins of certain cereals.During the course of the disease the mucosa loses its absorptive villi and hyperplasia of the enteric crypts occurs, leading to a diminished ability to absorb food. According to a study [1], the prevalence of the disease in the USA in not-at-risk groups was 1:133.

Endoscopy with biopsy is currently considered the gold standard for the diagnosis of celiac disease. However, in the past several techniques for enhanced celiac disease classification avoiding biopsies have been investigated, such as an immersion technique [2], chromoendoscopy [3] and zoom endoscopy [4].

In this paper, focus is on barrel-type distortions which are introduced by the wide-angle optics deployed in endoscopes. These distortions can be undone, by first estimating the distortion function and then applying the inverse of this function to the distorted images (Fig. 1). However, during distortion correction (DC) new issues arise as the images must be stretched especially in peripheral regions and thereby due to the lack of data points, these image regions are blurred. In a recent study [5], the effect of barrel-type distortions and distortion correction on the classification accuracy of computer aided celiac disease diagnosis has been investigated. Whereas in most cases the distortion correction leads to decreased classification accuracies, for some special cases stable improvements are

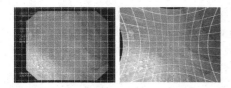

Fig. 1. This figure shows an original endoscopy image (left) and the distortion corrected version (right). The grid is artificially added for a better visualization of the distortion correction.

observed. We investigate the effect of barrel-type distortion correction on the classification performance of human experts. We separately analyze the effect on accuracy (in case of 2 and 4 classes), specificity and sensitivity. Furthermore, we compare the achieved rates with those achieved by computer based methods.

2 Materials and methods

The key issue of this paper is whether the correction of barrel-type distortions has a positive (or negative) impact on the classification performances of medical experts. We separately consider accuracy, specificity and sensitivity in the two-classes case as well as the accuracy in a four-classes case.

In case of the original barrel-type distorted images, peripheral regions appear distinctly smaller than central regions. This might be an issue during classification. However, a distortion correction, which is able to retrieve the geometrical correctness not necessarily enhances the classification rates. Medical experts are used to the wide-angle optics and potentially compensate the lens distortion mentally. Moreover, due to their practice they might be able to additionally compensate perspective distortions by considering the image properties. This process might be compromised in case of distortion correction. Moreover, as the images must be stretched during distortion correction, peripheral image regions are significantly blurred (due to a lack of data points). Especially this issue turned out to compromise some computer aided decision support techniques [5]. To estimate the effect of distortion correction on the human experts' classification performance, a first experiment (stage 1) is based on the complete endoscopic images. As the medical doctors are accustomed to these images, the straightforward investigation is to provide original and distortion corrected complete images which have to be manually classified.

Whereas human experts usually deal with these complete images, computer aided decision support systems are optimized for 128×128 pixel patches [6]. To get a ground-truth database, experts have manually extracted these patches. In order to be able to compare classification results of physicians with those of computer based methods, another experiment (stage 2) is based on such manually extracted patch images. Considering such image patches, the prior knowledge of the location in the complete image is removed and thereby it is no longer possible to mentally compensate the distortions.

Finally, we would like to know if the physicians are aware of the fact that the images suffer from lens distortions. Therefore, we provided 25 synthetically distorted checkerboard patterns (Fig. 2). The physicians should estimate the barrel-type distortions of typical endoscopes used for celiac disease diagnosis.

2.1 Experimental setup

The image test set used contains images of the duodenal bulb taken during duodenoscopies at the St. Anna Children's hospital using pediatric gastroscopes. First, we chose image patches which turned out to be hard to classify by computer based methods (to get larger differences between the classification performances). Then we added complete images from which these patches have been extracted.

Each of the 11 medical experts has classified 104 complete images and 144 image patches (Tab. 1). In each stage, the images are randomly permuted, separately for each physician. For each original image, the database additionally contains a corrected version. The group of human experts involved in this study consist of 9 pediatrics and 2 adult gastroenterologists. All of them are experts in the field of celiac disease diagnosis.

The condition of the mucosa should be estimated according to the modified Marsh classification scheme [7]. The experts had to assign one of the four labels Marsh-0 (healthy), Marsh-3A, Marsh-3B and Marsh-3C. As this four-classes (4C) case is highly difficult, we additionally evaluate the two-classes (2C) case. Therefore, the classes Marsh-3A, Marsh-3B and Marsh-3C are simply identified as Marsh-3. To generate the ground-truth, the condition of the mucosal areas covered by the images was determined by histological examination of biopsies from the corresponding regions.

For computer aided classification, we use the Shape Curvature Histogram [8] as feature extraction technique. Due to its compact dimensionality, this feature is optimally suited for the small datasets. In order to avoid overfitting, the parameters as proposed in [8] are utilized. For classification, we utilize the k-nearest neighbor classifier in combination with leave-one-patient-out cross validation. The classification accuracies for k reaching from 1 to 12 (12 corresponds to the minimal count of images per class) are averaged, to get stable and sound rates. For lens distortion correction, we deployed the method introduced in [9] (in combination with bi-linear interpolation), which is based on the division model [10]. This quite simple method proved to effectively rectify the geometrical image properties and is appropriate for a following feature extraction (as shown in [5]).

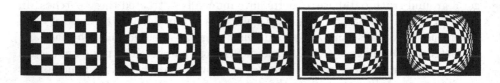

Fig. 2. Synthetically distorted checkerboard patterns. The framed image represents barrel-type distortions, typical for the used endoscopes.

Table 1. The test image databases used for the experiments.

Stage	1: Complete images	2: Image patches
Image size (pixels)	768 × 576 / 528 × 522	128 × 128
Number images: Marsh-0	26	36
Number images: Marsh-3 (3A, 3B, 3C)	26 (8, 8, 10)	36 (12, 12, 12)

3   Results

Figure 3 shows the 2C accuracy ((a) and (e)), the 4C accuracy ((b) and (f)), the (2C) specificity ((c) and (g)) and the (2C) sensitivity ((d) and (h)). The top sub-figures show the rates for each expert (x-axis). The physicians are ordered by their 2C accuracy (without DC). The bottom sub-figures show the cumulative average rates. To get these rates, for each x-axis value n we average the rates of the (ordered) experts from 1 to n. Thereby, we get mean rates of the best n physicians (where n corresponds to the x-axis value). We decided for this visualization strategy in order to get more stable and sound results. The gray horizontal line indicates the rate achieved with the computer based method (and the image patches). In the following we especially consider the accumulative rates (right sub-figures). Regarding these plots, we notice that the distortion correction (dashed lines) in general compromises the classification process. No matter if considering the 2C or the 4C case or the specificity, the dashed lines are always below the solid ones. Only the sensitivity in case of patch classification, seems to be similarly high of even slightly above in case of distortion correction.

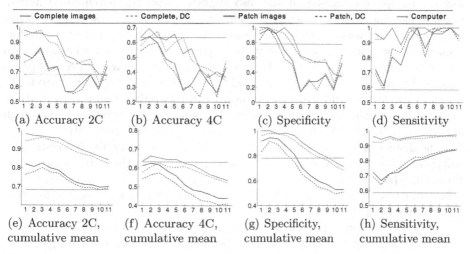

Fig. 3. These plots show the 2C and 4C accuracies as well as the specificities and the sensitivities. Whereas the top row ((a) - (d)) provides the rates for each individual expert, the bottom row ((e) - (h)) shows the cumulative rates.

4   Discussion

Obviously, diseased patients are slightly more likely to be detected in case of distortion corrected images. This diametric behavior might be due to the fact, that distortion correction leads to partly blurred images. Thereby the villi structure which indicates a healthy mucosa, might by hidden and thus false positives are provoked. However, to put it in a nutshell, distortion correction does not significantly enhance any of the classification properties and on average the classification accuracy drops.

Furthermore, some other quite interesting aspects can be deduced from the results. Considering image patches instead of complete images, the discriminative power in case of human experts significantly drops. Especially the sensitivity (Fig. 3(d)) of the best experts falls from about 90% to about 70% and below. Obviously for the physicians it is crucial not just to see a small texture patch, but to have knowledge of the whole image.

Moreover we notice that the highest overall accuracies are achieved by those medical doctors with the highest specificities. However, the highest sensitivities are achieved by those with lower accuracies. Seemingly the less experienced doctors (with lower accuracies) tend to less false negatives but more false positives.

Finally we consider the rates achieved by the computer aided method. In the two-classes case, in combination with the image patches (which are also used by the computer based method), the best 6 experts are able to outperform this method (Fig.3(a)). In case of the accustomed classification of complete images, the human experts are significantly better. In this scenario, all but one experts (partially significantly) outperform the computer based approach. On average (Fig.3(e), rightmost values), the computer based approach is significantly below the complete-image-based and also slightly below the patch-based human expert's classification accuracy. Considering the four-classes case, the computer aided approach turns out to be much more competitive compared to the performances of the human experts. Only two experts achieve higher accuracies with complete images and only one of the experts is similarly accurate in case of patch images. On average, the computer based approach significantly outperforms the human experts. It is not sensible to compare the specificity and the sensitivity of the computer aided method, as the used classifier is optimized to achieve high accuracies (and a balanced ratio between sensitivities and specificities).

The distortion estimation experiment (Fig. 2) reveals a quite interesting result. The majority of experts (7 persons) is not aware of the barrel-type distortions and chose the leftmost distortion-free image. The images chosen by the others (4 persons) are shown in Fig. 2 (second until fifth image). Each distorted pattern has been chosen once.

Obviously the majority of physicians are not aware of the barrel-type distortions introduced by the endoscopes. Seemingly this does not strongly affect their classification performance, as a distortion correction leads to worse results. However, in this work, we are not able to precisely estimate the effect of the lens distortions as the distortion correction leads to new inadequacies and there is nothing to prevent these distortions in the original endoscopic images.

5   Conclusion

This paper showed, that the human classification performance definitely does not benefit from barrel-type distortion correction. Quite the contrary, in almost all cases, the classification rates drop significantly. We also showed, that the computer based approach is highly competitive if considering the four-classes case. If considering the two-classes case, the human experts on average are more reliable. The human experts' performances significantly benefit from complete images instead of the smaller patches. Therefore, we encourage to develop a computer aided method, being based on the complete images to additionally exploit the (obviously important) larger image context.

Acknowledgement. This work is partially funded by the Austrian Science Fund (FWF) under Project No. 24366.

References

1. Fasano A, Berti I, Gerarduzzi T, et al. Prevalence of celiac disease in at-risk and not-at-risk groups in the United States: a large multicenter study. Arc Int Med. 2003;163(3):286–92.
2. Cammarota G, Cesaro P, Martino A, et al. High accuracy and cost-effectiveness of a biopsy-avoiding endoscopic approach in diagnosing coeliac disease. Aliment Pharmacol Ther. 2006;23(1):61–9.
3. Kiesslich R, Mergener K, Naumann C, et al. Value of chromoendoscopy and magnification endoscopy in the evaluation of duodenal abnormalities: a prospective, randomized comparison. Endoscopy. 2003;35(7):559–63.
4. Badreldin R, Barrett P, Wooff DA, et al. How good is zoom endoscopy for assessment of villous atrophy in coeliac disease? Endoscopy. 2005;37(10):994–8.
5. Gadermayr M, Liedlgruber M, Uhl A, et al. Evaluation of different distortion correction methods and interpolation techniques for an automated classification of celiac disease. Comput Methods Programs Biomed. 2013;112(3):694–712.
6. Hegenbart S, Kwitt R, Liedlgruber M, et al. Impact of duodenal image capturing techniques and duodenal regions on the performance of automated diagnosis of celiac disease. In: Proc ISPA; 2009. p. 718–23.
7. Oberhuber G, Granditsch G, Vogelsang H. The histopathology of coeliac disease: time for a standardized report scheme for pathologists. Eur J Gastroenterol Hepatol. 1999;11(10):1185–94.
8. Gadermayr M, Liedlgruber M, Uhl A. Shape curvature histogram: a shape feature for celiac disease diagnosis. In: Proc MICCAI-MCV; 2013. p. –. Accepted.
9. Melo R, Barreto JP, Falcao G. A new solution for camera calibration and real-time image distortion correction in medical endoscopy-initial technical evaluation. IEEE Trans Biomed Eng. 2012;59(3):634–44.
10. Fitzgibbon AW. Simultaneous linear estimation of multiple view geometry and lens distortion. In: Proc IEEE Comput Soc Conf Comput Vis Pattern Recognit; 2001. p. 125–32.

Clustering Socio-Demographic and Medical Attribute Data in Cohort Studies

Paul Klemm[1], Lisa Frauenstein[1], David Perlich[1], Katrin Hegenscheid[2],
Henry Völzke[2], Bernhard Preim[1]

[1]Otto-von-Guericke University Magdeburg, Germany
[2]Ernst-Moritz-Arndt University Greifswald, Germany
klemm@isg.cs.uni-magdeburg.de

Abstract. Longitudinal epidemiological studies like the Study of Health
in Pomerania (SHIP) analyze a group of thousands of subjects (a cohort)
by imposing a multitude of socio-demographic and biological factors.
Epidemiological findings rest upon hypotheses which yield a selection of
disease-specific cohort study parameters. They are then analyzed for significant interactions to identify risk factors. We propose an alternative
approach by incorporating clustering algorithms with a Visual Analytics
system to form subject groups which are the basis for an exploratory
analysis of the underlying parameter interactions. We investigated three
clustering techniques (k-Prototypes, DBSCAN and hierarchical clustering) for their suitability in these data sets. With our system, groups can
be automatically determined to provide insights into this complex data.

1 Introduction

Epidemiological long-term cohort studies like the Study of Health in Pomerania [1] comprise a large range of sociodemographic and medical attributes of
thousands of individuals to assess disease-specific risk factors. Knowledge about
disease-influencing factors may affect its prevention, diagnosis and treatment.
The resulting heterogeneous data space comprises several hundred variables
gathered with different epidemiological instruments like interviews, clinical examinations and medical imaging. Risk factors are assessed in a sequential
hypothesis-driven way by domain experts. Hypotheses formulation follows observations in clinical routine. To validate the hypotheses, an attribute list is
compiled and analyzed using regression analysis to check for statistical plausibility [2].

Visual Analytics methods integrate data analysis and visual exploration for
analyzing huge data spaces to generate and validate hypothesis. An important
technique for exploring heterogeneous data sets (data of different type) using Visual Analytics approaches is brushing over the subjects' attributes, which allows
for subject grouping. We aim to enhance the exploratory data analysis approach by automatically generating subject groups using clustering algorithms.
Our work is based on a data set that was compiled to analyze lower (lumbar)
back pain. Privacy protection of the participants is ensured by anonymization

of their personal data. Shape-based clustering of medical image data using spine detection models was carried out before [3]. Attributes of the lower spine canal, like curvature, torsion and vertebra positions, were extracted from the spine detection [4] to enhance the data set with shape-related parameters. Deterministic cluster results are a major requirement to ensure statistical resilience. Clustering subjects aims to reveal undiscovered correlations. Our main contributions are:

− Assessing three clustering methods (k-Prototypes, DBSCAN and hierarchical agglomerative clustering) for their suitability in cohort studies.
− Incorporating the clustering methods in a web-based Visual Analytics framework for browsing cohort study data.

2   Materials and methods

In this section, we describe the epidemiological data set we used, followed by a brief overview of the incorporated clustering methods.

2.1   The spine data set

A list of 77 attributes for 2333 subjects was compiled by domain experts at the University of Greifswald to analyze back pain. A finite element method was used to detect the lumbar spine in the MRI scans [4]. Curvature and torsion as well as the vertebra positions of the lumbar spine canal were extracted using the detection model. The data set is heterogeneous in terms of data types. A majority of 62 attributes are ordinal, i.e., results of multiple choice questionnaires related to lifestyle factors and medical background like back pain history. Body size measurements and parameters derived from the image data are covered from 17 scalar variables. A challenge when analyzing cohort studies are subjects with missing values for some attributes. Reasons for incomplete data range from medical/ethical to personal issues. The clustering workflow must account for missing data.

2.2   Clustering workflow

The clustering methods are embedded into a in-house developed Visual Analytics system, which comprises different views for ordinal and metric variables (Fig. 2.2). To trigger clustering, the user selects either all parameters of a data set or a subset from a list. Due to missing values, the system immediately displays the number of subjects that are omitted in the clustering step given the current attribute selection. The selection of the clustering method and its parameters closes this process, which returns computed groups that are rendered as seen in Fig. 2.2.

2.3   Clustering methods

Clustering methods divide the space spanned by data elements so that it maximizes the distance between groups and minimizes the within-groups variance.

Measurement of distance. Clustering heterogeneous data attributes at the same time requires distance measurements that consider different data types [5]. We calculated the similarity between numerical attributes using the Euclidean distance. Ordinal attribute values are compared in a binary fashion, having distance 0 when they are identical and distance 1 otherwise. The factor γ can be used to weight elements [5]. We applied three different clustering techniques.

K-means and k-prototypes. Dividing the data into k clusters using randomly generated centroids, each data point is iteratively attached to its closest centroid. K-Prototypes [6] enhances k-Means to allow for the clustering of ordinal and scalar attributes using the previously described weighted distance. The random initialization of centroids renders the k-Prototypes clustering results non-deterministic. This is not suitable for epidemiological applications where reproducibility of all results is required [2]. Therefore, the initial centroid positions are computed by placing centroids near values that are close to each other.

DBSCAN. Density-Based Spatial Clustering of Applications with Noise computes clusters based on object density. Elements are density-connected when they are reachable by a chain of dense objects. Density-connected elements form a cluster. Outliers are objects that are not associated to a cluster via density. DBSCAN is steered by parameters, which define the distance between neighbors

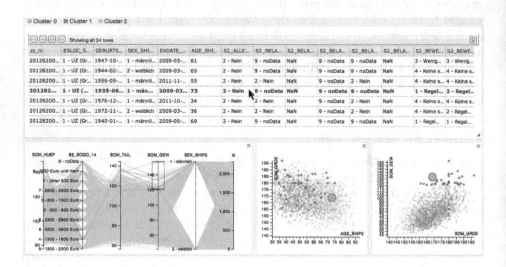

Fig. 1. Embedding a clustering result within the Visual Analytics framework. A k-Prototypes clustering with $k = 3$ results in three color-coded clusters. All subjects with body weight above 120 kg are brushed using parallel coordinates and highlighted in the scatterplots with red circles. One subject of cluster two is selected in the list view, which increases its opacity in the parallel coordinates and its radius in the scatterplots.

Table 1. Dice's coefficients for clustering results of k-Prototypes and DBSCAN.

Cluster Number	Algorithms	Dice's Coefficient
2	k-prototypes / DBSCAN ($\epsilon = 1.3$)	0.634
	k-prototypes / DBSCAN ($\epsilon = 1.4$)	0.655
	k-prototypes / DBSCAN ($\epsilon = 1.5$)	0.657
3	k-prototypes / DBSCAN ($\epsilon = 0.9$)	0.720
	k-prototypes / DBSCAN ($\epsilon = 1.1$)	0.644
	k-prototypes / DBSCAN ($\epsilon = 1.2$)	0.646
6	k-prototypes / DBSCAN ($\epsilon = 1.0$)	0.406

(ϵ) and the number of neighbors that a "dense"element must comprise ($minPts$). The method is independent of a predefined cluster number and accounts for outliers.

Hierarchical agglomerative clustering. The stepwise aggregation of the closest elements into a cluster yields a dendrogram whose levels represent clusters. By varying the minimum similarity, the desired number of clusters is obtained. The method is known to be outlier-prone.

3   Results

The difficulty of comparing cluster results in this application domain is twofold. First, we cannot measure the accuracy of a result due to missing ground truth. Second, the presented clustering methods have different parameters, which have a strong impact on their results. We tried to minimize the difference in the results by focussing on the same numerical and categorical parameters.

K-Prototypes was tested in a range of two to ten clusters. The cluster sizes range from 94 to 487 subjects. No overly large or small clusters are computed.

DBSCAN's parameter $minPts$ equals the minimum cluster size. Since epidemiologists are interested in larger groups of subjects, this value needs to be fairly high. Ester and colleagues argue that the impact of $minPts$ is little above a certain threshold [7]. We set this value empirically to 50, which produces size-balanced clusters. Parameter ϵ defines the size of an object's neighborhood. Set low, ϵ leads to many small outlier clusters, which we want to avoid–an ϵ value between 0.6 and 0.8 classifies 1602 subjects as outliers and is therefore not reasonable. Parameter ϵ set to 0.9 to 1.2 results in balanced clusters.

Hierarchical Agglomerative Clustering creates very unbalanced trees for our data. Many clusters only contain one element. Complete-Linkage produced the best results in terms of cluster size, but still yields one large cluster containing almost all subjects. Hence, this method was discarded for use on our data.

3.1 Comparison using Dice's coefficient

We used Dice's coefficient to compare the clustering results under use of different parameters [8]. It is defined as $\frac{2(A \cap B)}{|A|+|B|}$, where A and B are the clusters to compare and $A \cap B$ is the amount of elements in A and B. Dice's coefficient is 0 for disjunct and 1 for identical clusters. Since the hierarchical agglomerative clustering results are not plausible, we only compared k-Prototypes and DBSCAN. The results for clusters with size 2, 3 and 6 for DBSCAN with corresponding k-Prototypes results can be found in Tab. 1. While Dice's coefficient for 2 to 3 clusters is close to 0.65, it is only at 0.4 for 6 clusters. Cluster results are similar while there is a decreasing similarity for an increasing cluster number. This reflects the missing ground truth problem–these results are only an expression of similarity, not plausibility. The latter can only be determined in the context of epidemiological reasoning whether the groups represent meaningful correlations.

3.2 Visualization of clustering results

Enhancing the Visual Analytics framework by clustering capabilities for automatic grouping was a key motivation for this work. Each group is rendered using a different color and can therefore be differentiated in the linked plots (Fig. 2.2). We introduce an additional information window, which contains statistical information associated to each cluster (Fig. 2).

4 Discussion

We presented three methods for clustering epidemiological cohort study data to compute groups that capture data interactions. Linked to Visual Analytics systems, these methods provide an alternative way of gaining new insight into the complex interactions in these high-dimensional data sets. We found

Fig. 2. Information window for a clustering resulting from the k-Prototypes algorithm. The clustering parameters yield a reproducible clustering result. The distribution of metric parameters in the cluster is displayed using box plots. The most frequent value of each ordinal parameter is displayed using percentage statements.

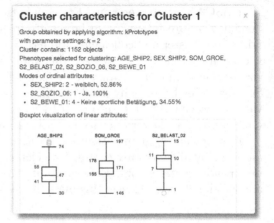

k-Prototypes and DBSCAN to be appropriate for our data. Hierarchical agglomerative clustering produced unbalanced cluster trees, yielding huge clusters containing almost all subjects and is therefore not suitable for our research. The clustering results are strongly dependent on the chosen variable types and the distance measure. Future extensions comprise better cluster group comparison to amplify hypothesis generation by highlighting influential parameters. Usability would benefit from automatic parameter designation using quality criteria. Missing data can be tackled with imputation [9]. For k-Prototypes, k could be derived by a knee function that plots the cluster number to a cluster quality measurement [10].

At the end, it falls to the user to validate the data for plausibility. A clustering-based automated grouping step can only highlight certain dependencies in the data set. It is no alternative to the classic epidemiological workflow, but rather an enhancement of the available tools, providing a different point of view. By combining both worlds, the huge cohort study data sets can be made tangible.

Acknowledgement. SHIP is part of the Community Medicine Research net of the University of Greifswald, Germany, which is funded by the Federal Ministry of Education and Research (grant no. 03ZIK012), the Ministry of Cultural Affairs as well as the Social Ministry of the Federal State of Mecklenburg-West Pomerania. This work was supported by the DFG Priority Program 1335: Scalable Visual Analytics.

References

1. Völzke H, Alte D, Schmidt C, et al. Cohort profile: the study of health in Pomerania. Int J Epidemiol. 2011;40(2):294–307.
2. Thew S, Sutcliffe A, Procter R, et al. Requirements engineering for e-science: experiences in epidemiology. Proc IEEE. 2009;26(1):80–7.
3. Klemm P, Lawonn K, Rak M, et al. Visualization and analysis of lumbar spine canal variability in cohort study data. Proc VMV. 2013; p. 121–8.
4. Rak M, Engel K, Tönnies KD. Closed-form hierarchical finite element models for part-based object detection. In: Proc VMV; 2013. p. 137–44.
5. Huang Z. Clustering large data sets with mixed numeric and categorical values. Proc PAKDD. 1997; p. 21–34.
6. Huang Z. Extensions to the k-means algorithm for clustering large data sets with categorical values. Data Min Knowl Discov. 1998;2(3):283–304.
7. Ester M, Kriegel HP, Sander J, et al. A Density-Based Algorithm for Discovering Clusters in Large Spatial Databases with Noise. Proc PAKDD. 1996; p. 226–31.
8. Dice LR. Measures of the amount of ecologic association between species. Ecology. 1945;26:297–302.
9. Donders ART, van der Heijden GJMG, Stijnen T, et al. Review: a gentle introduction to imputation of missing values. J Clin Epidemiol. 2006;59(10):1087–91.
10. Salvador S, Chan P. Determining the number of clusters/segments in hierarchical clustering/segmentation algorithms. Proc ICTAI. 2004; p. 576–84.

Urban Positioning Using Smartphone-Based Imaging

Deyvid Kochanov[1], Stephan Jonas[1], Nader Hamadeh[1], Ercan Yalvac[1],
Hans Slijp[2], Thomas M. Deserno[1]

[1] Dept. of Medical Informatics, Uniklinik RWTH Aachen, Aachen, Germany
[2] I-Cane Social Technologies, Sittard, Netherlands
sjonas@mi.rwth-aachen.de

Abstract. Orientation and navigation in a world dominated by visual
signs is still a major problem for blind and visually impaired people. The
Global Positioning System is of limited use due to its inaccuracy particularly in urban environments. Therefore, we propose a novel approach
of precise localization on predefined routes with the help of smartphones
and image processing techniques. From an initial acquisition of a given
route, a three-dimensional reconstruction is created. A query image is
submitted to the database and the location and direction of the camera
are calculated. Here, we demonstrate our approach on a evaluation-
dataset with a mean positioning error of 5.51 meters.

1 Introduction

According to global estimates, 15.5 million people in Europe are visually impaired [1]. The same study concludes that further growth is expected due to
the increase of diabetes and its effect on elder people. This emphasises the need
for reducing the impact or burden of sight loss by delivering improved support
through technology and innovation. Foremost, independency and mobility of
the blind and visually impaired has to be improved supporting free navigation
through unknown terrain. However, only very few technical advances towards
mobility, navigation and independence have been made since the introduction of
the white cane in the early 20th century.

New technological developments like the Global Positioning System (GPS) [2],
accelerometers and digital compasess provided novel opportunities to assist visually impaired blind people in the interpretation of environment and navigation
tasks. Moreover, satellite-based GPS positioning is not sufficiently accurate to
guide pedestrians through traffic, especially in urban environments. In particular, larger cities have tall buildings, which block or reflect satellite signals
reducing the accuracy to 34 meters [3].

Another approach uses the number of steps detected by an accelerometer,
reference-points and a mobile compass for navigation assistance. Fallah et al. [4]
presented a successful example of this method also with combining probabilistic
algorithms with natural capabilities of visual impaired persons to detect landmarks like corners with touch. However, this system is designed for indoor

environments, where maps are precisely defined by landmarks like corners and doors.

There is also supporting research that exploits stereo vision cameras or depth cameras like the Microsoft Kinect to navigate around obstacles [5]. However, the range of these devices is only a few meters and they are not fit for general navigation tasks that require localization.

Technologies that can be used in navigation systems today either have poor reliability in different conditions because of inaccuracies in measurement devices or are too expensive or too large to be integrated into mobile devices. Our system aims at using previously calculated 3D reconstruction and real time image processing on mobile phones to solve the accuracy problem while keeping the system affordable and easy to carry.

2   Materials and methods

Current three-dimensional (3D) reconstruction methods like structure from motion [6] can be used to generate city-scale models of real world scenes using unordered sets of 2D images. These reconstructions provide compact 3D models in the form of sparse point clouds (Fig. 1). The construction of these models is computationally expensive but it can be done off-line and incrementally.

Modern mobile devices like smartphones have sophisticated cameras and enough computational capacity to perform image processing tasks like feature extraction and detection. Free and open source libraries with implementations of the algorithms performing these tasks are readily available, for example MATLAB (The Mathworks[1]) and OpenCV[2].

---

[1] www.mathworks.com
[2] www.opencv.org

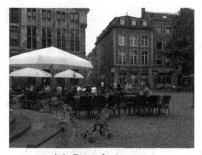
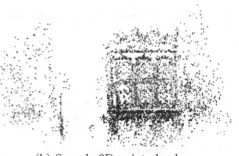

(a) Sample image   (b) Sample 3D point cloud

Fig. 1. Example 3D reconstruction of Aachen central market. The 3D reconstruction was created from a large dataset acquired for visualization reasons, not the evaluation dataset.

2.1 Reference acquistion

The images for the reference model are acquired while walking a route with a specialized smartphone application. The application records about one image per second along with other sensory data like GPS, accelerometer, magnetometer and gyroscope. The images and embedded metadata are buffered on the device and transferred to the server via the Internet connected by third (3G) or fourth (4G) generation mobile communication standards.

2.2 Model reconstruction

Image acquisition and processing for the 3D model construction is performed by first extracting image features with the scale invariant feature transform (SIFT) using MATLAB and OpenCV. Then, a 3D point cloud model is constructed using VisualSFM [7, 8]. This structure from motion methods also estimates the locations of the cameras in the initial set, which then can be used to construct navigation routes. The 3D model can be stored in a database of possible routes and used for localization of users identified by query images. Existing models can also be augmented by acquiring a route multiple times.

2.3 Query image localization

To estimate the location of the user, SIFT features are extracted from the image taken at the user's current position. Correspondences to the features of the points in the 3D point cloud are determined by calculating the distances between all features of the image against the point cloud and applying a threshold. The obtained matches are used to estimate the camera pose of the initial image with the following process. First, the camera matrix P is reconstructed. The camera matrix P maps the 3D world points X to their 2D image coordinates x within an unknown scaling factor λ

$$PX = \lambda x \tag{1}$$

In (1) P can be estimated from a set of corrspondences using the pseudoinverse.

$$PXX^T = \lambda x X^T \tag{2}$$

$$P = \lambda x X^T \left(X X^T \right)^{-1} \tag{3}$$

A more sophisticated and numerically stable method to estimate the matrix exists [9]. At least six correspondences are needed for the estimation of the camera matrix P. Howerver, noise caused by errors in the reconstruction and outlier matches can lead to errors in the estimation of the projection matrix.

To make the process more robust, random sample concensus (RANSAC) [9, 10] is used to discard outliers. RANSAC chooses a random sample from our set of correspondences, reconstruct the matrix and checks for consensus with the rest of the matches. Once a large enough set of inliers is found, the final camera matrix is computed. If no concensus is reached, the best model so far is returned. The camera position and orientation can be extracted from the camera projection matrix

$$P = K[R|t] \tag{4}$$

which is a composition of the projection matrix K and the camera motion matrix $[R|t]$ with R being a rotation matrix and t a translation vector. Because K is upper triangular matrix and R is orthogonal, QR decomposition can be used to compute the K and R from P. Thereby, the camera intrinsic parameters K and the relative camera position and orientation (R and t) are obtained [9]. After estimating a relative coordinates in the model, a real world position is computed by using real world locations of the cameras or keypoints in the initial dataset (e.g., GPS coordinates from a large number of cameras).

2.4   Evaluation

For ground truth data acquisition, an imaging protocol was set up. The protocol differs from the regular reference acquisitions by using a tripod to account for changes in height and making accurate measures of each camera location towards a reference point. This allows for easy reproduction of the set under different environmental conditions. The central marketplace of the city of Aachen was chosen as test location as it features both high buildings as well as pedestrians and other moving objects partly occluding the visual landmarks surrounding the buildings. Images at seven different locations and with three different angles were acquired with our acquisition app resulting in a total of 21 images (Fig. 2). In addition, a spreadsheets with the exact location of each camera towards a reference-point was created.

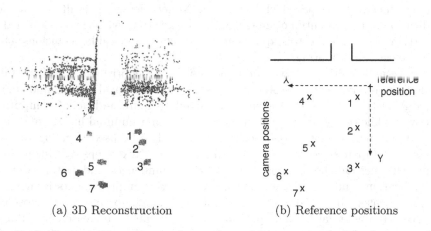

(a) 3D Reconstruction   (b) Reference positions

Fig. 2. Evaluation set 3D reconstruction and acquisition protocol of Aachen central market based on the complete evaluation set of 21 images. In the ground truth data, each camera position contains three shots in different direction (angulation of 30 degree).

Using a position-based leaving-one-out approach, six 3D models of the scene were created, each containing only 18 images from 6 locations. The remaining three images – all from the same position – were tested against the corresponding dataset. Since the 3D reconstructions itself can already contain errors, the distances of each query image towards the closest two positions, one in X and one in Y direction are used (Fig. 2(b)). Based on the ratio of these two distances and the supposed ratio, the positioning error was computed.

3   Results

Out of the 21 images used for the evaluation, one outlier localization was removed, which was more than 10 meters off. The average localization error of our system was 5.51 m (stdev 4.39 m).

4   Discussion

This work demonstrates that image guided localization is 2-5 times more precise than GPS-based localization which has an cummulated localization error of more than 30 m when relying to GPS only and more than 10 m with map-based correction [3]. Previous research suggest that from image base localization alone we can obtain localizations with error below 3 m with probabilty 0.75 and and below 18 m with probability 0.9 [10] which is compareable to our results. An increasing number of reference-images should furhter decrease the positioning error.

Another limitation of our evaluation is the quality of the reference images, as our evaluation images are acquired with a stable tripod while reference and query images are acquired while walking. Nonetheless, our results give a good indication of the potential of image-guided localization with smartphone cameras. further limitations of this approach are, of course, possible occlusions, changes in weather and lighting.

We aplied SIFT features and the RANSAC algorithm. Another approach that is often used in robotics is simultaneous localization and mapping (SLAM) [11]. However, the mapping would require additional computational power while our localization method can run on a minimal hardware setup.

Our smart camera-based positioning can then be used to navigate blind or visually impaired people on a predefined route. Next steps will focus on making the method more robust towards these influences and faster for realtime applications and a navigation prototype. Further improvements by using additional sensory data like GPS, accelerometer, magnetometer and gyroscope are currently investigated. The position accuracy can be increased by taking into account previous positions, current walking direction, and actual speed. Other benefits of image guided navigation, like depth calculation for the detection and warning of steps, gaps and other obstacles, will also be part of our future work.

Acknowledgement. This work was co-funded by the German Federal Ministry of Education and Research (BMBF, Grant No. 16SV5846) and the European Commission's Ambient Assisted Living (AAL) Joint Programme ICT for ageing well. (EU, Grant No. 810302758160 – IMAGO).

References

1. Resnikoff S, Pascolini D, Mariotti SP, et al. Global magnitude of visual impairment caused by uncorrected refractive errors in 2004. Bull World Health Organ. 2008;86(1):63–70.
2. Loomis JM, Golledge RG, Klatzky RL, et al. Navigation system for the blind: auditory display modes and guidance. Presence. 1998;7:193–203.
3. Modsching M, Kramer R, ten Hagen K. Field trial on GPS accuracy in a medium size city: the influence of built-up. Proc WPNC. 2006; p. 209–18.
4. Fallah N, Apostolopoulos I, Bekris K, et al. The user as a sensor: navigating users with visual impairments in indoor spaces using tactile landmarks. Proc SIGCHI. 2012; p. 425–32.
5. Filipe V, Fernandes F, Fernandes H, et al. Blind navigation support system based on Microsoft Kinect. Comp Sci. 2012;14:94–101.
6. Agarwal S, Snavely N, Simon I, et al. Building Rome in a day. Proc IEEE Int Conf Comput Vis. 2009; p. 72–9.
7. Wu C. Towards linear-time incremental structure from motion. Proc 3DV. 2013; p. 127–34.
8. Wu C, Agarwal S, Curless B, et al. Multicore bundle adjustment. Proc IEEE Comput Soc Conf Comput Vis Pattern Recognit. 2011; p. 3057–64.
9. Hartley RI, Zisserman A. Multiple View Geometry in Computer Vision. 2nd ed. Cambridge University Press; 2004.
10. Sattler T, Leibe B, Kobbelt L. Fast image-based localization using direct 2D-to-3D matching. Proc ICCV. 2011; p. 667–74.
11. Karlsson N, Di Bernardo E, Ostrowski J, et al. The vSLAM algorithm for robust localization and mapping. Proc IEEE ICRA. 2005; p. 24–29.

Quantification of the Aortic Morphology in Follow-Up 3D-MRA Images of Children

Stefan Wörz[1], Abdulsattar Alrajab[2], Raoul Arnold[3], Joachim Eichhorn[3],
Hendrik von Tengg-Kobligk[4], Jens-Peter Schenk[2], Karl Rohr[1]

[1]Dept. Bioinformatics and Functional Genomics, Biomedical Computer Vision Group,
University of Heidelberg, BIOQUANT, IPMB, and DKFZ Heidelberg
[2]Dept. Diagnostic and Interventional Radiology,
Div. Pediatric Radiology, University of Heidelberg
[3]Dept. Pediatric Cardiology, University of Heidelberg
[4]Institut für Diagnostische, Interventionelle und Pädiatrische Radiologie,
Inselspital, Universitätsspital Bern, Switzerland
s.woerz@dkfz.de

Abstract. The segmentation of the thoracic aorta and its main branches
from medical image data is an important task in vascular image analysis. We introduce a new model-based approach for the segmentation
of these vessels from follow-up 3D MRA images of children. For robust segmentation we propose an extended parametric cylinder model
which requires only relatively few parameters. The new model is used
in conjunction with a two-step fitting scheme for refining the segmentation result yielding an accurate segmentation of the vascular shape.
Moreover, we include a novel adaptive background masking scheme and
we use a spatial normalization scheme to align the segmentation results
from follow-up examinations. We have evaluated our proposed approach
using 3D synthetic images and we have successfully applied the approach
to follow-up 3D MRA images of children.

1 Introduction

The 3D geometric analysis of the aorta and its main branches from 3D medical
image data such as computed tomography angiography (CTA) and magnetic resonance angiography (MRA) is an important task in vascular image analysis. In
particular, the accurate segmentation and quantification of these vessels from images of children is important for early diagnosis and therapy planning of different
congenital diseases, for example, aortic coarctation and Marfan's syndrome [1].
However, compared to image data from adults, the automatic segmentation of
vessels in 3D images of children is more difficult since the vessels are smaller
and closer to each other, and in some cases image borders between neighboring vessels are barely visible (Fig. 1a, left arrow). In addition, different types
of pathologies such as aortic stenosis in the case of aortic coarctation need to
be coped with. Also, to minimize the exposure to radiation, in particular, in
follow-up examinations, usually MRA image data is acquired, which, however,
has typically a lower image resolution in comparison to CTA.

In previous work on vessel segmentation of the aorta different types of approaches have been used. For instance, approaches based on region growing [2], atlas registration [3], level sets [4], statistical shape models [5], and cylindric intensity models [6]. However, previous work has often only been applied to CTA image data [2, 3, 5] or aortic pathologies such as stenoses have not been considered [2, 4, 3, 5]. Furthermore, previous segmentation approaches are typically applied to image data from adults whereas work on image data of children and follow-up studies can hardly be found.

In this contribution, we introduce a new model-based approach for the segmentation of the thoracic aorta and its main branches from follow-up 3D MRA image data of children. The approach is based on cylindrical parametric intensity models in conjunction with a novel two-step fitting approach and a novel adaptive background masking scheme. Parametric intensity models have previously been used for the segmentation of the aorta [6] and also for other vessels [7], however, image data of children has not been considered. Applying such an approach [6, 7] to image data of children, however, leads partially to poor results because of the reasons mentioned above (vessels are smaller and closer to each other). First, the segmented centerline (and contour) often comprises a zigzag-like shape in the case of neighboring structures. Second, in difficult cases where neighboring vessels such as the pulmonary arteries are very close to the segmented vessel, tracking might prematurely terminate, which leads to a partial segmentation. The main reason in both cases is that neighboring structures are partly located within the 3D region-of-interest (ROI) used for model fitting, which negatively influences the segmentation result. To obtain more robust and accurate results, we introduce an extended 3D cylinder model and a novel two-step fitting scheme which uses prior information of the previous segments in the first step. In the second step, we refine the results by applying model fitting to the same vessel segment again but using a different model with elliptical cross-section and utilizing a smaller 3D ROI to accurately segment the shape of the vessel. Furthermore, we propose a novel adaptive background masking scheme to cope with interfering bright image structures (Fig. 1a, right arrow). More-

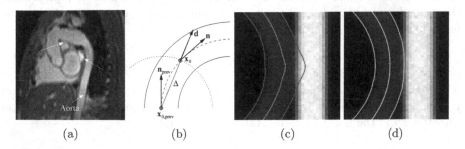

(a)   (b)   (c)   (d)

Fig. 1. (a) 2D section of a MR image of a thorax, (b) 2D sketch of the geometry of the current vessel segment $\mathbf{x}_0$ and the previous vessel segment $\mathbf{x}_{0,prev}$, and enlarged section of the segmentation result of a torus with a neighboring bright cylinder using (c) a weighting scheme [6] and using (d) the proposed adaptive masking scheme.

over, we use a normalization scheme to combine the segmentation results from follow-up examinations. We have successfully applied the proposed approach to segment the aorta and its main branches in follow-up 3D MRA images of children.

2   Methods

In this section, we first introduce our new extended cylinder model which incorporates information from preceding vessel segments. Then, we present a two-step model-based fitting scheme for robust and accurate vessel segmentation, which includes a novel adaptive background masking scheme. Finally, we describe a normalization scheme to combine the results of follow-up examinations.

2.1   Extended cylinder model

The proposed extended cylinder model $g_{\mathrm{M,Cylinder}}$ is based on a 3D parametric intensity model $g_{\mathrm{Cylinder}}(\mathbf{x}, R, \sigma)$ with $\mathbf{x} = (x, y, z)^T$ and can be written as

$$g_{\mathrm{M,Cylinder}}(\mathbf{x}, \mathbf{p}) = a_0 + (a_1 - a_0)\, g_{\mathrm{Cylinder}}(\mathcal{R}(\mathbf{x}), R, \sigma) \qquad (1)$$

where R is the radius of the circular cross-section, σ denotes the standard deviation of Gaussian image smoothing, a_0 and a_1 are the intensity levels of the background and vessel, respectively, and $\mathcal{R}(\mathbf{x})$ is a 3D rigid transform which represents the 3D position and orientation. In previous work [6], the used rigid transform was determined without using prior information, which, however, can lead to a zigzag-like shape of the centerline. The idea of our new approach is to constrain the 3D rigid transform by using information from the previous vessel segment (3D position $\mathbf{x}_{0,\mathrm{prev}}$ and 3D normal $\mathbf{n}_{\mathrm{prev}}$, Fig. 1b). The current centerline position $\mathbf{x}_0$ is located on a sphere (dotted circle) with radius Δ (fixed distance between two centerline positions) and can be expressed by spherical coordinates θ (inclination) and ϕ (azimuth). The goal is to align the normal $\mathbf{n}$ of the current cylinder with the direction of the tangent of a circle representing the curved centerline (dashed circle). This can be achieved by introducing the following 3D rigid transform

$$\mathcal{R}(\mathbf{x}, \theta, \phi) = \mathbf{R}_{\theta,\phi}(\mathbf{x} - \mathbf{x}_0(\theta, \phi)) \qquad (2)$$

where the 3D rotation matrix $\mathbf{R}_{\theta,\phi}$ is given by $\mathbf{R}_{\theta,\phi} = (\mathbf{p}_1, \mathbf{p}_2, \mathbf{n})^T$. $\mathbf{p}_1$ and $\mathbf{p}_2$ denote the principal directions orthogonal to the normal $\mathbf{n}$. The principal directions and the normal can be stated using θ and ϕ

$$\mathbf{n} = \begin{pmatrix} \sin\theta\cos\phi \\ \sin\theta\sin\phi \\ \cos\theta \end{pmatrix}, \qquad \mathbf{p}_1 = \begin{pmatrix} \cos\theta\cos\phi \\ \cos\theta\sin\phi \\ -\sin\theta \end{pmatrix}, \qquad \mathbf{p}_2 = \begin{pmatrix} -\sin\phi \\ \cos\phi \\ 0 \end{pmatrix} \qquad (3)$$

The 3D position $\mathbf{x}_0(\theta, \phi)$ can be computed using the normal $\mathbf{n}$

$$\mathbf{x}_0(\theta, \phi) = \mathbf{x}_{0,\mathrm{prev}} + \Delta \mathbf{d} = \mathbf{x}_{0,\mathrm{prev}} + \Delta \left(\mathbf{n}_{\mathrm{prev}} + \mathbf{n}\right) \left|\mathbf{n}_{\mathrm{prev}} + \mathbf{n}\right|^{-1} \qquad (4)$$

Using the prior information, the rigid transform $\mathcal{R}$ in (2) comprises only two free parameters θ and ϕ, whereas in previous work four to six parameters have been used [7, 6]. Therefore, the extended model in (1) comprises in total only six parameters $\mathbf{p} = (R, a_0, a_1, \sigma, \theta, \phi,)^T$, which increases the robustness and allows segmentation even in the case of neighboring structures.

2.2 Two-step fitting scheme

With the extended cylinder model introduced above, a robust segmentation of the centerline is obtained, however, the accuracy of the segmented shape might be reduced in difficult regions. To improve the result we use a two-step scheme. In the first step, we use the extended model to obtain a robust segmentation. In a second step, we apply model fitting to the same vessel segment again. In this step, we use a different model with elliptical cross-section and utilize a smaller 3D ROI to accurately segment the shape of the vessel. For initialization we use the estimated parameters from the first step.

2.3 Adaptive background masking

To mask out bright image structures that might disturb model fitting we use an image mask $0 \leq g_{\mathrm{mask}}(\mathbf{x}) \leq 1$ where voxels $\mathbf{x}$ belonging to bright structures are assigned a low value close to zero. In our approach, we adapt the intensity level of masked voxels based on the local background intensity level. Consequently, masked voxels are treated as background, whereas in previous schemes they are not explicitly treated but left out in the fitting. For example, in the experiment shown in Fig. 1c,d a mask has been used for the bright cylinder. Segmenting the

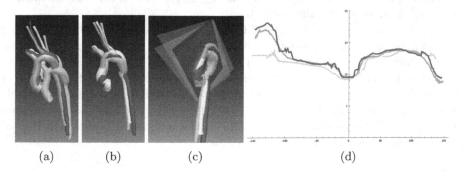

(a)   (b)   (c)   (d)

Fig. 2. Segmentation results of the aorta and its main branches for four different MRA images in a follow-up examination without normalization (a), with normalization (b), and with visualized fitted planes (c), as well as (d) the estimated radius along the centerline of the aortic arch for the follow-up examination shown in (b).

curved cylinder using a standard weighting scheme (c) yields a poor result since the contour extends into the bright cylinder. Using the new adaptive scheme (d) yields a more accurate result. To compute the mask we use image clipping to detect bright structures (Fig. 1a, right arrow).

2.4   Normalization scheme for follow-up examinations

To combine the results from follow-up examinations where the MRA image data has been obtained using different MR scanners with different image resolution and different coordinate systems, we perform a spatial normalization to align the coordinate systems. Based on the segmentation results, we use the centerlines to compensate 3D translations. Furthermore, we perform a least-squares plane fitting to compensate different 3D orientations. For example, Fig. 2a shows the segmentation results of the aorta and its main branches for four different MRA images in a follow-up examination without normalization. After correction of the translation (b), it can be seen that the shapes are much better aligned. Fig. 2c shows fitted planes for correction of different orientations.

3   Experimental results

We have applied our approach to 3D synthetic images and to follow-up 3D MRA image data of children. We have used different types of 3D synthetic images comprising straight and curved tubular structures of varying radii with closely neighboring objects of different contrasts and with additive Gaussian noise. For example, we have generated 100 different 3D images of a torus with a neighboring bright cylinder (Fig. 1c). Our new approach successfully segmented all tori with low mean and maximal errors of the centerline position of $\bar{e}_{x_0} = 0.10$ and $e_{x_0,max} = 0.26$ voxels, respectively. In contrast, using a previous approach [6] with standard weighting scheme the segmentation prematurely terminates in 34 cases because of the neighboring cylinder. For the remaining 66 images, the previous approach yielded $\bar{e}_{x_0} = 0.39$ and $e_{x_0,max} = 2.85$ voxels. Thus, the new approach is more robust and accurate.

We have also successfully applied our approach to segment the aorta and its main branches in ten follow-up 3D MRA images of children. In addition to determining the 3D centerline and 3D contour, our approach also quantifies, for example, the radius and curvature along the centerline and the volume of the aortic arch. As an example, Fig. 2b shows an overlay of the normalized 3D segmentation result for four different MRA images in a follow-up examination. The estimated radius along the centerline of the aortic arch is shown in Fig. 2d for the four segmentation results in Fig. 2b.

4   Discussion

We have introduced a new model-based approach for the segmentation of the thoracic aorta and its main branches from follow-up 3D MRA image data of children. The approach is based on model fitting of parametric intensity models with cylindrical shape. For robust segmentation of vessels even in difficult cases, we proposed a new extended cylinder model which requires only relatively few parameters. The new model is used in conjunction with a two-step fitting scheme for refining the segmentation result yielding an accurate segmentation of the vascular shape. Moreover, we included a novel adaptive background masking scheme and we use a spatial normalization scheme to align the segmentation results from follow-up examinations. We have evaluated our proposed approach using different 3D synthetic images and we have successfully applied the approach to follow-up 3D MRA image data of children.

Acknowledgement. This work has been funded by the Joachim Siebeneicher-Stiftung.

References

1. Eichhorn J, Fink C, Delorme S, et al. Rings, slings and other vascular abnormalities – ultrafast computed tomography and magnetic resonance angiography in pediatric cardiology. Z Kardiol. 2004;93(3):201–8.
2. Taeprasartsit P, Higgins WE. Method for extracting the aorta from 3D CT images. Proc SPIE. 2007;6512.
3. Isgum I, Staring M, Rutten A, et al. Multi-atlas-based segmentation with local decision fusion – application to cardiac and aortic segmentation in CT scans. IEEE Trans on Med Imaging. 2009;28(7):1000–10.
4. Zhao F, Zhang H, Wahle A, et al. Congenital aortic disease: 4D magnetic resonance segmentation and quantitative analysis. Med Image Anal. 2009;13(3):483–93.
5. Zheng Y, John M, Liao R, et al. Automatic aorta segmentation and valve landmark detection in C-arm CT for transcatheter aortic valve implantation. IEEE Trans on Med Imaging. 2012;31(12):2307–21.
6. Wörz S, von Tengg-Kobligk H, Henninger V, et al. 3D quantification of the aortic arch morphology in 3D CTA data for endovascular aortic repair. IEEE Trans on Biomed Eng. 2010;57(10):2359–68.
7. Noordmans HJ, Smeulders AWM. High accuracy tracking of 2D/3D curved line structures by consecutive cross-section matching. Pattern Recognit Lett. 1998;19(1):97–111.

Adapted Spectral Clustering for Evaluation and Classification of DCE-MRI Breast Tumors

Sylvia Glaßer, Sophie Roscher, Bernhard Preim

Department for Simulation and Graphics, OvG-University Magdeburg
glasser@isg.cs.uni-magdeburg.de

Abstract. Classification of breast tumors in perfusion DCE-MRI solely based on dynamic contrast enhanced magnetic resonance data is a challenge. Many studies employ grouping of voxels into regions via clustering for further analysis. However, the clustering result strongly depends on the chosen clustering algorithm and its parameter settings. In this paper, we explain how spectral clustering can be adapted to breast tumor data and suggest how the clustering parameters can be automatically derived such that no pre-defined user input, e.g., cluster number, is necessary. The presented spectral clustering approach has the great advantage of generating spatially connected regions. Furthermore, it can be enabled for automatic classification and yields similar results as previous approaches.

1 Introduction

For the evaluation of breast tumors, conventional X-ray mammography is in some cases not sufficient or not diagnostically relevant, in particular in younger woman where the dense breast tissue does not reveal pathologic masses. To confirm the malignancy or benignity of such unclear lesions as well as to detect small metastasis in case of a known primary tumor, dynamic contrast enhanced magnetic resonance imaging (DCE-MRI) is applied. DCE-MRI has a high sensitivity when compared to X-ray, however, the specificity is only moderate. Thus, in clinical research, the automatic classification of breast lesions based on their DCE-MRI-based contrast enhancement and morphology is an active research area [1]. In clinical practice, the radiologist defines a region of interest (ROI) in the most suspect part of the tumor and analyzes the average relative contrast enhancement (RE) over time of this ROI. Based on washin and washout characteristics from the RE curve as well as analysis of the tumor's morphology, the radiologist carries out a diagnosis. The manual ROI placement suffers from intra- and inter-observer variability which can strongly hamper the diagnostic result since a tumor is as malignant as its most malignant part. Furthermore, when a ROI covers benign and malignant tumor tissue, the ROI's average RE curve may be not appropriate to assess the tumor's malignancy. In spite of these shortcomings, determination of the most suspect ROI and thus the most suspect tumor part is important for further diagnosis like core needle biopsy. To solve these problems, we introduce a spectral clustering approach to group voxels into homogeneous regions and to maintain spatial connectivity of these regions. Then, the most suspect ROI can be identified and employed for automatic tumor classification.

Our approach is based on our previous work [2], where density-based clustering is employed to breast DCE-MRI lesions. Then, a most suspect region is extracted that serves as ROI for further analysis. Similarly, region merging is employed to group and identify suspect regions of DCE-MRI tumors in [3]. The results were employed for automatic breast tumor classification based on tumor heterogeneity by Preim et al. [4], yielding an increased heterogeneity for malignant tumors. However, the spatial connectivity of the resulting regions can be improved by our approach and we achieve similar or even better classification results. Also related to our work is the study of Chen et al. [5]. They apply fuzzy c-means clustering and extract the most characteristic RE curve for breast tumor classification but they can not automatically determine a most suspect ROI.

2 Material and methods

2.1 Tumor data

We tested our approach with a database consisting of 68 breast lesions from DCE-MRI data. From the 68 lesions, 31 tumors are classified as benign lesions and 37 as malignant lesions. The classification of the lesions was confirmed by histopathology (60 cases) or follow-up examination after 6 – 9 months (8 cases). The database only contains tumors that have been detected in MRI and that cannot be detected in conventional x-Ray mammography. The identification and delineation of the lesion from background was conducted by an experienced radiologist. The MR image parameters include an in-plane resolution of $\approx 0.67 \times 0.67\,\mathrm{mm}^2$ with an image matrix of $\approx 528 \times 528$, ≈ 100 slices with a slice gap of $1.5\,\mathrm{mm}$ acquired at five or six time steps, i.e. one pre-contrast and four to five post-contrast images. MRI perfusion data sets suffer from motion artifacts due to breathing and patient's movement. Thus, an elastic registration was carried out for motion correction [6]. The signal intensities values SI_t of the data sets at time step t were normalized with the pre-contrast signal intensity SI_0 to extract relative enhancement RE_t values; $RE_t = (SI_t - SI_0)/SI_0 \times 100$. For each voxel, the following descriptive perfusion parameters were extracted:

- $\mathrm{Max_{RE}}$, the maximum of the RE values ,
- $\mathrm{T_{Max}}$, the point in time when RE_t equals $\mathrm{Max_{RE}}$,
- washin, the value of RE_2, where $t = 2$ is the first time step after the early post-contrast phase,
- washout, the normalized difference between the last time step $t = n$ and $t = 2$, i.e. $(RE_n - RE_2)/(n - 2)$.

For further characterization, we assign each voxel's RE curve to an 3TP class, based on the three-time-point (3TP) method [7]. The 3TP method defines three types of initial RE enhancement (slow, intermediate and fast) and three types of curve shapes (washin, plateau, washout) yielding 9 classes (Fig. 1). It involves three well chosen time steps: t_a, the first point in time before the contrast agent injection, t_b, 2 min after t_a and t_c, 4 min after t_a. Since our study contains five to six time steps due to different scanning parameters, we assign the third time t_3 step to t_b and the last time step t_n to t_c. The selection of parameters and the adaption of the 3TP method is based on our previous work [2].

Fig. 1. Nine classes according to the 3TP method [7].

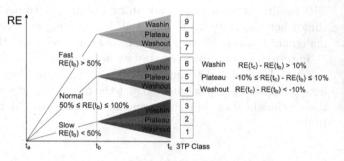

2.2   Methods

Our approach consists of two steps: the adoption of spectral clustering for each tumor and the feature extraction on which the classifier will be learned.

Step 1: Clustering in the spectral space We apply a spectral clustering method to divide each tumor into homogeneous and spatially continuous clusters based on the normalized (via z-scoring) perfusion parameters Max_{RE}, T_{Max}, washin, and washout.

Spectral clustering employs graph cuts such that edges between different groups (clusters) have very low weights and edges within the same cluster have high weights. Such a graph cut can be easily found by using the eigenvectors and eigenvalues of a specific matrix – the Laplacian matrix – to map the original data points to a low dimensional space [8]. In this new representation, clusters can be easier separated (regarding the high-dimensional space) by applying simple clustering techniques like k-means. A weighted, undirected graph is constructed from the initial data set. Each node represents a data point and each edge the similarity between two points with a symmetric and non-negative similarity function. Based on this affinity matrix, a Laplacian matrix is constructed and an eigenvalue decomposition is performed. The eigenvalues and eigenvectors are used to map the original data points to the k dimensional vectors of the spectral domain. For a more detailed review, we refer to [8].

We use the Ng-Jordan-Weiss Algorithm [8] to directly partition the data into k groups. The similarity graph is constructed based on the descriptive perfusion parameters. Each node of the graph represents a voxel of the corresponding breast tumor. Hence, the tumor data are represented in an regular orthogonal 3D grid and each node is connected to its adjacent nodes within a 26-neighborhood. We use the Gaussian similarity function [8]

$$s(x_\mathrm{i}, x_\mathrm{j}) = \exp\left(-\frac{d(x_\mathrm{i}, x_\mathrm{j})}{2\sigma^2}\right)$$

to represent the local neighborhood relationships. The distance $d(x_\mathrm{i}, x_\mathrm{j})$ between two points is measured by using the cosine similarity of the corresponding perfusion parameter values [8]. The scaling parameter σ describes how rapidly the affinity decreases with the distance between x_i and x_j. Instead of manually selecting σ, we use the approach described in [9] to calculate a local scaling parameter for each data point. Although we still have to select the n number of neighbors that should be considered to compute this scale, this selection is independent of scale [9]. We applied three internal cluster validation measurements [10]: the Davies-Bouldin index, the Dunn index, and the Calinski-Harabasz index to empirically find an n that provides the best clustering result. We varied n in the range of [3..11] and analyzed the corresponding validation indices yielding the best result for $n = 3$. In spectral clustering, we also have to specify the number of clusters k. For the presented method, the three validation indices are applied again. Then, the best k is chosen via majority voting based on the values of the validation indices. If no majority exists, we employ the Davies-Bouldin index. For each data set, the spectral clustering is computed several times with different clusters k ($k = \{3..9\}$) and the optimal k is selected according to the validation indices. In summary, the distance function $d(x_\mathrm{i}, x_\mathrm{j})$ detects similar descriptive perfusion parameter values and the 26-neighborhood yields the spatial connectivity of voxels in a cluster. This is an advantage in comparison to the density-based clustering approach presented in [2].

Step 2: Feature extraction for classification Based on the spectral clustering result, we extract features to compare the discriminative power of our clustering result. Based on our previous work [2], we choose one cluster as most suspect region. Therefore, we analyze the 3TP class of the clusters averaged RE curve and again employ the 3TP class ranking: 7, 9, 8, 4, 6, 5, 1, 3, 2. Thus, if three clusters exist, with average curves of 3TP classes 7, 4 and 8, we choose the cluster with average RE curve classified as 3TP class 7.

We employ the following features for each tumor to learn a classifier:

- biological features, i.e. age and tumor size in mm^3,
- features of the chosen cluster and it's average RE curve, i.e. washin, washout, and 3TP class, as well as the per centaged cluster size (when compared to the whole tumor), and
- features characterizing the whole tumor clustering result, i.e. the number of clusters, the separability (the inter-cluster variance), the homogeneity (the averaged intra-cluster variance), and the similarity measures Purity, Jaccard index and F1 score based on the comparison of the clustering result and the 3TP method classification of all tumor voxels.

Fig. 2. Learned decision tree: the attributes at the upper part of the tree are the most important ones.

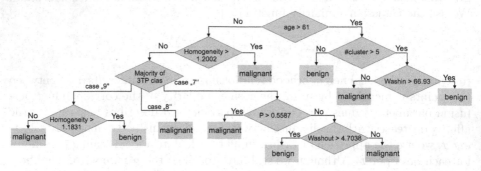

The classifier was created with the Weka library, a Java software library that encompasses algorithms for data analysis and predictive modeling [11]. Based on our previous work [2], a decision tree was trained with the C4. 5 classification algorithm [12]. It automatically selects features with high discriminative power. It performs 10-fold cross validation and requires at least two instances (two tumors) for each tree leaf. The best tree result is depicted in Fig. 2.

3   Results

For the automatic classification of our database, we learned the decision tree, depicted in Fig. 2. It correctly classifies 56 of 68 tumors, i.e. 82.24%. Inherent to decision trees, the most important features are at top levels, i.e. closer to the root, since the splitting a larger set of tumors. Hence, the feature patient age was employed as most important feature, however all other attributes characterize the tumor's heterogeneity and kinetic contrast enhancement behavior. Due to the specialty of our database (only suspicious or malignant lesions but no typical benign ones were included), we do not consider specificity or sensitivity, but the number of correctly classified tumors. The results are similar to our previous work [2], but we do only employ 10-fold cross validation instead of 5 folds. However, the benefit is the improved identification of the most suspect ROI w.r.t. the spatial connectivity (Fig. 3). Hence, no outliers are produced. Nevertheless, the identified most suspect cluster has similar discriminating power when applied for automatic classification as previous results [2].

4   Discussion

In this paper, we explained how spectral clustering can be successfully adapted to breast DCE-MRI tumors. We carried out k-means in the spectral domain and provide automatic parameter choices for the input parameters. The clustering result produces spatially connected homogeneous regions as well as a most suspect ROI, and achieves similar classification results as proposed in literature. Our results are in particular promising, since the employed database comprises only tumors that are very hard to differentiate into benign and malignant ones. Hence, only histopathologic evaluation or follow-up could confirm the diagnosis. For future work, a bigger study, 5-fold cross validation and the combination with morphologic features should be carried out.

Acknowledgement. We thank Myra Spiliopoulou and Uli Niemann for fruitful discussions. This work was supported by the DFG project SPP 1335 "Scalable Visual Analytics".

References

1. Schnall MD, Blume J, Bluemke DA, et al. Diagnostic architectural and dynamic features at breast MR imaging: multicenter study. Radiology. 2006;238(1):42–53.
2. Glaßer S, Niemann U, Preim B, et al. Can we distinguish between benign and malignant breast tumors in DCE-MRI by studying a tumors most suspect region only? Proc CBMS. 2013; p. 59–64.
3. Glaßer S, Preim U, Tönnies K, et al. A visual analytics approach to diagnosis of breast DCE-MRI data. Comput Graph. 2010;34(5):602–11.
4. Preim U, Glaßer S, Preim B, et al. Computer-aided diagnosis in breast DCE-MRI: quantification of the heterogeneity of breast lesions. Eur J Radiol. 2012;81(7):1532–8.
5. Chen W, Giger ML, Bick U, et al. Automatic identification and classification of characteristic kinetic curves of breast lesions on DCE-MRI. Med Phys. 2006;33(8):2878–87.
6. Rueckert D, Sonoda L, Hayes C, et al. Nonrigid registration using free-form deformations: application to breast MR images. IEEE Trans Med Imaging. 1999;18(8):712–21.
7. Degani H, Gusis V, Weinstein D, et al. Mapping pathophysiological features of breast tumors by MRI at high spatial resolution. Nat Med. 1997;3:780–2.
8. Von Luxburg U. A tutorial on spectral clustering. Stat Comput. 2007;17(4):395–416.
9. Zelnik-Manor L, Perona P. Self-tuning spectral clustering. Adv Neural Inf Process Syst. 2004; p. 1601–8.
10. Rendon E, Abundez I, Arizmendi A, et al. Internal versus external cluster validation Indexes. Int J Comput Commun. 2011;5(1):27–34.
11. Holmes G, Donkin A, Witten IH. WEKA: a machine learning workbench. Proc IIS. 1994; p. 357–61.
12. Quinlan JR. C4.5: Programs for Machine Learning. Morgan Kaufmann Publishers; 1993.

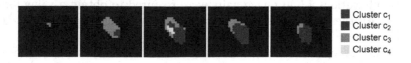

Cluster c_1
Cluster c_2
Cluster c_3
Cluster c_4

Fig. 3. Five slices showing the clustering result for a small breast tumor.

Simultaneous Segmentation and Registration for FAIR Perfusion Imaging

Christian Siegl[1], Jana Martschinke[1], Rolf Janka[2], Roberto Grosso[1]

[1]Chair for Computer Graphics, Friedrich-Alexander-Universität Erlangen-Nürnberg
[2]Institute of Radiology, Universitätsklinikum Erlangen
christian.siegl@cs.fau.de

Abstract. Renal perfusion might be the key factor in controlling the systemic blood pressure. While up to no now, there is no way to measure renal perfusion non-invasively, a promising technique might be MR-imaging with arterial spin labeling. This technique was developed to measure brain perfusion. In contrast to the brain the kidney is moving due to breathing, which makes post processing of the acquired images a demanding issue. In this work, we present a tool that supports a physician in performing kidney perfusion analysis using this technique. To accommodate this, we will show a custom tailored segmentation and registration approach that can cope with the challenges of this technique. By using this tool, the physician can analyze kidney perfusion using less images which enhances usability in clinical day to day application.

1 Introduction

Hypertension is a widespread disease in the developed countries and it is one of the main risk-factors of arteriosclerosis. Big efforts are done to adjust blood pressure. Most newer drugs interact with the so called renin-angiotensin system that controls the kidney perfusion. Another interesting approach is renal nerval ablation. By improving renal perfusion this has an impact on the renin angiotensin system. Hence, renal perfusion might be the key factor in manipulating the blood pressure. It is not easy to measure renal perfusion non-invasively. One interesting approach is MR-imaging with arterial spin labeling, which means the normal flowing blood gets labeled and acts like a "contrast medium" to measure kidney perfusion. This technique was developed to measure brain perfusion. In contrast to the brain, the kidney is moving due to breathing which makes breath-hold imaging mandatory. To acquire images with a reasonable temporal resolution and signal to noise ratio the patient has to hold breath for about 10 seconds per perfusion image (which consists of two images, Sect. 2.1). In previous publications 13-40 image pairs were required to obtain a value for the perfusion. All these images have to be reviewed, segmented and registered for further processing.

In this work we present a software tool that supports the physician in the process of analyzing series of perfusion images. With a semi-automatic segmentation that is required for only one image and a hybrid segmentation/registration for the rest of the images, we offer an easy to use and fast tool for perfusion analysis and evaluation. Our method is also capable of sorting out images that do not show the required quality, which relieves the physician of the error prone process of examining all images. We will furthermore show that it is possible to reduce the number of images required for reliable perfusion results, which shortens the acquisition sequence for the patient as well as the subsequent analysis.

2   Previous work

2.1   FAIR true-FISP perfusion imaging

FAIR (flow-sensitive alternating inversion-recovery) True-FISP (fast imaging with steady-state precession) perfusion imaging was first introduced by Martirosian et al. [1] in 2004. To get one perfusion image, three images have to be acquired. A M0 image for normalization, a global inversion image and a slice inversion image. Based on these three images, a perfusion value per pixel can be calculated [1].

Martirosian et al., Fenchel et al. [2], and Artz et al. [3] show that FTFP-imaging is a very promising technique. They demonstrated that FTFP-imaging yields perfusion results that are comparable to those obtained with commonly accepted and currently used methods. FTFP-imaging delivers also an intra- and inter-visit reproducibility of the perfusion values.

However, techniques known to date use a large number of image pairs (13-40 slice and global images, i.e. a total of up to 82 images) that is averaged to reduce signal to noise ratio and other errors due to the acquisition process. Our goal is to reduce the number of image pairs required for the sake of usability in a clinical day to day application.

2.2   Kidney segmentation

There are multiple publications that deal with the subject of kidney segmentation. The most advanced approaches towards automatic kidney segmentation use either an active shape model [4], graph cuts [5] or the EM-algorithm which requires prior information [6]. All these methods perform well, but there are cases where they do not produce reliable results, which makes theses methods problematic for MR-image based perfusion in real clinical applications.

3   Materials and methods

For our evaluation tool we opted for Matlab. Matlab offers a very convenient, platform independent rapid prototyping environment for our image processing application. Furthermore an easy to use functionality for building graphical user interfaces is offered. Performance problems can easily be solved by using the MEX − C interface.

For our experiments we had access to real patient data. Every acquisition series consists of 9 images: One M0 image and 4 slice/global inversion image pairs.

3.1   Segmentation

The first stage of our pipeline is the segmentation of the kidney in one of the images. There are automatic approaches for segmenting kidneys (Sec. 2). However, our experience shows that they are not reliable enough for our data. In our pipeline, the segmentation of the kidney in only one image is required, but this one has to be precise. With this in mind we decided on the semi-automatic segmentation approach introduced by Mortensen and Barret [7]: intelligent scissors.

Using this method, the user has to define points along the contour of the kidney that are connected using the Dijkstra-Algorithm. This step is very efficient and gives the user an immediate response to mouse inputs which helps in placing the reference points on the contour. In order to emphasize the edges in the image, we propose the following cost function per pixel for the Dijkstra algorithm

$$f_{cost} = f_{Laplace} + f_{MagGradient} + f_{DirGradient} \tag{1}$$

Where $f_{Laplace}$ is 0 at the zero-crossings of a Laplace filtered image and 1 otherwise. $f_{MagGradient}$ is the inverse magnitude of the gradient scaled from 0 to 1. The term $f_{DirGradient}$ decreases the cost if one moves perpendicular to the direction of the gradient. Furthermore, in $f_{DirGradient}$ pixels with consistent gradient direction are favored.

This approach allows for a kidney segmentation with only 3-6 clicks depending on how well the boundary of the kidney is visible in the image.

3.2   Registration

Starting with our semi-automatic segmentation, which is carried out in only one single image, the remaining images (in our case at least 8) have to be processed

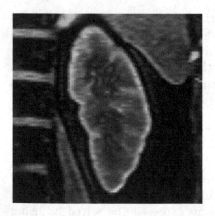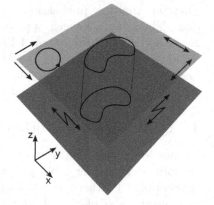

Fig. 1. Kidney segmentation using our semi-automatic approach (left). The outline from segmentation is mapped onto a plane, the image that has to be registered on another plane. The plane with the outline can be translated, rotated, scaled and sheared. The outline is then projected onto the plane with the image (right).

Fig. 2. Two kidney segmentation/registrations on top and bottom. The first column shows the segmentation, the second column the initial projection into another image, the last column the registration result. In the first row, the registration works very well and mainly translation is applied. In the second row the registration also works well, but due to patient movement it is no longer possible to correctly match the outline.

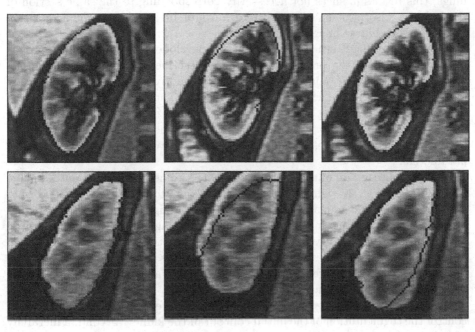

automatically. Therefore, the registration stage has to efficiently accomplish two things: correctly register kidneys and perform segmentation for the remaining images.

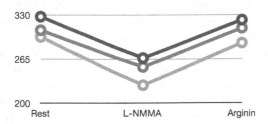

Fig. 3. Graph showing the drop-off in perfusion due to medication with L-NMMA for three patients. After giving Arginin, perfusion fully recovers in all three cases.

The correct registration of the image series we are working with is especially problematic because of the acquisition scenario. As described in Sect. 1, the images are acquired with the patient holding breath for around 10s. In a series of 9 images, taken at different times, with the kidney moving together with the lungs, this results in slices not necessarily corresponding to the same section of the kidney. Also patients often start to move or breath during the acquisition which leads to blurry images.

With this difficult situation in mind we developed a registration approach that can tackle all the problems previously described. Our algorithm implements a very stiff non-rigid registration that is motivated by movements likely to happen during image acquisition (Fig. 1, left). The kidney can be translated due to the patient holding breath at a different point in the breathing cycle (two translational parameters). As the plane of kidney movement does not coincide with the acquisition plane, we added one rotation, two scaling and two shearing parameters.

In our approach an outline of the segmented kidney is mapped onto a plane (outline plan, Fig. 1, right). The image we want to register is mapped onto a second plane (image-plane). In the starting configuration these two planes are identical. By projecting the outline onto the image-plane we have an initial segmentation of the image. We can now apply the transformations mentioned above to the outline-plane to register the two images.

To optimize the image registration we propose an adapted version of the cost function used for the segmentation. The cost function was modified as follows. First, we no longer require the gradient direction information used to control the segmentation of the initial contour of the kidney. Second, a hierarchy of subsampled cost-images is used to reduce the effect of local minima in the optimization. Pixels with low cost along the kidney contour are emphasized in the image hierarchy by applying a minimum-filter subsampling. The cost image and hierarchy are computed for the image-plane and are evaluated along the projected outline, giving us an objective function for optimization. To get a coarse alignment and favor rigid transformation we start out with one purely rigid optimization pass (only translation).

This registration approach has two very important benefits. First, it combines registration with segmentation and uses a similar cost function as it was proposed in the segmentation step. The registration considers basically only the outline of the kidney and delivers the segmentation for free. The second benefit is the possibility to discard images if the registration fails or the results are not satisfactory. The transformations allowed in the registration mimics the movements and deformations which might occur during the acquisition of the image series. With these physically motivated degrees of freedom, we have the benefit of being able to assess the resulting values. We are able to sort out images for which the non-rigid transformation required by the registration is too high. Additionally, we can detect a failed registration if the accumulated cost value of the projected outline is too high (Fig. 2, right). At the beginning of the whole process of segmentation of a first single image and the subsequent automatic registration and segmentation of the complete image series, the physician has to select a starting image from the sequence. The method proposed so far allows us to detect if the physician has selected a particularly bad first image for segmentation. In this case, the image will badly align with the rest of the series and we can advise to start over with another image. By using these mechanisms, we can greatly assist the physician in getting results that are as accurate as possible.

4 Results

For evaluating our developed tool we had access to datasets of 10 healthy patients, each consisting of three image series. One series as baseline, one series after giving a medication that is known to reduce kidney perfusion (L-NMMA) and one with recovered perfusion by administering Arginin to the patient. Our experiments showed that we are able to obtain reasonable perfusion values for all image series. The drop-off in perfusion due to L-NMMA can be seen for all 10 patients (Fig. 3). Half of the series contained at least one image that did not show sufficient image quality or was shifted too severely and had to be sorted out automatically by our pipeline. Without this step, the resulting perfusion values are not accurate.

5 Discussion

We have shown that we are able to build a tool that enables a physician to conveniently analyze FAIR True-FISP perfusion images. Experiments with real data based on only 4 images pairs have produced promising results. In future work the software tool will be tested on more patient data with focus on the interpretation of the resulting perfusion images.

References

1. Martirosian P, Klose U, Mader I, et al. FAIR true-FISP perfusion imaging of the kidneys. Magn Reson Med. 2004.
2. Fenchel M, Martirosian P, Langanke J, et al. Perfusion MR imaging with FAIR true FISP spin labeling in patients with and without renal artery stenosis: initial experience. Radiology. 2006.
3. Artz NS, Sadowski EA, Wentland AL, et al. Reproducibility of renal perfusion MR imaging in native and transplanted kidneys using non-contrast arterial spin labeling. J Magn Reson Imag. 2011.
4. Spiegel M, Hahn DA, Daum V, et al. Segmentation of kidneys using a new active shape model generation technique based on non-rigid image registration. Comp Med Imag Graph. 2009.
5. Ali AM, Farag AA, El-Baz A. Graph cuts framework for kidney segmentation with prior shape constraints. Lect Notes Comput Sci. 2007.
6. Yuksel SE, El-Baz A, Farag AA, et al. A kidney segmentation framework for dynamic contrast enhanced magnetic resonance imaging. J Vib Control. 2007.
7. Mortensen EN, Barrett WA. Interactive segmentation with intelligent scissors. Proc CVGIP. 1998.

Atlasbasierte Feature-Registrierung zur automatischen Einstellung der Standardebenen bei mobilen C-Bogen CT-Daten

Michael Brehler[1], Joseph Görres[1], Ivo Wolf[2], Jochen Franke[3],
Jan von Recum[3], Paul A. Grützner[3], Hans-Peter Meinzer[1], Diana Nabers[1]

[1]Abteilung für Medizinische und Biologische Informatik, DKFZ Heidelberg
[2]Institut für Medizinische Informatik, Hochschule Mannheim
[3]Berufsgenossenschaftliche Unfallklinik, Ludwigshafen
m.brehler@dkfz-heidelberg.de

Kurzfassung. Das Standardvorgehen bei der Behandlung von Calcaneusfrakturen ist eine Osteosynthese. Mit Hilfe der intraoperativen Bildgebung wie dem mobilen C-Bogen CT kann der Chirurg das Repositionsergebnis noch im Operationssaal verifizieren und wenn nötig korrigieren. Die Mobilität des C-Bogen CT hat jedoch zur Folge, dass Informationen über die Orientierung des Patienten zum Gerät verloren gehen. Dadurch kann keine Standard-Ausrichtung der dreidimensionalen Daten an die Anatomie erfolgen. Eine manuelle Einstellung des Volumendatensatzes durch den Chirurgen ist damit unabdingbar. Dies ist ein zeitaufwendiger Schritt und kann bei einer unpräzisen Einstellung zu Fehlern bei der Beurteilung der Daten führen. In diesem Paper stellen wir zwei automatische Methoden zur Einstellung der Standard-Ebenen auf mobilen C-Bogen CT Daten vor. Die automatischen Methoden rekonstruieren die Standard-Ebenen in zwei Schritten: als Erstes werden SURF-Keypoints (2D und neu eingeführte Pseudo-3D-Punkte) für das Bildvolumen berechnet, in einem zweiten Schritt wird eine Atlas-Punktwolke auf diese Merkmale registriert und die Parameter der Standard-Ebenen transformiert. Die Genauigkeit unserer Methoden wurde an 51 klinischen mobilen C-Bogen CT Bildern mit manuell eingestellten Standard-Ebenen evaluiert. Die Referenzdaten wurden von drei Chirurgen mit unterschiedlichem Erfahrungsstand erstellt. Die durchschnittlich benötigte Zeit der Experten (46 s) unterscheidet sich von der des fortgeschrittenen Benutzers (55 s) um neun Sekunden. Die Berechnungszeit des 2D-Surf Ansatzes beträgt 10 Sekunden und liefert bei 88% der Ebenen der Referenzdaten eine korrekte Einstellung. Der Pseudo-3D Ansatz liefert die besten Ergebnisse mit einer Genauigkeit von 91% und einer Berechnungszeit von nur 8 Sekunden.

1 Einleitung

Das Standardvorgehen bei der Behandlung von Calcaneusfrakturen ist eine Osteosynthese, eine Reposition der Knochenfragmente und ihre Fixierung mit

Schrauben und, falls notwendig, einer Calcaneus-Platte [1]. Die Benutzung des mobilen C-Bogen CTs, eines intraoperativen bildgebenden Verfahrens, eröffnet den Chirurgen die Möglichkeit, noch während der Patient in Narkose liegt, das Repositionsergebnis und die Position der eingesetzten Implantate direkt zu verifizieren. Die Bildqualität des mobilen C-Bogen CT Scans hängt dabei von der Knochenqualität, der Anzahl und Größe der eingesetzten Metallimplantate sowie von dem Body Mass Index des Patienten ab [2]. Die Mobilität des Geräts hat jedoch zur Folge, dass Informationen über die Orientierung des Patienten zum Gerät verloren gehen. Insbesondere bei unfallchirurgischen Fällen bei denen oft starke Deplatzierungen anatomischer Strukturen auftreten ist dies der Fall. Dadurch können die Standard-Ebenen nicht automatisch ausgerichtet werden und müssen von den Chirurgen manuell durch Rotation und Translation an einer Workstation im Operationssaal eingestellt werden. Die Bildebenen werden so orientiert, dass sie die zu beurteilenden anatomischen Strukturen schneiden. Für den Calcaneus sind dies die Gelenkflächen zum Talus und zum Cuboid-Knochen (Abb. 1). Um das Arthroserisiko für den Patienten zu minimieren, ist eine exakte Abbildung der Gelenkflächen für die Rekonstruktion des Calcaneus sehr wichtig [1]. Deswegen ist es besonders wichtig die Standard-Ebenen für eine gute Visualisierung der Gelenkflächen bestmöglichst einzustellen. Insbesondere für ungeübte Benutzer ist das Einstellen der Standard-Ebenen ein zeitaufwendiger Prozess, der für den Patienten eine verlängerte Zeit unter Narkose bedeutet und gleichzeitig durch die Interaktion mit der Workstation die Sterilität gefährdet. Wir stellen zwei automatische Methoden vor, welche mit Hilfe einer atlasbasierte Feature-Registrierung die Standard-Ebenen von mobilen C-Bogen CTs einstellt. Da bei unserem Verfahren keine Interaktion benötigt wird, ist das Verfahren für den operativen Eingriff geeignet. Nach unserem besten Wissen existiert keine andere Arbeit, die sich mit der Einstellung der Standard-Ebenen auf C-Bogen CT Bildern bisher befasst hat.

2   Material und Methoden

Durch die nicht standardisierte Einstellung der Bildebenen in den mobilen C-Bogen CT Volumendaten, werden im Folgenden die Bildebenen als A-, B- und C-Ebene mit dazugehörigen Richtungen entlang der Normalen $\mathbf{d}_i, i \in \{A, B, C\}$ durch das Bildvolumen mit $\mathbf{d}_A \perp A$, $\mathbf{d}_B \perp B$ und $\mathbf{d}_C \perp C$ bezeichnet.

2.1   Referenzdaten

Als Referenzdatensatz haben wir klinische C-Bogen CT Bilder von 51 Patienten verwendet. Auf jedem dieser Bilder ist der Calcaneus vollständig abgebildet. Die Bildebenen wurden von drei Ärzten mit unterschiedlichem Erfahrungsstand (zwei Experten und ein fortgeschrittener Benutzer des C-Bogen CT Systems) manuell eingestellt. Die A-Ebene wurde parallel zu der Calcaneus-Platte orientiert oder, falls diese im Bildvolumen nicht vorhanden ist, entlang der größten Ausdehnung des Calcaneus (Abb. 1). Die B- und C-Ebene wurden orthogonal zu den Gelenkflächen zu Talus und zum Cuboid-Knochen ausgerichtet. Die für die Einstellung benötigten Positionen, Winkel zwischen den Ebenen und Zeit, wurden gemessen.

2.2 Methoden zur automatischen Einstellung der Standard-Ebenen

Das erste Verfahren zur automatischen Einstellung der Standard-Ebenen nutzt die Detektion eindeutiger 2D-Features im Calcaneus-Bild. Das zweite fasst Agglomerate der 2D-Features zu sogenannten Pseudo-3D-Features zusammen und nutzt so eine dezimierte und robustere Anzahl von Features. Nach der Feature-Detektion werden die Feature-Punkte eines im Vorfeld erzeugten Atlas mit eingestellten Standard-Ebenen auf die neu erzeugten Feature-Punkte registriert. Dies erlaubt eine Transformation der Standard-Ebenen des Atlas auf das Bild. Als Features haben wir die Speeded Up Robust Features (SURF) Keypoints von Bay et al. [3] verwendet. Die SURF-Features sind invariant gegenüber Translation, Rotation und Skalierung, und somit für die vorliegenden Daten geeignet.

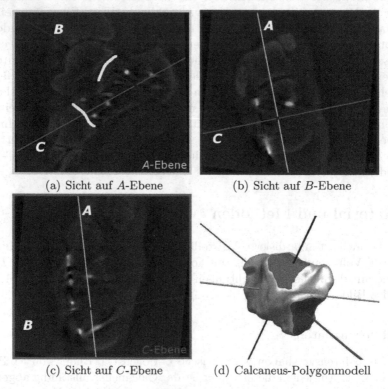

(a) Sicht auf A-Ebene   (b) Sicht auf B-Ebene

(c) Sicht auf C-Ebene   (d) Calcaneus-Polygonmodell

Abb. 1. (a), (c) und (b) zeigen eine Ebenenperspektive des Bildvolumens mit manuell eingestellten Ebenen. Die B- und C-Ebene sind orthogonal zu den Gelenkflächen (gelbe Linien) eingestellt und die A-Ebene parallel zu der Calcaneus-Platte. (d) Polygonmodell eines manuell segmentierten Calcaneus mit hervorgehobenen Gelenkflächen (rot) und eingestellten Ebenen.

2D SURF-Keypoints. Die SURF-Keypoint-Detektion erfolgt durch einen fast multi-scale Hessian Keypointdetektor. Durch Approximation der Hesse-Matrix mit Hilfe von Box-Filtern auf Integralbildern wird eine schnelle Berechnung gewährleistet [3, 4]. Durch Iteration über alle Bildschichten des Bildvolumens in einer Richtung (d_A, d_B oder d_C) berechnen wir 2D-Feature-Punkte für jede einzelne Bildschicht. Die Feature-Punkte von allen Schichten entlang einer Richtung bilden eine 3D-Punktwolke, welche das gesamte Volumenbild repräsentiert. Abb. 2(b) zeigt die berechneten 2D-Features von allen drei Richtungen in einem Datensatz.

Pseudo-3D. Der Pseudo-3D Ansatz basiert auf den Ergebnissen der 2D-SURF-Keypoints. Der Input sind die erhaltenen 2D-SURF-Keypoints von allen drei Richtungen (d_A, d_B und d_C) des vorliegenden Bildvolumens (Abb. 2(b)). Pseudo-3D-Keypoints werden mit einer Nachbarschaftsradiussuche berechnet: Für jeden detektierten Feature-Punkt p wird eine Kugel mit einem Radius von 0.5 mm um p zentriert. Wenn die Kugel mindestens einen Merkmalspunkt aus jeder Richtung (d_A, d_B und d_C) enthält, wird der Schwerpunkt von allen innen-liegenden Punkten berechnet und als Pseudo-3D-Feature-Punkt definiert.

Atlasbasierte Registrierung. Der Atlas wurde aus dem Referenzdatensatz generiert und besteht aus den entsprechenden Feature-Punkten (2D oder Pseudo-3D) und den durch die Experten eingestellten Standard-Ebenen (Abschn. 2.1). Durch eine rigide Registrierung mit dem Iterative Closest Point Algorithm (ICP) werden die Feature-Punkte des Atlas auf die Feature-Punkte des Eingabebildes bestmöglich abgebildet. Als Abbruchkriterien wurde eine maximale Anzahl von 500 Iterationen und ein root-mean-square error (RMSE) von 10^{-3} verwendet. Anschließend werden die Standard-Ebenen des Atlas unter Verwendung der von

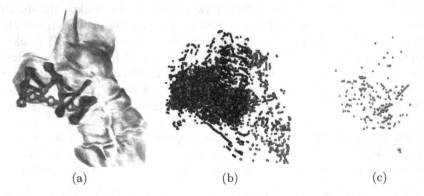

(a)   (b)   (c)

Abb. 2. Beispiel eines volumengerenderten Calcaneus C-Arm CT mit Implantaten (rot) (a), die korrespondierende Punktwolke besteht aus drei 2D-Feature-Punktmengen generiert entlang der orthogonalen Richtungen d_A, d_B und d_C (grün, blau und rot) (b). Die aus (b) generierten Pseudo-3D-Feature-Punkte sind in (c) zu sehen.

Tabelle 1. Evaluierung der Orientierung der Standard-Ebenen auf den Referenzdaten in Bezug auf die Gelenkflächen.

	2D: d_A	2D: d_B	2D: d_C	pseudo-3D
Korrekt orientierte Ebenen	81%	88%	83%	91%

der Registrierung erhaltenen Transformation auf das Eingabebild transformiert. Der Atlas besteht aus Feature-Punkten von einem einzigen Volumenbild. Ausgewählt wurde der Atlas mit dem kleinsten durchschnittlichen Ausrichtungsfehler bei einer Registrierung auf alle anderen verfügbaren Referenzdaten.

3 Ergebnisse

Die Bilddaten wurden mit einem ARCADIS Orbic 3D® mobilen C-Bogen CT (Siemens Healthcare, Erlangen) erzeugt, das ein $\{256\}^3$ Voxel Volumenbild aus 100 2D-Projektionen rekonstruiert. Die durchschnittliche Zeit, die die beiden Experten für die Einstellung verwendet haben, liegt bei 46 s ± 11 s und unterscheidet sich um neun Sekunden von der Bearbeitungszeit des fortgeschrittenen Benutzers 55 s ± 15 s). Für die Evaluierung der automatischen Methoden haben wir die 2D-Features von A, B und C und die Pseudo-3D-Features miteinander verglichen. Der beste Atlas für den Referenzdatensatz wurde durch eine leave-one-out Validierung ermittelt. Für eine zuverlässige Ground-truth wurden die Gelenkflächen manuell von einem medizinischen Experten in jedem Bild segmentiert. Für die Evaluierung wurde die Ausrichtung der automatisch eingestellten B- und C-Ebene zur Gelenkfläche bewertet (Abb. 1). Tab. 1 zeigt die Ergebnisse der automatischen Methoden. Die 2D-Features entlang der Richtung d_B lieferten das beste Ergebnis der 2D-Strategie mit 88% korrekt geschnittenen Gelenkflächen. Der Pseudo-3D-Ansatz liefert allerdings die besten Ergebnisse mit 91% korrekten Schnitten. Der Ansatz ignoriert die Feature-Punkte, die durch Artefakte oder Rauschen im Bild entstanden sind (Abb. 2). Die Gesamtanzahl der Feature-Punkte wird dadurch deutliche reduziert: durschnittlich 275 Punkte für Pseudo-3D und d_A : 3801, d_B : 3952 und d_C : 3594 für die 2D-Features. Ein einziges Bild konnte aufgrund seiner stark abweichenden Intensitätswerte im Vergleich zu den anderen Bildern nicht korrekt registriert werden. Die Berechnungszeit der 2D-Features in einer Richtung (256 Bildschichten) dauerte ungefähr zwei Sekunden und die Registrierung mit einem Atlas acht Sekunden. Der Pseudo-3D-Ansatz ($3 \times 2 s = 6 s$) mit der Registrierung ($2 s$) insgesamt acht Sekunden[1]. Die vorgestellten Verfahren wurden in C++ implementiert und in das Medical Imaging Interaction Toolkit (MITK, www.mitk.org, [5]) integriert.

---

[1] Die Berechnung wurden mit C++ Code auf einem CPU-Kern von einem Intel® Core i7™ CPU 860 at 2.8 GHz durchgeführt.

4   Diskussion

Zwei Methoden zur automatischen Einstellung der Standard-Ebenen von mobilen C-Bogen CT Bildern wurden vorgestellt. Unsere Methoden liefern gegenüber der manuellen Einstellung der Standard-Ebenen eine deutliche Zeitersparnis. Für ein System, welches in einem intraoperativen klinischen Umfeld benutzt wird, sind die Berechnungszeit und die Genauigkeit die wichtigsten Faktoren. Wir behandeln diese Probleme durch die Verwendung von SURF-Keypoints welche signifikant weniger Berechnungszeit mit fast der gleichen Genauigkeit wie andere Methoden zur Merkmalsgenerierung z.b. dem SIFT Algorithmus liefern [3, 6]. Die Verlässlichkeit der eingestellten Standard-Ebenen von unseren Ansätzen hängt direkt von der Genauigkeit der Registrierung der generierten Feature-Punkte ab. Da das C-Bogen CT hauptsächlich für knöcherne Strukturen verwendet wird und der Fuß bei der Operation immer annähernd gleich ausgerichtet wird, sind Rotation, Translation und Skalierung die auftretenden Bildtransformationen und eine rigide Registrierung ist ausreichend. Die Benutzung der Pseudo-3D-Features reduziert drastisch die Anzahl der Feature-Punkte für die Registrierung, was zusätzlich die Berechnungszeit verkürzt und das Rauschen durch Artefakte im Vergleich zur Benutzung von nur einer einzigen Richtung (2D-SURF) verringert. Die Genauigkeit kann weiter gesteigert werden, indem Artefakte in den C-Bogen CT Daten in einem Vorverarbeitungsschritt reduziert bzw. komplett herausgefiltert werden. Durch das entwickelte System können sich die Chirurgen in Zukunft ohne Zeitverlust und ohne die Sterilität zu beeinträchtigen auf die Diagnose der Gelenkflächen konzentrieren.

Danksagung. Die Autoren möchten sich bei Dr. Karl Barth und Dr. Gerhard Kleinszig für den technischen Support und die bereitgestellten Informationen über das C-Bogen CT System bedanken. Dieses Projekt wurde von Siemens Healthcare, X-ray Products teilfinanziert.

Literaturverzeichnis

1. Von Recum J, Wendl K, Vock B, et al. Intraoperative 3D C-arm imaging: state of the art. Unfallchirurg. 2012;115(3):196–201.
2. Franke J, von Recum J, Suda AJ, et al. Intraoperative three-dimensional imaging in the treatment of acute unstable syndesmotic injuries. J Bone Joint Surg Br. 2012;94(15):1386–90.
3. Bay H, Ess A, Tuytelaars T, et al. SURF: speeded up robust features. Comput Vis Image Underst. 2008;110(3):346–59.
4. Viola P, Jones M; IEEE. Rapid object detection using a boosted cascade of simple features. Proc IEEE Comput Soc Conf Comput Vis Pattern Recognit. 2001;1:I-511–8.
5. Nolden M, Zelzer S, Seitel A, et al. The medical imaging interaction toolkit: challenges and advances. Int J Comput Assist Radiol Surg. 2013;8(4):607–20.
6. Lowe DG; IEEE. Object recognition from local scale-invariant features. Proc IEEE Int Conf Comput Vis. 1999;2:1150–7.

Segmentierung von Zellkernen für Hochdurchsatz-DNA-Bildzytomerie

David Friedrich[1], Christoph Haarburger[1], Adrian Luna-Cobos[1],
Dietrich Meyer-Ebrecht[1], Alfred Böcking[2], Dorit Merhof[1]

[1]Lehrstuhl für Bildverarbeitung, RWTH Aachen
[2]Institut für Pathologie, Krankenhaus Düren
david.friedrich@lfb.rwth-aachen.de

Kurzfassung. Krebs lässt sich durch das Vermessen des DNA-Gehaltes morphologisch auffälliger Zellkerne frühzeitig diagnostizieren. Die manuelle Erfassung von Zellkernen ist sehr arbeitsaufwändig, lässt sich jedoch durch ein virtuelles Mikroskop und ein Mustererkennungssystem beschleunigen. Die Umstellung auf die Hochdurchsatz-Variante erfordert eine neuartige Zellkern-Segmentierung, die effizient und präzise sein muss und möglichst wenige irrelevante Objekte segmentiert. Zu diesem Zweck wurde ein dreistufiges Verfahren entwickelt: Pixel werden anhand ihrer Farbwerte mittels eines Maximum-Likelihood-Ansatzes oder durch einen kNN, SVM oder Adaboost-Klassifikator klassifiziert und bilden eine initiale Segmentierung. Irrelevante Objekte werden anhand schnell zu berechnender Merkmale ausgeschlossen. Ein weiteres Merkmal wird berechnet, um zu entscheiden, ob die Kontur einer Verbesserung bedarf. Falls erforderlich geschieht dies durch ein parametrisches Aktives Konturmodell. Auf einem Testset von 80 annotierten Sichtfeldern erreicht die Segmentierung mittels kNN-Klassifikator die beste Performance. Zellkerne werden mit einer Sensitivität von 98.9% detektiert. Im Vergleich zum bisherigen Vorgehen werden bis zu 33% weniger Objekte segmentiert, die keine Zellkerne sind. Nach der Verbesserung wird ein Dice-Koeffizient von 0,908 und eine Hausdorff-Distanz von $0{,}721$ μm erreicht.

1 Einleitung

Die DNA-Bildzytometrie ist ein Verfahren zur Krebsfrühdiagnose, welches auf der Messung des DNA-Gehaltes morphologisch auffälliger Zellkerne beruht. Für die DNA-Messung werden eine spezielle Färbetechnik, ein Mikroskop, eine Kamera und dedizierte Messalgorithmen verwendet. Ein Pathologe identifiziert hunderte bis tausende auffällige Zellkerne, wählt sie per Mausklick im Live-Bild am PC für die Messung aus und analysiert schließlich deren DNA-Verteilung. Lässt sich die DNA-Verteilung nicht durch Proliferation gesunder Zellen erklären (DNA-Aneuploidie), liegt Krebs vor. Da die Diagnose auf einem Messergebnis eines validen Biomarkers beruht [1], sind die Reproduzierbarkeit und diagnostische Genauigkeit höher als bei herkömmlichen Verfahren [2], bei denen subjektiv die Morphologie von Zellen oder Geweben bewertet wird. Durch die Diagnose auf Zellebene wird eine frühzeitige Diagnose ermöglicht: Es sind sieben Fälle von Mundkrebs dokumentiert, bei denen Krebs bis zu zwei Jahre vor der konventionellen Herangehensweise diagnostiziert wurde [3].

Allerdings ist eine manuelle DNA-Bildzytometrie sehr arbeitsaufwändig: Es werden über 40 Minuten benötigt, um die erforderliche Anzahl an Zellkernen zu identifizieren. Durch ein virtuelles Mikroskop für die automatische Digitalisierung und ein Mustererkennungssystem für die Identifikation relevanter Zellkerne kann der manuelle Arbeitsaufwand um den Faktor 8 reduziert werden [4]. Der bisher verwendete Segmentierungsalgorithmus trennt durch ein Schwellwertverfahren im HSV-Raum den weißen Hintergrund von rosa eingefärbten Zellkernen [5]. Wendet man diesen Algorithmus auf ein ganzes Sichtfeld an, werden jedoch auch viele irrelevante Objekte wie Schmutzpartikel oder Kernsegmente segmentiert, da sie sich ebenfalls vom Hintergrund abheben. Diese Objekte hätte der Benutzer in der manuellen Variante nicht ausgewählt. In der automatischen Variante, bei der bis zu 150.000 Objekte pro Fall verarbeitet werden müssen, erhöhen Sie unnötigerweise den Aufwand für die Klassifikation. Entdeckt der Benutzer eine unpräzise Segmentierung, so lässt sich diese manuell oder automatisch korrigieren [6]. Geschieht dies nicht, so kann der DNA-Gehalt nicht genau gemessen werden und es kommt zu Fehlklassifikationen von Zellkernen, was möglicherweise eine Fehldiagnose zur Folge hat.

Eine nur auf Schwellwerten basierende Segmentierung ist daher nicht ausreichend im Rahmen des Hochdurchsatz-Szenarios. MacAuley et al. verwenden zur Konturverbesserung ein iteratives Verfahren basierend auf morphologischer Bildverarbeitung auf alle Zellkerne an [7]. Der Beitrag unserer Arbeit ist ein mehrstufiges Verfahren, welches irrelevante Objekte eliminiert und die aufwändigen Verbesserungsalgorithmen nur auf schlecht segmentierten Zellkernen durchführt: Zunächst wird eine initiale Segmentierung durch die Klassifikation der Farbwerte erstellt. Irrelevante Objekte, die sich nicht anhand der Farbinformation von Zellen unterscheiden lassen, werden anhand schnell zu berechnender Merkmale entfernt. Schließlich wird geprüft, ob eine Verbesserung der Kontur nötig ist und falls erforderlich durch ein Aktives Konturmodell durchgeführt.

2   Material und Methoden

2.1   Bildgebung und Goldstandard

Für die Bildgebung wurde ein Motic BA 410 Mikroskop mit $40\times$ Objektiv sowie eine MotiCam 285A RGB-Kamera (1360×1024 Pixel, 8 Bit) verwendet. Für diese Kombination entspricht ein Pixel im Bild $0.18\,\mu m$ auf dem Objektträger. Helligkeitsunterschiede im Bild wurden durch eine Shading-Korrektur behoben. Zellproben aus vier Modalitäten (Gebärmutterhals- und Mundschleimhautabstrich, Körperhöhlenerguß-Punktion, Prostata-Biopsie) wurden durch die Reaktion nach Feulgen proportional zu ihrem DNA-Gehalt eingefärbt. Als Farbstoff kam dabei Pararosanilin zum Einsatz, was zu einer rosaroten Kolorierung der Zellen führt. Zum Trainieren der Farbwerte wurden 25.307 Zellkerne von acht

Patienten verwendet, die von einem Pathologen für das Training von Mustererkennungssystemen annotiert wurden und deshalb nur Zellkerne mit visuell präziser Segmentierung enthalten. Weiter wurden die Artefakte in diesen Daten in Unterklassen aufgeteilt, welche sich ohne Mustererkennungssystem von Zellen trennen lassen. Dazu gehören große Schmutz-Partikel, Zellkerne die kleine Schmutzpartikel enthalten, Zellkernfragmente aus sich auflösenden Zellkernen sowie kleine Haarrisse im Mikroskop-Objektträger. Abb. 1 gibt einen Überblick über die extrahierten Artefakte und zeigt exemplarisch die auftretenden Zellkernklassen. Um die Detektionsperformance und Präzision der Segmentierung zu testen wurden 1133 Zellen in 80 Bildausschnitten manuell segmentiert (Material von acht weiteren Patienten). Die Berechnungen wurden auf einem Core i5 mit 2,80 GHz unter Matlab (Mathworks) durchgeführt.

2.2   Initiale Segmentierung

Beim Maximum-Likelihood-Ansatz (MLE) werden Pixel im Hinblick auf ihre Auftretenswahrscheinlichkeit klassifiziert: Im Farbtrainingsset gehören 37,62% der Pixel zu Zellen und 62,38% zu Artefakten oder Hintergrund. Für jede RGB- oder HSV-Farbwert-Kombination wird berechnet, wie häufig sie im Trainingsset innerhalb der jeweiligen Klasse auftritt. Liegt der Anteil in Zellkernen über 37,62%, so wird diese Kombination als Zelle segmentiert, sonst als Hintergrund.

Allerdings hat dieses Vorgehen den Nachteil, dass Farbwerte die nicht im Trainingsset auftreten als Hintergrund klassifiziert werden. Hier ist es wünschenswert, Trennlinien zwischen den Farbwerten von Zellen und Hintergrund beziehungsweise Artefakten zu finden, welche die Zuordnung generalisieren. Deshalb wurden für den Klassifikationsansatz ein k-Nächste-Nachbar-Klassifikator

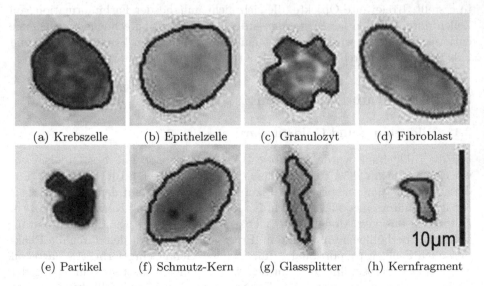

(a) Krebszelle   (b) Epithelzelle   (c) Granulozyt   (d) Fibroblast

(e) Partikel   (f) Schmutz-Kern   (g) Glassplitter   (h) Kernfragment

Abb. 1. Beispiele für Zellkernobjekte (a–d) und Artefakte (e–h).

(kNN), ein Adaboost-Klassifikator und Support Vector Machines auf den Farbwerten trainiert. Für kNN wurde die Euklidische Distanz und $k=11$, 21, 31 oder
41 gewählt. Als schwacher Klassifikator für das AdaBoost-Verfahren wurde der lineare Klassifikator eingesetzt. Um die Optimierung während des SVM-Trainings
zu beschleunigen wurden beim Training für jedes Objekt jeweils nur Median-
Werte für Hintergrund und Zelle in jedem Farbkanal berücksichtigt. Die Klassi-
fikatoren wurden im RGB- und HSV-Farbraum (8 Bit pro Kanal) trainiert.

Um den Zeitaufwand für die initiale Segmentierung zu reduzieren, werden die
Klassifikationsergebnisse für alle 256^3 auftretenden Farbwertkombinationen in einer Lookup-Table gespeichert. Vor der Segmentierung wird das Bild mit einem
Median-Filter der Größe 1.25 μm gefiltert. Nach der initialen Segmentierung werden zur Glättung morphologisches Opening und Closing (Strukturelement Kreis
mit Radius 0.36 μm) und zum Schließen von Löchern eine Flood-fill Operation
durchgeführt. Alle Objekte kleiner als 5 μm^2 werden entfernt.

2.3 Ausschluss anhand von Objektmerkmalen

Im Gegensatz zu großen Schmutzpartikeln oder Glassplittern lassen sich Zellkerne mit kleinen Schmutzpartikeln (Abb. 1(f)) und Zellkernfragmente (Abb. 1(h))
nicht durch die Farbwerte von Zellkernen trennen. Der Ausschluss solcher Objekte geschieht durch schnell zu berechnende Zellmerkmale: Schmutzpartikel schwächen das einfallende Licht in allen Kanälen stark, während Zellkerne das Licht
vor allem im Rot- und Grünkanal absorbieren. Deshalb wird auf dem Blaukanal-
nal, wo die Schwächung bei Schmutzpartikeln stark und bei Zellen gering ist,
eine Filterung mit einem rechteckigen Filterelement durchgeführt (Kantenlänge
0.54 μm). Die minimale Filterantwort innerhalb eines Objektes wird zur Diskri-
minanz von Zellen mit und ohne Schmutzpartikel verwendet. Zellkernfragmente hingegen sind kleiner und heller als Zellkerne. Deshalb werden sie über die
Objektgröße und den mittleren Intensitätswert im Grünkanal über einen quadratischen Klassifikator von Zellkernen getrennt. Sowohl der Schwellwert für die
Trennung von Zellkernen mit Schmutz als auch der quadratische Klassifikator
wurden auf dem Trainingsset trainiert.

2.4 Konturverbesserung

Um die segmentierte Kontur zu verbessern und Fehler in der Segmentierung zu
korrigieren wird in ausgewählten Fällen eine Konturverbesserung durchgeführt.
Bei schlecht segmentieren Zellkernen unterscheiden sich die Farbintensitäten im
segmentierten Bereich nur wenig von der Farbintensität innerhalb der konvexen

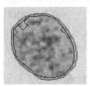

Abb. 2. Beispiel für die Konturverfeinerung eines Zellkerns. Blau:
Initiale Segmentierung, Schwarz: Konvexe Hülle, Rot: nach Verbesserung. Die Hausdorff-Distanz zur Goldstandard-Segmentierung verringert sich von 1.41 μm auf 0.649 μm.

Tabelle 1. Performance der Segmentierungsverfahren. Neben den Statistiken aus Abschnitt 2.5 ist für jedes Verfahren die beste Parameterkombination angegeben.

Verfahren	Parameter	Sens. (%)	PPV (%)	Dice	Hausdorff (μm)
Referenz [5]	HSV	99,9	47,4	0,89	0,756
MLE	HSV	98,2	56,2	0,90	0,816
kNN	HSV, k=41	98,9	56,7	0,91	0,725
SVM	HSV	97,6	57,0	0,89	0,874
Adaboost	HSV	98,8	52,8	0,91	0,698

Hülle und außerhalb des segmentierten Bereiches. Ist das Verhältnis dieser Intensitäten zu gering, wird die Segmentierung über ein parametrisches Aktives Konturmodell („Snakes") verfeinert. Dieses Modell liefert schnell eine verfeinerte Kontur [6]. Da oft nur geringe Fehler korrigiert werden müssen und die Laufzeit gering gehalten werden soll, werden nur 50 Iterationen durchgeführt. Die Parameter für die Aktiven Konturen wurden der Optimierung von [6] entnommen. Abb. 2 zeigt ein Beispiel zur Verbesserung einer initialen Segmentierung.

2.5   Evaluierung

Für die Evaluierung wurden die entwickelten Algorithmen auf dem Testset angewendet. Für die Erfassung der Detektionsperformance wurden die Sensitivität (Anteil der gefundenen Zellen) sowie der positive Prädiktionswert (PPV, Anteil Zellkerne an segmentierten Objekten) berechnet. Die Präzision der Segmentierung wird durch den Dice-Koeffizienten sowie die Hausdorff-Distanz quantifiziert.

3   Ergebnisse und Diskussion

Die Detektionsperformance nach der initialen Segmentierung und dem Ausschluss durch Objektmerkmale ist in Tab. 1 angegeben. Stets erreichte die initiale Segmentierung im HSV-Raum eine bessere Performance, im Schnitt ist der Dice-Koeffizient um 0.02 höher als bei RGB. Die beste Gesamt-Performance erreicht die Segmentierung basierend auf dem kNN-Algorithmus, deshalb wird dieser Algorithmus im Folgenden weiter analysiert: Es werden 98,94% aller Zellen segmentiert, was leicht niedriger ist als beim Referenz-Algorithmus. Allerdings befinden sich unter den segmentierten Objekten auch bedeutend weniger unnötig segmentierte Objekte, was sich durch einen höheren positiven Prädiktionswert ausdrückt. Beim kNN-Algorithmus wurden im Durchschnitt 10,7 Nicht-Zellkern-Objekte pro Bildausschnitt segmentiert, im Vergleich zu 15,68 für das Referenzverfahren. Für eine Hochdurchsatz-DNA-Bildzytometrie werden ungefähr 4000 Sichtfelder analysiert, so dass bei dieser Performance die Mustererkennung circa 20.000 Objekte weniger klassifizieren muss. Bei den unnötig segmentierten Objekten handelt es sich meist um Artefakte wie überlagernde Zellkerne, die durch das dahinter geschaltete Mustererkennungssystem erkannt werden müssen. Die konditionale Verbesserung der Kontur wird auf 12,5% der Zellkerne durchgeführt und erreicht einen Dice-Koeffizienten von 0,908 und eine Hausdorff-Distanz von 0,721 μm. Betrachtet man nur die verfeinerten Zellkerne, so liegt die Hausdorff-Distanz vor der Verbesserung bei $1,05\,\mu$m und nachher bei $0,91\,\mu$m. Dies zeigt erstens, dass sich durch das auf der konvexen Hülle basierende Merkmal schlecht segmentierte Zellkerne identifizieren lassen, da die Hausdorff-Distanz der verfeinerten Zellkerne überdurchschnittlich hoch ist. Zweitens verbessert die Anwendung des vorgeschlagenen Konturverbesserungsalgorithmus die Präzision deutlich. Die durchschnittliche Laufzeit dieses Algorithmus liegt bei 1,51 Sekunden pro Sichtfeld (initiale Segmentierung: $0,67\,\mathrm{sec}$, Ausschluss irrelevanter Objekte: $0,14\,\mathrm{sec}$, Konturverbesserung: $0,70\,\mathrm{sec}$).

Als zukünftige Arbeit sollte eine automatische Anpassung an die Färbeintensität sowie Verfahren für berührende Zellkerne entwickelt werden: Die Färbeintensität bei DNA-Bildzytometrieproben kann zwischen verschiedenen Objektträgern schwanken. Bei den nicht segmentierten Zellen handelt es sich vor allem um blasse Zellkerne. Um auch diese erfolgreich zu segmentieren, sollten gezielt Daten von blassen Präparaten in das Trainingsset aufgenommen werden. Durch einen Algorithmus, der sich nach der Segmentierung einiger Sichtfelder adaptiv an die Färbung anpasst wird im Fall von starken Färbungen verhindert, dass zu viele blasse Nicht-Zellkern-Objekte segmentiert werden. Bei Segmentierungen, die stark von der Referenzsegmentierung abweichen, handelt es sich meistens um berührende Zellkerne, die als ein Objekt segmentiert werden. Entfernt man diese Art der Fehlsegmentierung, die im Testset 34 mal auftritt und sich mit Hausdorff-Distanzen bis zu $10,8\,\mu$m in der Statistik niederschlägt, so verbessert sich die durchschnittliche Hausdorff-Distanz auf $0,628\,\mu$m. Deshalb sollte dieser Fall ebenfalls durch ein schnell zu berechnendes Objektmerkmal detektiert und ein Trennalgorithmus angewandt werden.

Literaturverzeichnis

1. Rajagopalan H, Lengauer C. Aneuploidy and cancer. Nature. 2004;432:338–41.
2. Nguyen VQH, Grote HJ, Pomjanski N, et al. Interobserver reproducibility of DNA-image-cytometry in ASCUS or higher cervical cytology. Anal Cell Pathol. 2004;26(3):143–50.
3. Böcking A, Sproll C, Stöcklein N, et al. Role of brush biopsy and DNA cytometry for prevention, diagnosis, therapy and followup care of oral cancer. J Oncol. 2011; p. 1–7.
4. Friedrich D, Chen J, Zhang Y, et al. Identification of prostate cancer cell nuclei for DNA-grading of malignancy. Proc BVM. 2012; p. 334–9.
5. Höck L. Entwicklung robuster Verfahren für die automatische Segmentierung und Identifikation geeigneter Zellkerne in der DNA-Bildzytometrie. Diplomarbeit, RWTH Aachen; 2008.
6. Friedrich D, Luna-Cobos A, Biesterfeld S, et al. Konturverfeinerung über Fourierdeskriptoren. Proc BVM. 2013; p. 211–6.
7. MacAulay C, Palcic B. An edge relocation segmentation algorithm. Anal Quant Cytol Histol. 1990;12(3):165.

Ultraschallsimulation für das Training von Gallengangspunktionen

Julian Schröder[1], Andre Mastmeyer[1], Dirk Fortmeier[1,2], Heinz Handels[1]

[1]Institut für Medizinische Informatik, Universität zu Lübeck
[2]Graduiertenschule für Informatik in Medizin und Lebenswissenschaften, Universität zu Lübeck
mastmeyer@imi.uni-luebeck.de

Kurzfassung. Ultraschalluntersuchungen sind ein wichtiger Bestandteil der modernen Medizin. Ein Anwendungsgebiet ist zum Beispiel die Ultraschallkontrolle während einer Gallengangspunktion. Die Deutung von Ultraschallbildern ist schwierig, sodass dieses über einen langen Zeitraum am Patienten erlernt werden muss. Eine Alternative ist eine virtuelle Trainingsumgebung mit Ultraschallsimulation. In diesem Beitrag wird die Ultraschallsimulation innerhalb eines Punktionssimulators vorgestellt, mit der Gallengangspunktionen unter Ultraschallkontrolle trainiert werden können. Die Ultraschallsimulation nutzt unbearbeitete 3D CT-Daten und beruht darauf, Reflexionen entlang eines Strahlenfächers ausgehend von der Sonde zu berechnen. Dabei werden Reflexion, Transmission und Absorption berücksichtigt. Zur Erhöhung des Lerneffekts kann der Anwender je nach Schwierigkeit dem simulierten Bild zusätzliche Visualisierungen hinzufügen, zum Beispiel eine Umrandung der Zielstruktur oder ein nachgebildetes Doppler-Ultraschall. Im Ergebnis können unter Benutzung partiell segmentierter CT-Daten in Echtzeit realistische Ultraschallbilder simuliert werden.

1 Einleitung

Der Erfolg von ultraschallgestützten Nadelpunktionen ist stark von den Fähigkeiten des Arztes abhängig. Die erfolgreiche Punktion kann im klinischen Alltag schwer erlernt werden. Daher bietet ein VR-Simulator eine optimale Trainingsumgebung, um ohne Gefährdung realer Patienten Punktionseingriffe zu trainieren und zu planen. In diesem Beitrag wird die Implementierung einer Ultraschallsimulation auf Grafikhardware (CUDA) vorgestellt. Diese wurde in den vorhanden Punktionssimulator integriert, um das Training ultraschallgestützter Punktionen zu ermöglichen. Für die Simulation des virtuellen Patienten werden 3D/4D CT Aufnahmen genutzt, welche vorab partiell semi-automatisch segmentiert werden, sodass jederzeit eine akkurate Lokalisierung der Ziel- und Risikostrukturen gewährleistet ist. Die Interaktion mit den simulierten Werkzeugen, z.B. Punktionsnadel, US-Sonde oder Palpationstool, erfolgt mit Hilfe eines haptischen Geräts. Die durch Werkzeuge hervorgerufenen Deformationen im Gewebe werden algorithmisch abhängig von Gewebeeigenschaften berechnet und visualisiert [1]. Während einer Simulation können neben dem Patienten und dem US-Bild noch verschiedene Schnittbilder der CT Daten und eine simulierte Röntgenaufnahme mit Kontrastmittelverlauf dargestellt werden, um zusätzliche Hilfestellungen zu geben.

Die Ultraschallsimulation orientiert sich an den Methoden von Reichl et al. [2], Wein et al. [3] und Karamalis [4]. Der Ansatz von Bürger et al. [5] nutzt voll segmentierte CT-Daten und Oberflächenmodelle, sodass er für unseren Simulator mit partiell segmentierten Daten nicht geeignet ist.

2 Pipline der Ultraschallsimulation

Die Ultraschallsimulation kann in sieben Schritte unterteilt werden (Abb. 1).

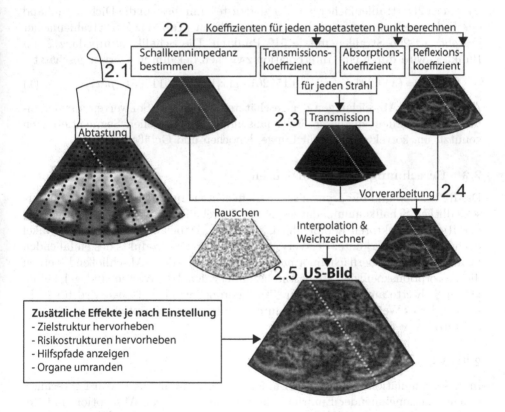

Abb. 1. Visualisierung der einzelnen Schritte, angefangen bei der Abtastung des CT-Bildes bis zum simulierten US-Bild. Die Nummern entsprechen den folgenden Unterkapiteln im Text.

Tabelle 1. Fallunterscheidung für die Umrechnung von HU Werten in Dichte [6].

HU Bereich	Formel
HU > 100	$\rho = 1.017 + 0.592 \cdot 0.001 \cdot HU$
$100 \leq HU > 22$	$\rho = 1.003 + 1.169 \cdot 0.001 \cdot HU$
$22 \leq HU > 14$	$\rho = 1.03$
$14 \leq HU > -99$	$\rho = 1.018 + 0.893 \cdot 0.001 \cdot HU$
$-99 \leq HU$	$\rho = 1.03091 + 0.0010297 \cdot HU$

2.1 Abtastung der 3D CT-Daten und Berechnung der Schallkennimpedanz

Im ersten Schritt der Simulation werden mit Hilfe von CUDA Hounsfield-Werte auf einem 2D-Strahlenfächer parallel abgetastet, um diese in die Dichte ρ anhand der Fallunterscheidungen in Tab. 1 umzurechnen (Tab. 1). Der Strahlenfächer besteht aus 256 Strahlen mit je 512 Punkten. Die Schallkennimpedanz Z im Punkt x_i wird durch eine Interpolation zwischen bekannten Werten geschätzt

$$Z = (349.281 \cdot \rho(x_i) - 0.151261 \cdot \rho(x_i)^2 + 0.00117651 \cdot \rho(x_i)^3) \qquad (1)$$

Aufgrund von Abweichungen der geschätzten Werte von Sollwerten aus der Literatur [7] werden an dieser Stelle falls nötig die partiellen Segmentierungen genutzt, um korrekte Werte für Lunge, Knochen und Gefäße zu setzen.

2.2 Berechnung der Koeffizienten

Die Reflexions- und die Transmissionskoeffizienten sind abhängig von den unterschiedlichen Schallkennimpedanzen Z am Gewebeübergang und werden mittels der Richtungsvektoren der Strahlen berechnet. Dabei kann der Einfallswinkel nach Reichl et al. [2] unter der Verwendung des Skalar-Produkts des einfallenden Strahls mit der Oberflächennormalen berechnet werden. Abschließend werden die Absorptionskoeffizienten bestimmt, indem den HU-Werten und gelabelten Daten Sollwerte aus der Literatur [7] zugeordnet werden. Dabei wird für nicht segmentiertes Weichteilgewebe ein durchschnittlicher Absorptionskoeffizient von $0, 55$ dB/cm verwendet [7].

2.3 Berechnung der Transmission

In dieser Simulation wird mit einer ursprünglichen Intensität I_0 von 1 gerechnet, welche mit zunehmender Eindringtiefe vom Gewebe durch Absorption und Reflexion abgeschwächt wird. Um alle 256 Strahlen parallel zu berechnen, wird auf der GPU ein Block mit 256 Threads erzeugt. Die noch vorhandene Energie $I_i(x_i)$ wird rekursiv für jeden Punkt auf einem Strahl tiefenabhängig berechnet, sodass die reflektierte Intensität $I_r(x_i)$ mit dem Reflexionskoeffizienten bestimmt werden kann. In der Simulation wird angenommen, dass die reflektierte Intensität auf dem gleichen Weg zurück zur Sonde gelangt und die empfangene Intensität $I_e(x_i)$ erneut vom Gewebe abgeschwächt wird.

2.4 Tiefenabhängige Verstärkung (Time Gain Control, TGC)

Nachdem die Signale von der Sonde empfangen wurden, findet eine Vorverarbeitung statt. Je größer die Entfernungen der Reflexionen von der Sonde sind, desto stärker sind Signale durch das Gewebe abgeschwächt worden. Ziel ist es, dass gleiche Gewebeübergänge unabhängig von der Entfernung zur Sonde und der Abschwächung vom Gewebe dargestellt werden. Um den Entfernungsunterschied auszugleichen, wird eine tiefenabhängige Verstärkung durchgeführt, um die TGC-Verstärkung eines US-Gerätes zu simulieren. Die verwendete Verstärkungsfunktion $f(d)$ berücksichtigt die Frequenz f und kann durch den Parameter c vom Anwender über die GUI eingestellt werden

$$f(d) = \exp(-c \cdot d \cdot f/10.0)^2 \qquad (2)$$

Somit kann das verstärkte Signal $I(x_i)$ mit der Entfernung d zur Sonde berechnet werden

$$I_v(x_i) = \frac{I_e(x_i)}{f(d)} \cdot I_0 \qquad (3)$$

Durch die als konstant angenommene Abschwächung findet hinter schwach absorbierendem Gewebe eine Aufhellung im Bild statt. Dies geschieht zum Beispiel hinter einer gefüllten Harnblase, aufgrund eines geringen Abschwächungskoeffizienten von ca. $0.0002\,\mathrm{dB/cm}$ [7].

2.5 Darstellung des US-Bildes

Die Zusammensetzung des Fächerbildes orientiert sich an der von Karamalis [4] vorgestellten gewichteten Bildkomposition und kann wie alle Parameter über die GUI eingestellt werden. Abschließend wird dem Bild ein künstliches Perlin-Rauschen hinzugefügt und es wird mit einem Weichzeichenfilter gefaltet. Dem fertig simulierten Bild können vom Anwender weitere Hilfsvisualisierungen, wie

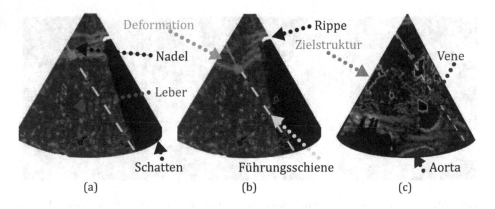

Abb. 2. Veranschaulichung der Deformationen beim Einstich in die Leber in Abb. (a), (b) und verschiedener weiterer Hilfsvisualisierungen in Abb. (c).

zum Beispiel die farbige Umrandung von Risiko- oder Zielstrukturen der Punktion, hinzugefügt werden. Dafür wird ein Kantenfilter auf die parallel ausgelesenen Label Informationen der 3D Daten angewendet. Weiterhin kann der Eindruck eines Doppler-Ultraschalls erzeugt werden, sodass auch kleine Blutgefäße sichtbar werden. Die Nadel der Punktion wird im Ultraschallbild weiß-grau eingezeichnet.

3 Ergebnisse

Abb. 2 stellt ein simuliertes US-Bild der Leber mit verschiedenen Hilfsvisualisierungen dar, sodass Gefäße und Zielstrukturen eindeutig differenziert werden können (Abb. 2). Die simulierten Deformationen durch die Nadel an Gewebegrenzen werden in Abb. 2(b) am Beispiel einer Punktion der Leber verdeutlicht (Abb. 2). Auch die simulierte Schattenbildung hinter Knochen wird deutlich. In unserer PTCD-Simulation wird eine Führungsschiene an der US-Sonde simuliert, um eine Punktion in der US-Ebene zu ermöglichen. Der Einstichpfad anhand der Führungsschiene wird im simulierten US-Bild mit einer gelben gestichelten Linie dargestellt.

Abb. 3 stellt ein reales US-Bild der Niere einem mit der vorgestellten Methode simuliertem US-Bild gegenüber. Die Form der Niere ist auf beiden Bildern gut erkennbar, jedoch hat das reale Bild weichere Kanten und weist eine radiale Unschärfe auf. Weiterhin ist die Niere durch ihr lokales US-Rauschen erkennbar. Dies wurde in der Simulation nicht berücksichtigt und erschwert somit etwas die Differenzierung verschiedener Gewebe.

4 Diskussion

In diesem Beitrag wurde die echtzeitfähige Simulation von Ultraschallbildern basierend auf CT-Bildern und Teilsegmentierungen für einen existierenden Gallengangspunktionstrainer vorgestellt. Die Berechnung der Ultraschallsimulation

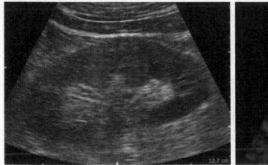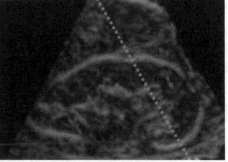

Abb. 3. Beispiel eines realen (links) und eines simulierten (rechts) Ultraschallbildes der Niere. In beiden Bildern ist die Niere eindeutig erkennbar (Quelle US-Bild: Urologie Marburg, http://www.urologie-marburg.de/uploads/images/niere_normal.gif).

benötigt 8, 017 ms mit einer NVIDIA Quadro 4000 und kann maximal 124 Bilder pro Sekunde ausgeben. Um ein US-Bild der Größe 256 mal 256 Pixel auszugeben, werden 256 Strahlen mit jeweils 512 Punkten auf der Grafikkarte berechnet. Die ultraschalltypische Abschattung im Gewebe durch Reflexion und Absorption kann erfolgreich simuliert werden, des Weiteren kommt es hinter schwach absorbierendem Gewebe durch die tiefenabhängige Verstärkung zu einer Aufhellung. Zusätzlich können Hilfsvisualisierungen, z.B. nachgebildetes Doppler-US, dem US-Bild hinzugefügt werden. Eine Doppler-US Nachbildung ist nötig, da eine Doppler-Ultraschallsimulation aufgrund fehlender Blutflussinformationen mit den vorhanden Datensätzen nicht möglich ist.

Mehrfachreflexionen und Speed-Displacement sind in diesem Ansatz noch nicht berücksichtigt und könnten vielleicht bei einer Integration des Raytracing frameworks CUDA Optix und zusätzlicher Informationen, zum Beispiel Mesh-Modells, hinzugefügt werden. Mittels CUDA Optix und Mesh-Modells kann auch versucht werden, die Brechung der Strahlen für die Darstellung ultraschalltypischer Artefakte zu simulieren.

Die vorgestellte Simulation ermöglicht das realitätsgetreue Training und die effektive Planungsunterstützung für die ultraschallgestützte Gallengangspunktion. Bisher wurde die Simulation mit 3D CT-Daten getestet, eine Nutzung von 4D CT-Daten ist nahtlos möglich und führt durch die Bewegung zu noch realistischeren Bildern. In Zukunft kann außerdem versucht werden, die Simulation für 3D Ultraschallbilder methodisch zu erweitern. Dafür könnten im einfachsten Fall mehrere 2D-Bilder aufgenommen werden, um einen 3D Fächer abzutasten. Aus diesen Volumenaufnahmen kann ein 3D Ultraschallbild rekonstruiert werden.

Danksagung. Diese Arbeit wird von der DFG gefördert (DFG-HA 2355/10-1).

Literaturverzeichnis

1. Fortmeier D, Mastmeyer A, Handels H. Image-based soft tissue deformation algorithms for real-time simulation of liver puncture. Curr Med Imaging Rev. 2013;9:154–65.
2. Reichl T, Passenger J, Acosta O, et al. Echtzeit-Ultraschallsimulation auf Grafik-Prozessoren mit CUDA. Proc BVM. 2009.
3. Wein W, Brunke S, Khamene A, et al. Automatic CT-ultrasound registration for diagnostic imaging and image-guided intervention. Med Image Anal. 2008;12(5):577–85.
4. Karamalis A. GPU Ultrasound Simulation and Volume Reconstruction; 2009.
5. Buerger B, Bettinghausen S, Radle M, et al. Real-time GPU-based ultrasound simulation using deformable mesh models. IEEE Trans Med Imaging. 2013;32(3):609–18.
6. Schneider U, Pedroni E, Lomax A. The calibration of CT Hounsfield units for radiotherapy treatment planning. Phys Med Biol. 1996;41(1):111.
7. Bushberg JT, Seibert JA, Leidholdt EM, et al. The Essential Physics of Medical Imaging. Wolters Kluwer Health; 2011.

Tracking von Instrumenten auf fluoroskopischen Aufnahmen für die navigierte Bronchoskopie

Teena Steger[1,2], Wissam El-Hakimi[2], Stefan Wesarg[1]

[1]Fraunhofer Institut für Graphische Datenverarbeitung IGD, Darmstadt
[2]Graphisch-Interaktive Systeme, Technische Universität, Darmstadt
teena.steger@igd.fraunhofer.de

Kurzfassung. Intraoperative C-Bogen-Fluoroskopie dient bei der bronchoskopischen Biopsie zur Lokalisation des Bronchoskops und der Biospiezange innerhalb des Patiententhorax. Bei bekannter C-Bogen Pose ist es möglich, aus der 2D-Position der Instrumentenspitze auf der Fluoroskopie deren 3D-Position innerhalb des Bronchialbaums zu berechnen. Während die Pose mit Hilfe einer Markerplatte auf dem Patiententisch bestimmt werden kann, fehlt bisher eine automatische Verfolgung der Instrumentenspitze auf der kontinuierlichen Fluoroskopie. In dieser Arbeit wird eine solche Tracking-Methode vorgestellt und evaluiert. Erste Experimente an einem Bronchialbaum-Phantom lieferten sehr robuste und präzise Ergebnisse und auch die Echtzeitfähigkeit konnte gezeigt werden.

1 Einleitung

Bei der Bronchoskopie wird ein biegsamer Schlauch mit einer eingebauten Kamera an der Spitze (Bronchoskop) in die Bronchien des sedierten Patienten eingeführt. So können Biopsieinstrumente durch den Schlauch an der verdächtigen Stelle positioniert und eingesetzt werden. Zusätzlich behilft sich der Arzt intraoperativer C-Bogen-Aufnahmen, um sich zu orientieren. Den zweidimensionalen C-Bogen-Bildern fehlt aber die räumliche Tiefe, die für eine schnelle und präzise Navigation des Bronchoskops benötigt wird. Indem dem Arzt eine dreidimensionale Lokalisation des Bronchoskops innerhalb der Bronchien geboten wird, kann die Instrumentenführung erheblich erleichert werden. In [1] wird ein System zur trackerlosen bronchoskopischen Navigation vorgestellt. Mit Hilfe einer Markerplatte auf dem Patiententisch wird dabei die C-Bogen Pose berechnet, um die Position des Bronchoskops, welches in der C-Bogen-Aufnahme abgebildet wurde, durch einen virtuellen Röntgenstrahl in das CT-Volumen zu projizieren. Die aktuelle Position des Bronchoskops ist dann der Schnittpunkt mit dem Bronchialbaum im CT. Diese Position kann dann in einem 3D-Bronchialbaum visualisiert werden. Wesentlich für dieses Konzept ist die automatische Detektion und Verfolgung der Instrumentenspitze in der kontinuierlichen C-Bogen-Fluoroskopie. In der Literatur gibt es zahlreiche Arbeiten zur Detektion von kurvenförmigen Strukturen auf Fluoroskopiebildern [2]. Dabei können dies zwar sowohl anatomische Strukturen, wie z.B. Gefäße [3], als auch medizinische Werkzeuge, wie z.B. Katheter [4] oder Führungsdrähte [5], sein, aber bronchoskopische Instrumente, insbesondere Biopsiezangen, wurden bisher weder automatisch detektiert noch getrackt. In dieser Arbeit kommt eine weitere Schwierigkeit hinzu: es sollen nicht alle auf dem Bild sichtbaren Werkzeuge detektiert werden, sondern nur die relevanten Instrumente innerhalb des Bronchialbaums. Die entwickelte Methode basiert deshalb auf einer Katheterdetektionsmethode [6], ist aber auf den speziellen Anwendungsfall der bronchoskopischen Navigation angepasst.

2 Material und Methoden

Während der Bronchoskopie bedient sich der Arzt der kontinuierlichen Fluoroskopie, um die aktuelle Position der Spitze des Bronchoskops oder der Biopsiezange innerhalb des Thorax zu visualisieren. Es wurde eine Methode entwickelt, um das automatische Verfolgen dieser Spitze auf den Fluoroskopieaufnahmen zu ermöglichen. Dabei stellten sich mehrere Herausforderungen, die berücksichtigt wurden: Unterschiedliche Formen und Größen von Bronchoskop- und Biopsiezangenspitzen, nicht-bronchoskopische Operationswerkzeuge auf dem Bild, überdeckende anatomische Strukturen, Atmungsbewegung des Patienten und die Forderung nach Echtzeitfähigkeit beim Tracking. Abb. 1(a) zeigt beispielhaft eine Fluoroskopieaufnahme, auf der einige dieser Schwierigkeiten zu erkennen sind. Um diesen Anforderungen, vor allem der Echtzeitfähigkeit, gerecht zu werden, wurde ein zweistufiger Algorithmus gewählt. Der erste Teil ist aufwändiger und wird einmalig am Beginn, bei jeder C-Bogen-Bewegung und zur Korrektur ausgeführt. Der zweite Schritt hingegen ist echtzeitfähig und wird auf den folgenden Frames zum Tracking angewendet. Im ersten Schritt werden alle auf dem Bild sichtbaren Spitzen von schlauchartigen Instrumenten detektiert und irreführende, nicht bronchoskopische Instrumente ausgeschlossen. Die daraus resultierende Bronchoskop- oder Biopsiezangenspitze wird im zweiten Schritt verwendet, um ein Konturenmodell zu generieren, welches dann für das darauffolgende Tracking genutzt wird. Da somit sowohl der Suchbereich als auch das zu suchende Konturenmodell verkleinert werden, kann dieser Schritt sehr schnell erfolgen.

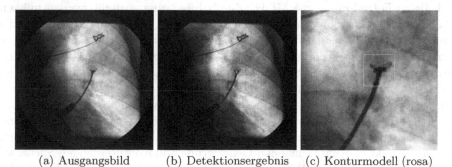

(a) Ausgangsbild   (b) Detektionsergebnis   (c) Konturmodell (rosa)

Abb. 1. Beispiel einer intraoperativen Fluoroskopie-Aufnahme mit Bronchoskop und Biopsiezange sowie nicht-bronchoskopischen Operationswerkzeugen.

2.1 Detektion

Um das Tracking der Instrumentenspitze auf mehreren Frames zu vereinfachen und damit zu beschleunigen, wird zunächst auf einem einzelnen Frame ein geeignetes Template und die Ausgangsposition des Werkzeugs detektiert. Dazu wird die Spitze mit einem etwas aufwändigeren Verfahren auf dem gesamten Framebild gesucht. Abb. 1(b) (grün) zeigt beispielhaft eine so detektierte Spitze. Diese Detektion der Bronchoskop- bzw. Biospiezangenspitze erfolgt in drei aufeinanderfolgenden Schritten. Im ersten Schritt wird der Suchbereich auf den abgebildeten (projizierten) Bronchialbaum eingeschränkt, da bronchoskopische Instrumente sich nur innerhalb der Bronchien befinden können. Dazu wird die C-Bogen Pose, die nach jeder Bewegung des Systems mit Hilfe einer Markerplatte berechnet wird [1], genutzt, um den im präoperativen CT segmentierten Bronchialbaum auf das aktuelle Fluoroskopie-Frame virtuell zu projizieren. Dieser Bereich definiert dann den Suchbereich für die folgenden beiden Schritte. Zuvor werden auch die Marker der Platte virtuell abgebildet und danach die tatsächlich abgebildeten Marker aus dem aktuellen Frame mit einer Inpainting-Methode entfernt [7]. Ansonsten würden die Marker der Platte die Detektionsmethode irreführen. Die Instrumentenspitze erscheint stets etwas dunkler, d.h. blobartiger, als der Instrumentenschlauch und wird deshalb mit einer Blob-Detektionsmethode basierend auf der Determinante der Hesse-Matrix nach [6] gefunden. Schlauchartige Strukturen werden mit Hilfe des sogenannten mittleren Krümmungsbildes unter Verwendung der gerichteten 1. und 2. Ableitungen des Gauss-Kernels erkannt (Abb. 1(b) (blau)). Im letzten Schritt werden die Spitzen- und Schlauchkandidaten, unter Beachtung bestimmter Kriterien bezüglich Winkel und Länge, zusammengefügt. Falls mehrere längliche Strukturen und deren Spitzen detektiert wurden, muss der Arzt die korrekte Spitze manuell auswählen.

2.2 Tracking

Nun können die Kontur und Position der detektierten Spitze verwendet werden, um eine nächstgelegene und möglichst ähnliche Struktur auch auf den folgenden Frames zu erkennen und somit zu verfolgen. Es ist zu beachten, dass auch auf diesen Folge-Frames die Marker durch Inpainting entfernt werden müssen. Da sich deren Position aber nicht verändert hat, können die entsprechenden Bereiche einfach kopiert werden. Dabei auftretende Ungenauigkeiten aufgrund der Atembewegung beeinflussen das Tracking nur geringfügig. Auch in diesem Schritt kann zudem der Suchbereich auf die virtuelle Bronchialbaum-Projektion reduziert werden. Das Verfolgen der Instrumentenspitze erfolgt modellbasiert, d.h., es wird zunächst ein Konturenmodell der vorher detektierten Spitze erstellt und dann in einem kleinen Suchbereich um die aktuelle Position herum nach einer möglichst ähnlichen Struktur gesucht. Auf diese beiden Komponenten des Verfahren, Konturenmodell-Generierung und Konturenmodell-Suche, soll nun eingegangen werden. Während die Generierung einmalig zu Beginn erfolgt, wird die Suche danach auf jedem Frame erneut durchgeführt.

Konturenmodell-Generierung Aufgrund der bekannten aktuellen Position der Spitze wird ein Bereich um diesen Punkt generiert, welcher möglichst viel der Spitze und einen kleinen Teil der Umgebung, aber möglichst wenige andere Strukturen, beinhaltet. Dazu wird zunächst eine Schwellwertfilterung in einer kleinen quadratischen Umgebung um die detektierte Spitze ausgeführt. Eventuell vorhandene Hohlflächen in dem binären Ergebnisbild werden aufgefüllt und das Ganze nun kreisförmig dilatiert. Die resultierende Bereich wird nun verwendet, um eine Region aus dem Originalbild auszuschneiden, welche dieselbe Form besitzt. Innerhalb dieser Region werden nun aufgrund lokaler Grauwertdifferenzen (Grauwertkonstrast) die Punkte ausgewählt, die signifikante Merkmale der relevanten Struktur darstellen. Es findet also letztlich eine Trennung zwischen Instrumentenspitze und Hintergrund statt. Die resultierende Kontur der Instrumentenspitze wird nun als Konturenmodell im Folgenden verwendet (Abb. 1(c)).

Konturenmodell-Suche Bevor die eigentliche Suche beginnt, wird ein quadratischer Bereich um die aktuelle Spitzenposition ausgewählt, in dem nach dem vorher erstellten Konturenmodell gesucht werden soll. Dieser Bereich wird nach jeder erfolgreichen Suche an der neuen gefundenen Position orientiert. Für jeden Frame wird das Suchfenster also in seiner Positionierung angepasst. Bei der Suche werden auch mögliche Rotationen des Modells berücksichtigt. Die Position der Struktur, die am besten auf das Konturenmodell passt, wird dann mitsamt einer Bewertung und des Rotationswinkels des Modells zurückgegeben. Die Bewertungszahl dient als Maß dafür, welcher Anteil des Konturenmodells im Bild gefunden wurde. Der zurückgelieferte Rotationswinkel wird dazu verwendet, um das Suchfenster im nächsten Frame entsprechend zu drehen.

3   Ergebnisse

Die vorgestellte Methode zur Detektion und Verfolgung einer Bronchoskopspitze wurde an einem Bronchialbaum-Phantom aus Polyurethan getestet. Das Bron-

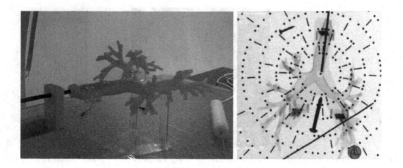

Abb. 2. Links: C-Bogen mit Bronchialbaummodell auf Markerplatte, Bronchoskop und weiteren metallischen Objekten im Bildbereich. Rechts: Erstes Frame der kontinuierlichen Fluoroskopie des Versuchsaufbaus.

chialbaum-Modell wurde mitsamt eines Gestells auf der Markerplatte platziert, welche wiederum auf dem Patiententisch eines Ziehm RFD C-Bogens mit Flachbettdetektor positioniert wurde. In der Nähe des Modells wurden auch einige metallische Objekte positioniert, um nicht-bronchoskopische Operationswerkzeuge zu simulieren. Dann wurde ein Bronchoskop etwa 15 cm in die Trachea des Bronchialbaum-Modells eingeführt und wieder unter C-Bogen-Durchleuchtung herausgezogen. Die gesamte Bronchoskopbewegung wurde so in einem Fluoroskopie-Video festgehalten. Der Versuchsaufbau ist in Abb. 2(a) zu sehen. Das erste Frame des Videos (Abb. 2(b)) wurde nun verwendet, um die C-Bogen Pose aufgrund des abgebildeten Markermusters zu bestimmen. Diese Pose wurde für die Generierung einer virtuellen Bronchialbaumprojektion (Abb. 3(b)) und die Entfernung der Marker aus dem Bild (Abb. 3(a)) genutzt.

Im nächsten Schritt wurde eine automatische Detektion der Bronchoskopspitze durchgeführt. Das Ergebnis ist in Abb. 3(c) (grün) zu sehen. Nach Starten des Videos wurden die Marker auf jedem der 400 folgenden Frames entfernt. Hierzu wurde aber nicht erneut durch die Inpainting-Methode interpoliert, sondern einfach das Inpainting-Ergebnis des ersten Frames übernommen. Dies ist möglich, da die Position der Marker sich nicht und ihre Umgebung sich nur sehr wenig verändert haben. Auf diese Weise kann die Ausführungszeit erheblich reduziert werden. Nach Entfernung der Marker wurde ausgehend von der initialen Detektion, die Bronchoskopspitze nach der beschriebenen Methode weiterverfolgt. Dabei wurde in jedem Frame die aktuelle Position durch ein grünes Rechteck um die Spitze herum gekennzeichnet (Abb. 4). So konnte visuell beurteilt werden, auf welchen Frames das Tracking erfolgreich war. Die visuelle Inspektion ergab, dass die Bronchoskopspitze kontinuierlich korrekt verfolgt werden konnte. Auch an schwierigen Stellen, an denen Überlagerungen durch das Bronchialbaum-Gestell auftraten (Abb. 4(c)), hat das Tracking erfolgreich funktioniert. Die Ausführungszeit des Tracking-Schritts für die einzelnen Frames betrug im Schnitt 29, 5 ms auf einem Intel Core i7 2.93 GHz-Rechner. Damit ist mit einer möglichen Framerate von über 30 fps Echtzeit-Verarbeitung gewährleistet.

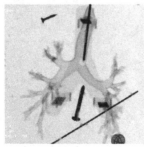 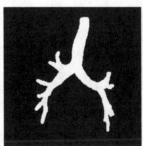 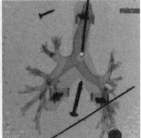

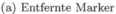 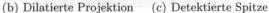

(a) Entfernte Marker   (b) Dilatierte Projektion   (c) Detektierte Spitze

Abb. 3. Vorverarbeitungsschritte des ersten Frames der kontinuierlichen Fluoroskopie.

Abb. 4. Tracking der Bronchoskopspitze (grün) auf kontinuierlicher Fluoroskopie.

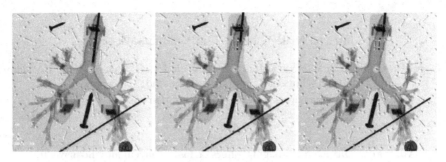

4 Diskussion

Die Ergebnisse des Experiments am Bronchialbaummodell zeigen, dass die Methode prinzipiell sowohl robust und genau als auch echtzeitfähig ist. Die Methode konnte auch eine Vielzahl falscher Instrumente, die ebenfalls auf dem Bild sichtbar waren, automatisch ausschließen. Das Tracking der Spitze funktionierte schnell und präzise. Die nur oberflächlich entfernten Marker auf der Fluoroskopie haben das Tracking-Ergebnis nicht merklich negativ beeinflusst.

Es wurde eine Methode zur Detektion und Verfolgung von Operationsinstrumenten auf kontinuierlicher Fluoroskopie vorgestellt, die erstmals an die Anforderungen einer bronchoskopischen Navigation angepasst ist und die Berechnung der C-Bogen Pose nutzt. Diese Methode stellt den letzten Baustein für das Bronchoskopie-Navigationssystem ohne EM-Tracker dar und komplettiert dieses somit. Im nächsten Schritt muss die Methode als auch das gesamte System auf klinischen Daten getestet und evaluiert werden.

Literaturverzeichnis

1. Steger T, et al. Navigated bronchoscopy using intraoperative fluoroscopy and preoperative CT. Proc IEEE Int Symp Biomed Imaging. 2012; p. 1220–3.
2. Bismuth V, et al. Curvilinear structure enhancement with the polygonal path image–application to guide-wire segmentation in X-ray fluoroscopy. Med Image Comput Comput Assist Interv. 2012;15:9–16.
3. Sun K, et al. Morphological multiscale enhancement, fuzzy filter and watershed for vascular tree extraction in angiogram. J Med Syst. 2011;35:811–24.
4. Yatziv L, et al. Toward multiple catheters detection in fluoroscopic image guided interventions. IEEE Trans Inf Technol Biomed. 2012;16(4):770–81.
5. Honnorat N, et al. Guide-wire extraction through perceptual organization of local segments in fluoroscopic images. Med Image Comput Assist Interv. 2010;13:440–8.
6. Ma Y, et al. Real-time x-ray fluoroscopy-based catheter detection and tracking for cardiac electrophysiology interventions. Med Phys. 2013;40(7):071902.
7. Steger T, et al. Marker Removal for C-arm Pose Estimation based Bronchoscope Navigation using Image Inpainting. Biomed Tech (Berl). 2013.

Enhanced Shadow Detection for 3D Ultrasound

Matthias Noll[1,2], Julian Puhl[1], Stefan Wesarg[1]

[1]Cognitive Computing & Medical Imaging, Fraunhofer IGD, Darmstadt, Germany
[2]GRIS, Technische Universität Darmstadt, Germany
matthias.noll@igd.fraunhofer.de

Abstract. Ultrasound imaging offers a fast, convenient and save instrument to conduct patient examinations for various medical scenarios. However, depending on the target region, occluding bone segments and other materials cause large and undesirable shadowing artifacts. Thus, the experience of the ultrasound operator is crucial for obtaining an ultrasound without artifacts for patient diagnosis. Even more so, when applying automated image processing algorithms. We therefore like to introduce our automatic 3D ultrasound shadow detection method that employs scan line energy and local image entropy information. Applying the method can help to prevent low quality image acquisitions with large shadowing artifacts by indicating shadow occurrences.

1 Introduction

Ultrasound is a widespread medical imaging system that provides a fast, non-invasive and non-hazardous way to obtain patient anatomy information. However, in dealing with ultrasound, challenges like speckle, a poor signal-to-noise ratio and various imaging artifacts have to be addressed [1]. Ultrasound shadow artifacts are a particularly interesting problem. They occur at interfaces that reflect and/or absorb a significant portion of the ultrasound beam. The appearance of a shadow artifact is usually a black cone shaped region, distal to the interface and contains no valid tissue information. Ideally, their occurrence should be prevented during image acquisition, which can be achieved by indicating shadow areas and accordingly repositioning of the ultrasound transducer. If this is not feasible, image post-processing algorithms should indicate or remove shadow areas from the region of interest. This is especially desirable when applying automated ultrasound analysis algorithms, because considering shadow regions during calculation can improve processing results. In the literature, relatively few methods were proposed that deal with ultrasound shadows. Recent publications are [2, 3] where random walks and adaptive thresholding are utilized to detect shadows. In [4], the authors have proposed a shadow detection method using a combination of an image noise model and a signal rupture criterion along transducer scan lines. We have adopted and modified this 2D approach for 3D ultrasound images. During the adoption the processing result was further enhanced by adding additional ultrasound shadow characteristics.

2   Materials and methods

2.1   Transducer model extraction

To achieve the detection of ultrasound shadow artifacts we have implemented a basic 3D ultrasound scan line simulation model. Ultrasound transducer beams are spatial and expand, when out of scan focus. For the simulation model we assume a linear increase in the transducer beam circumference. This model behavior was introduced by using a scan line radius that depends on the total number of simulated scan lines. The radius is chosen so that neighboring scan lines will not overlap after an initial depth of $2 - 3\,cm$, which is equivalent to the ultrasound near-field and thus commonly comprised of artifacts. Starting with a new 3D ultrasound data set (Fig. 1 (d)) and an unknown transducer setup, we first extract the ultrasound tissue mask from the recorded volume to omit background pixels with no tissue information. Afterward, the transducer surface points are extracted through top-down volume iteration until arriving at the tissue mask. For 3D acquisitions this procedure must be applied to each volume slice to cover the entire concave transmission surface of curved ultrasound transducers. The probe geometry is then derived from the detected transducer surface points. By applying the transducer geometry, arbitrary scan lines can be emitted into the general ultrasound propagation directions, thereby simulating transducer beams (Fig. 1 (e)). During simulation, the scan line values are extracted by calculating the median value of the image neighborhood given by the beams circumference at each scan line index.

2.2   Shadow detection

Following the transducer geometry computation we apply a 3D adaption of the statistical shadow detection method described in [4]. Applying the methods local symmetric entropy criterion $\mathcal{R}$ (rupture criterion) to each simulated scan line we find all signal ruptures, where each rupture is a possible shadow start location. For the rupture detection, a sliding window of 5 pixels proved to be a

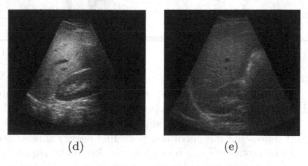

(d)   (e)

Fig. 1. An ultrasound acquisition (d) and a scan line simulation with 150 transducer scan lines (e) shown for the XY image direction of a 3D ultrasound.

sound search range. Analogue to it's 2D implementation the data set is divided into three dimensional blocks of $5 \times 5 \times 5$ pixels, which increases the local tissue information and reduces the variance between all σ estimation results. The final shadow detection test, $(V)(u_f) < \mathbb{E}(u_f) \cdot \sigma^2$ with $\mathbb{E}(u_f)$ being the mean and $(V)(u_f)$ being the variance of the scan line intensities after a detected rupture, is then performed for each previously detected ruptures. The result of the method is a 3D gray scale image analog to the original 2D method, where tissue is set to intensity value 255, shadow respectively to 0 (Fig. 2 (c)).

A weakness of the approach is, that the shadow detection test only fails, if the remaining scan line signal does not contain any further tissue information. This assumption holds for fluids and the core shadow (center line of e.g. strong rib shadow) but not for shadow artifacts in general. Neighboring transducer beams usually introduce some information to shadow regions through ultrasound wave dispersion. An example of this behavior can be seen in Fig. 2 (a) and (c). Here, the rib shadow (left side) starts at near surface depth. But tissue information can still be found at some distance below the kidney. Only then, the shadow test fails in close proximity of the lower image border (Fig. 2 (c)).

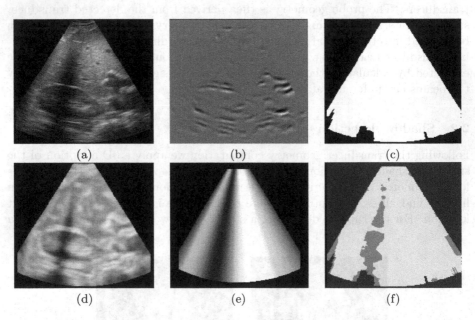

Fig. 2. (a) shows a rib shadow occurring in an eFAST kidney scan. Visible are the kidney (bottom left) and liver with vessels (top). (b) visualizes the smoothed rupture criterion calculated for 150 simulated scan lines. (c) is the detected shadow mask applying the adopted shadow detection approach [4]. (d) shows the local entropy feature image. (e) represents the maximum scan line energy image, derived from the accumulated scan line intensities. (f) represents the improved shadow detection mask of the proposed method with gray values being newly detected shadow regions.

2.3   Detection enhancement

To improve the detection result, we need an additional criterion to enlarge the shadow region (0) or reduce the tissue region (255). First we introduce a new value (127), which marks a possible shadow candidate.

In [5], the authors showed that the local entropy can be used to differentiate between ultrasound tissue regions with different brightness. We've adopted the findings of Zimmer et al. and compute the local entropy image (Fig. 2 (d)) of the input data. For the calculation we use a neighborhood radius of 3 pixels and a Rayleigh probability distribution function. Additionally the maximum possible entropy value is calculated to obtain percentaged entropy thresholds. Now, simple thresholding is not the ideal approach because we either generate undersegmentation in shadow regions or oversegmentation in tissue regions, as can be observed in Fig. 3. Thus, additional adjustments are required.

Further examining the simulated scan line intensity values, we see a significant intensity reduction for scan lines residing in a core shadow or its circumference. Thus, introducing an additional feature for low intensity scan lines and adapting the algorithm output accordingly should improve the shadow detection result. A good measure for low intensity scan lines is the image energy. We have integrated an energy measure to the transducer model by calculating the accumulated intensity profile for each scan line. Investigating the simulated scan line data, we only consider the last accumulation value, providing the total energy of each scan line (Fig. 2 (e)). Following the energy calculation, possible shadow regions are separated from viable regions by applying an additional threshold step with the median of all total energy values.

After the successful region separation, we are able to apply two additional information thresholds to the entropy image. In regions where the ultrasound image intensity is above the median energy we apply a relaxed threshold of 13%, otherwise 16%. Generally speaking in low energy regions, more entropy information is utilized to enlarge shadow regions. The result (Fig. 2 (f)) clearly offers allot more shadow information compared to the original method (Fig. 2 (c)). The applied thresholds were determined using brute force methods on all available ultrasound images. Therefore, the threshold should be adjusted to work well for other ultrasound devices.

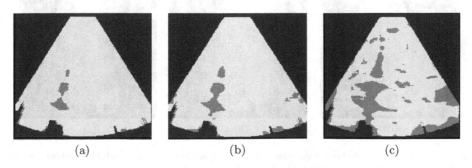

(a)   (b)   (c)

Fig. 3. The entropy based shadow relaxation for 13% (a), 14% (b), and 16% (c).

3   Results

Fig. 4 shows our shadow detection method for 3D ultrasound images. Representatively, we have selected one image for each of three major shadow artifact classes: minor (a), medium (b) and severe (c). The first row shows the recorded ultrasound that serves as the input for the shadow detection algorithm. The second row represents the shadow detection result employing our method, with white (255) being useful tissue information, gray (127) being (presumably) additional shadow areas, that should be prevented or excluded during image processing, and black (0) being explicit shadow areas.

The introduced enhancement algorithm produced all gray (127) mask values, thereby providing new shadow information ((d), (e) and (f)). Prior to the enhancement the original method just detected tissue (255) values (Fig. 2(c) and (f)). One can clearly see, that for all of the three classes shown in Fig. 4 and the algorithm pipeline overview in Fig. 2, a significant improvement in shadow detection was achieved. In some areas of medium and severe shadow images a slight over segmentation can be observed. We believe this can be reduced by further tuning the algorithm parameters. Qualitative evaluation was further performed on 4 data sets using the segmentation assessment in [6]. We compared all segmented shadow regions of our method and the original method to a ground truth segmentation. While all results increased slightly for our method, we dramatically improvement the average relative absolute volume difference, with 0 being a perfect segmentation (Tab. 1). To note, using different process-

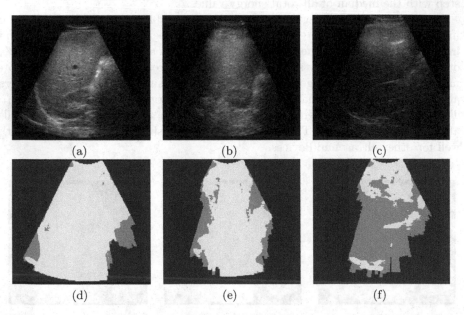

(a)   (b)   (c)

(d)   (e)   (f)

Fig. 4. Detection matrix with the input ultrasound (a)–(c) and the detection results (d)–(f) of the proposed method for minor, medium and severe shadow artifacts.

Table 1. Ground truth evaluation of the proposed method. For the first 5 entries a zero value is equivalent to a perfect segmentation result.

Method ∅	Original	Proposed
Volumetric Overlap Error [%]	19.4796	17.3241
Relative Absolute Volume Difference[%]	18.3091	-0.6448
Average Symmetric Surface Distance [mm]	0.3153	0.2462
RMS Symmetric Surface Distance [mm]	0.5403	0.4030
Maximum Symmetric Surface Distance [mm]	3.9013	3.2374
MICCAI Average Score	63.6917	79.3417

ing parameters the proposed method can still be applied to 2D ultrasound data and offers real time performance with an average of 24 fps.

4   Discussion

We have presented a 3D adaption of a literature 2D shadow detection method that was further enhanced by a combination of scan line energy and local image entropy information. A transducer model was derived automatically from the algorithm input data. Transducer scan lines were simulated using the presented enhancement method to enable shadow detection. Experiments showed a significantly improved shadow detection that outperforms the adopted literature approach. Future work will investigate further detection enhancement by distinguishing fluids from shadows in possible shadow areas.

References

1. Loizou C, Pattichis CS, Istepanian R, et al. Ultrasound image quality evaluation. IEEE Inf Technol Appl Biomed. 2003; p. 138–41.
2. Karamalis A, Wein W, Klein T, et al. Ultrasound confidence maps using random walks. Med Image Anal. 2012;16(6):1101–12.
3. Basij M, Moallem P, Yazdchi M, et al. Automatic shadow detection in intra vascular ultrasound images using adaptive thresholding. Proc IEEE Int Conf Syst Man Cybern. 2012; p. 2173–7.
4. Hellier P, Coupe P, Meyer P, et al. Acoustic shadows detection, application to accurate reconstruction of 3D intraoperative ultrasound. Proc IEEE ISBI. 2008; p. 1569–72.
5. Zimmer Y, Akselrod S, Tepper R. The distribution of the local entropy in ultrasound images. Ultrasound Med Biol. 1996;22(4):431–9.
6. van Ginneken B, Heimann T, Styner M. 3D segmentation in the clinic: a grand challenge. Proc MICCAI. 2007;10:7–15.

Respiratory Motion Estimation Using a 3D Diaphragm Model

Marco Bögel[1,2], Christian Riess[1,2], Andreas Maier[1], Joachim Hornegger[1], Rebecca Fahrig[2]

[1]Pattern Recognition Lab, FAU Erlangen-Nürnberg
[2]Department of Radiology, Lucas MRS Center, Stanford University, Palo Alto, CA, USA
marco.boegel@informatik.stud.uni-erlangen.de

Abstract. Long acquisition times of several seconds lead to image artifacts in cardiac C-arm CT. These artifacts are mostly caused by respiratory motion. In order to improve image quality, it is important to accurately estimate the breathing motion that occurred during image acquisition. It has been shown that diaphragm motion is correlated to the respiration-induced motion of the heart. We present a method to estimate an accurate three-dimensional (3D) model of the diaphragm and its compression motion field from a set of C-arm CT projection images acquired during free breathing. First results on the digital XCAT phantom are promising. The method is able to estimate the motion field amplitude exactly. The boundaries of the estimated compression motion field are estimated within 3 mm accuracy.

1 Introduction

C-arm CT enables reconstruction of 3D images during medical procedures. However, long acquisition times of several seconds, during which the heart is beating and the patient might breathe, may lead to image artifacts, such as motion blurring or streaks. A widely used technique to reduce breathing motion is the single breath-hold scan. The physician instructs the patient to hold his breath after expiration. Projection images are acquired during a single breath-hold. Although this approach is widely used, multiple studies have shown that breath-holding does not eliminate breathing motion entirely and there is significant residual motion. Monitoring the position of the right hemidiaphragm during breath-hold, Jahnke et al. observed residual breathing motion to a certain extent for almost half their test group [1]. Therefore, it is necessary to develop methods to estimate and compensate for respiratory motion in cardiac C-arm CT.

There are many ways to estimate respiratory signals. Many are based on additional hardware, e.g. Time of Flight- or stereo vision-cameras. Other techniques aim to extract the respiratory signal directly from the projection images. Image-based respiratory motion extraction often relies on tracking of fiducial markers in the projection images [2, 3]. Wang et al. have shown that the motion of the diaphragm is highly correlated to respiration-induced motion of the

heart [4]. Sonke et al. propose to extract a 1D breathing signal by projecting diaphragm-like features on the cranio-caudal axis and to select the features
with the largest temporal change [5]. Similar techniques using diaphragm tracking in projection images have been proposed recently [6, 7]. Motion estimation
approaches based on the diaphragm motion are limited as they only take into
account the motion at the diaphragm top. With the presented approach we aim
to use the whole diaphragm surface to measure respiratory motion.

2 Materials and methods

We propose a method to estimate diaphragm motion as a compression motion
field in two optimization steps. First we do an initial estimation which will yield
a reconstruction with reasonably good diaphragm-lung contrast, which is then
used to segment the diaphragm. The acquired diaphragm model is utilized in the
second step to register the model to the projection images. For reconstruction
we use a voxel-driven motion-compensated reconstruction algorithm by Schäfer
et al. [8]. A flow diagram of the proposed method is provided in Fig. 1.

2.1 Initial estimation

In this method we assume that respiratory diaphragm motion can be modelled
as a compression motion field. During inspiration the diaphragm is compressed,
however respiratory motion is limited by a fixed lower plane where no motion
occurs. Therefore, to lower parts of the diaphragm surface less motion is applied
than to the diaphragm top. The top of the diaphragm at expiration state defines
an upper border for the compression field.

In order to estimate a compression motion field, we need to estimate a lower
and upper border of the motion field, as well as the motion amplitude that is
measured at the upper border. We use a diaphragm-tracking algorithm from
previous work [7] to acquire some prior information. We can get the 3D position of the diaphragm top for each projection by triangulation of the diaphragm

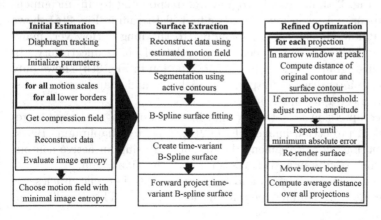

Fig. 1. Diagram of the proposed algorithm.

vertices, as well as a 1D motion signal using only the z-coordinates of the triangulated points. Additionally we also get a segmentation of the diaphragm in 2D projection space.

Afterwards, the 1D motion field that was acquired through diaphragm tracking is processed to determine the indices of inspiration and expiration. Then, the signal is normalized to a maximum range of $[-1.0, 1.0]$. Additionally, we choose the upper border of the compression field as the triangulated 3D world coordinate position of the diaphragm during expiration. To account for triangulation errors we choose the upper plane slightly above the triangulated point.

Optimizing the motion field requires a large number of reconstructions using different motion fields. In order to reduce computation time we choose to reconstruct very small volumes of 128^3 voxels, with a resolution of $2.0\,\frac{mm}{voxel}$. As we show in this work, this is sufficient to evaluate the diaphragm and lung contrast using image entropy.

Using prior knowledge we reduce the search space for the optimal scale to a small window of $10\,mm$ around the absolute maximum magnitude of the triangulated signal. The search space for lower borders can be narrowed down based on the visibility of the diaphragm in the projections. We chose a relatively large step size of approximately 10% of the volume size for the lower border.

In order to assess the image quality we chose an ROI centered around the diaphragm top. We measure how badly the diaphragm-lung interface is blurred using the image entropy. We choose a relatively narrow ROI of $4\,cm$ diameter. The height of the ROI spans the lower half of the volume. For the proposed 128^3 voxel volume with $2.0\,\frac{mm}{voxel}$ resolution, this results in an ROI of $40 \times 40 \times 128\,mm$. The center of this ROI is the triangulated top of the diaphragm at expiration state. The Shannon entropy is a measure of uncertainty

$$H(X) = -\sum_{i=1}^{N} p(x_i) \cdot \ln(p(x_i)) \tag{1}$$

In order to get the probabilities $p(x_i)$ for each intensity value x_i, a histogram over the intensities in the ROI is computed. In our implementation we chose to use 100 bins. Fig. 2 shows two histograms corresponding to an uncompensated and a compensated reconstruction. The first histogram in Fig. 2(a) shows one large peak at low intensities corresponding to the lungs. However, many intensities are similarly frequent, which means relatively high uncertainty. In comparison, the histogram of the correct reconstruction in Fig. 2(b) shows only two large peaks at intensities corresponding to lungs and diaphragm. Thus, there is very low uncertainty in the image.

We use the compression field that results in the best image entropy to reconstruct the set of projection images of the 2D segmented diaphragm. Based on this reconstruction we can segment the diaphragm using an active contour segmentation, which results in a 3D surface mesh of the diaphragm.

In order to get a smooth surface and reduce segmentation inaccuracies, we approximate the mesh as a uniform cubic surface B-spline. This B-spline representation allows us to use very efficient projection algorithms to speed up the registration process in the next step.

2.2   Refined optimization

While the initial motion field estimation provided relatively good results, we limited our approach to very small reconstruction volumes in order to reduce computational effort. Our estimation algorithm was able to find a good approximation of the motion field, however, close to the correct motion field, the results of our image entropy measurements are very similar, which is in part caused by the smoothing effect of our small volumes and the relatively large step size we used in the estimation of the lower compression field border. With the following method we aim to refine our estimated compression motion field, using a registration approach.

First, we create a time variant surface B-spline by adding the compression motion field to the B-spline control points. In order to get a good time-resolution a surface B-spline is created in this way for each projection. Afterwards, we want to compute forward projections of this time-variant surface B-spline, using the GPU [9]. With this approach we are able to create one forward projection of our B-spline in approximately $20 - 40$ ms.

Our aim is to register the forward projection of the diaphragm B-spline model to the original projection images that include the respiratory motion, using a very quick contour-based approach. Due to the fact that our new forward projections only contain the diaphragm, contour detection is trivial. With the contours available, we separately estimate the motion magnitude and the lower border of the compression field.

Estimation of motion amplitude. First, we adjust the motion amplitude, so that the tops of the two contours are aligned. In order to determine how to adjust the magnitude, we measure the average distance of the two contours in a narrow window of 40 pixels around the top. If the average distance exceeds a predefined threshold, we adjust the motion field magnitude for this surface B-spline. For the XCAT phantom we chose a threshold of 1 pixel. We can adjust the amplitude either iteratively with a predefined step size, or we can re-project the top points of both contours onto the plane that passes through the

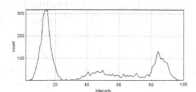
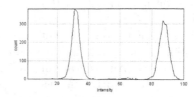

Fig. 2. Histograms of the intensities in the ROI around the diaphragm top of an uncompensated (left) and an optimized (right) reconstruction.

3D diaphragm top of the initial diaphragm tracking and that is parallel to the detector. We can then update the motion field magnitude using the difference of the 3D spline top position and the 3D position of the tracked diaphragm.

Estimation of compression border. After updating the motion field magnitude, the updated time-variant surface B-spline is forward projected again. The peaks of the original and spline contours are now aligned. Now, the slope of the B-spline contour is either too steep or too flat. This can be adjusted by lifting or lowering the lower border of the compression field. We can determine in which direction the lower border has to be moved by looking at the average error distance over all projection images. The lower border is moved by an arbitrary step size in each iteration, until the average error is below a predefined threshold.

3   Results

We evaluated our estimated motion fields on the digital XCAT phantom using projections of a breathing thorax. An acquisition protocol of four seconds with a full respiration cycle with 24 mm diaphragm amplitude was simulated to create 200 projection images of size 640×480 pixels with a resolution of $0.616 \frac{mm}{pixel}$. The compression motion field used in the phantom had the lower boundary placed at -98 mm and the upper diaphragm boundary at -38 mm.

We evaluated the initial estimation on lower boundaries ranging from -179 mm to -75 mm, with a step size of 26 mm. The correct minimum for the motion amplitude was found at 24 mm. We also observed similarly low image entropy at scales close to 24 mm even for incorrect lower borders. The optimal border detected by the initial estimator is located at -101 mm. Using smaller steps of 2 mm, we are not able to further increase the accuracy.

Refining the motion field in this case yields only slight changes at individual projections. Fig. 3 shows reconstruction results for two coronary slices through the two hemidiaphragms. Image contrast at the diaphragm is considerably improved as we observe very clear diaphragm contours, even at the sides.

4   Discussion

As results on the XCAT phantom show, our method allows us to estimate a compression motion field of the diaphragm based on free-breathing C-arm CT projection data. We are able to estimate the amplitude of the diaphragm motion as well as the lower boundary of the compression field. Studies have shown that the motion of the diaphragm is highly correlated to respiration-induced motion of the heart [4]. An accurate motion signal of the diaphragm can be used as a surrogate signal to drive an elastic respiratory motion model of the heart.

The presented method works well with reconstructions of low resolution in order to reduce computational effort. Our initial optimization-based on image entropy works very well, and might possibly be accurate enough in many cases

Fig. 3. Image quality of two coronary slices (left, roght) of a compensated (top) and uncompensated (bottom) reconstruction of the XCAT phantom.

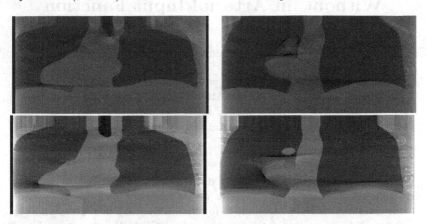

without further refinement, as it is able to estimate the motion amplitude accurately, and the compression boundaries within 3 mm accuracy.

Future work will deal with the interpolation of the diaphragm motion vector field with a respiratory heart motion model, in order to compensate residual breathing motion in breath-hold scans.

References

1. Jahnke C, Paetsch I, Achenbach S, et al. Coronary MR imaging: breath-hold capability and patterns, coronary artery rest periods, and beta-blocker use. Radiology. 2006;239:71–8.
2. Wiesner S, Yaniv Z. Respiratory signal generation for retrospective gating of cone-beam CT images. Proc SPIE. 2008;6918:691817–1–12.
3. Marchant TE, Price GJ, Matuszewiski BJ, et al. Reduction of motion artefacts in on-board cone beam CT by warping of projection images. Br J Radiol. 2011;84:251–64.
4. Wang Y, Riederer S, Ehman R. Respiratory motion of the heart: kinematics and the implications for spatial resolution in coronary imaging. Magn Reson Med. 1995;33:716–9.
5. Sonke JJ, Zijp L, Remeijer P, et al. Respiratory correlated cone beam CT. Med Phys. 2005;32:1176–86.
6. Chen M, Siochi RA. Diaphragm motion quantification in megavoltage cone-beam CT projection images. Med Phys. 2010;37(5):2312–20.
7. Bögel M, Hofmann HG, Hornegger J, et al. Respiratory motion compensation using diaphragm tracking for cone-beam C-arm CT: a simulation and a phantom study. Int J Biomed Imaging. 2013;2013:1–10.
8. Schäfer D, Jandt U, Carroll JD, et al. Motion compensated reconstruction for rotational X-ray angiography using 4D coronary centerline models. Proc Fully 3D. 2007; p. 245–8.
9. Maier A, Hofmann H, Schwemmer C, et al. Fast simulation of X-ray projections of spline-based surfaces using an append buffer. Phys Med Biol. 2012;57(19):6193–210.

Model-Based Parameterestimation in DCE-MRI Without an Arterial Input Function

Constantin Heck[1], Lars Ruthotto[2], Jan Modersitzki[1], Benjamin Berkels[3,1]

[1]Institute of Mathematics and Image Computing, Universität zu Lübeck
[2]Department of Earth, Ocean and Atmospheric Sciences, UBC Vancouver
[3]AICES Graduate School, RWTH Aachen University
constantin.heck@mic.uni-luebeck.de

Abstract. Analysis of DCE-MRI data is often carried out by fitting parametric models. However, one major factor of uncertainty is the determination of the arterial input function (AIF). We introduce a novel approach to estimate kinetic parameters in DCE-MRI without an AIF. An existing method by Riabkov et al., where the AIF is introduced as an additional unknown, is extended by the addition of spatial diffusive regularization of the parameter maps and a control term for the scale of the AIF. We validate our method on artificial data, where it significantly reduces the relative error as compared to the original method by Riabkov. Additionally, we present first promising results on real data.

1 Introduction

The glomular filtration rate (GFR) describes the renal filtration capacity and is thus one of the central parameters for quantifying kidney function and diseases [1]. Therefore, proper measurement of the GFR is of utmost importance. A conventional approach to determine the GFR is via the measurement of serum creatinine [1]. Unfortunately, this approach can only specify one GFR for both kidneys. Dynamic contrast-enhanced (DCE) MRI is a very promising alternative as it enables to measure the GFR for each kidney individually [2, 3]. In order to extract physiological parameters from the data, pharmacokinetic models have proven to be very successful [4]. Here, the contrast agent uptake is modelled as a function parameterized by only a few physiological parameters [4] and a global arterial input function (AIF) describing the concentration of contrast agent in the bloodplasma. Among the parameters usually are the amount of vascularization and the filtration capacity. In this paper, we propose a new method to compute a voxel-wise map displaying the GFR. Although our method can deal with a variety of pharmacokinetic models, for ease of presentation and computation we focus on the so-called Patlak model [5]. The Patlak model has been shown to describe the contrast agent uptake in the kidney in a small time window after injection reasonably well [2]. A well-known challenge of this model fitting approach lies in the dependence of the model on the AIF [6]. As the AIF is also an unknown, it has to be estimated using additional measurements or by introducing an additional model [2, 4, 7]. A different approach to address this issue was proposed in [8], where the AIF was introduced as a further unknown. In this paper, we suggest to extended the approach [8] by adding a diffusion regularizer on the parameter maps as well as a normalization constraint on the AIF and thereby add spatial information. We validate the new regularized method using simulated data where ground truth is available and show its improved robustness against noise as compared to the unregularized method in [8]. Finally, we present first promising results on real data courtesy of Jarle Rørvik from the Haukeland University Hospital in Bergen, Norway.

2 Methods

2.1 Pharmacokinetic modelling

In this paper, we focus on two-compartment pharmacokinetic models [4] and in particular on the Patlak model. Here, one compartment is the blood plasma and the other the extracellular-extravascular space. It is assumed that no outflow takes place. The governing equation of the Patlak model [2] is

$$C(t) = p\, C_{\text{AIF}}(t) + q \int_0^t C_{\text{AIF}}(\tau)\, \mathrm{d}\tau \tag{1}$$

where $p \geq 0$ describes the amount of vascularization, $q \in \mathbb{R}_0^+$ the clearance, i.e. the flow from plasma to extracellular-extravascular space, and $C_{\text{AIF}} : \mathbb{R}_0^+ \to \mathbb{R}_0^+$ is the AIF. One of the difficulties is that the observation starts at a time $t_0 > 0$. We bypass this difficulty by introducing the delay parameter $d := \int_0^{t_0} C_{\text{AIF}}(\tau)\, \mathrm{d}\tau$, such that (1) yields our model

$$C(t) = p\, C_{\text{AIF}}(t) + qd + q \int_{t_0}^t C_{\text{AIF}}(\tau)\, \mathrm{d}\tau =: M(p, q, d, C_{\text{AIF}}, t), \quad t \geq t_0 \tag{2}$$

Note that conceptually, the delay d depends on C_{AIF}. However, as we are only interested in C_{AIF} for $t \geq t_0$, we can confine to a simple scalar parameter instead. A well-known property of most two-compartment models is their dependency on scale [8]: rescaling C_{AIF} and d by some parameter f, and q and p by $1/f$ leads to the same observation C. Without additional knowledge it is thus impossible to uniquely recover p, q, d and C_{AIF} from a given C. We will address this issue in more detail in the next section.

2.2 Parameter estimation

We assume that discrete measurements of C are available. More precisely, we have a time-series of K different MRI measurements at time points t_k and n locations x_i. Let $T = (t_0, \ldots, t_{K-1})$ denote the vector of time points, then for each voxel x_i, we want to find parameters such that $C(x_i, T) \approx M(p_i, q_i, d, A, T)$, where $C(x_i, T)$ denotes the time discrete measurements at voxel x_i, p_i and q_i

denote the spatially dependent Patlak-parameters, d as above, and $A := C_{AIF}(T)$ is the global time discrete AIF. As for all compartment models, it is assumed that there is one global AIF for all compartments. Following the approach in [3], we neglect local delays in the arrival time and assume the AIF to be constant for all voxels. Note that we also replace the integration in (2) by a trapezoidal rule, assuming the AIF to be sufficiently smooth. The goal is to minimize the objective function $J : \mathbb{R}^n \times \mathbb{R}^n \times \mathbb{R} \times \mathbb{R}^K \to \mathbb{R}$

$$
J(p,q,d,A) := \sum_{i=1}^{n} \|C(x_i, T) - M(p_i, q_i, d, A, T)\|^2 \\
+ \alpha_1 \|\nabla p\|^2 + \alpha_2 \|\nabla q\|^2 + \alpha_3 (I(d, A) - 1)^2
$$

(3)

subject to $p, q, d, A \geq 0$ (non-negativity constraints). The first summand is the data fitting term, the second and third term are regularizations enforcing smooth parameter maps and the last term enforces the discrete integral of the AIF to be one. We use an L_2-type data fitting term as we expect a Gaussian type noise in the data. Due to a relatively low spatial resolution, partial volume effects, and additional motion blur of our data we assume the smoothed regularization to be appropriate. To account for the scale dependency mentioned in the final remark of Section 2.1, we added the penalty on $I(r, A)$. Of course, various modifications of this model are possible. For explicit computations we use the trapezoidal rule, $I(r, A) = d + \sum_{k=1}^{K-1} (A_k + A_{k-1})(t_k - t_{k-1})/2$. We implemented the minimization of (3) with a standard Gauss-Newton optimization with Armijo line search. In addition, the non-negativity constraints were implemented as projections onto the set of feasible points.

3   Results

In a first step, we show results for a controlled environment, where the true solution is known. Here, we use a software phantom to create numerical data from given parameter maps and added various amounts of white Gaussian noise, as expected in the data. With the arithmetic mean $\mu(C)$ and the noise standard deviation σ_{Noise}, we use $SNR := \mu(C)/\sigma_{Noise}$ as an indicator of quality. We compared our results by the following relative error and relative standard deviation $RE(q) := \|q_{true} - q\|_2 / \|q_{true}\|_2$, $SD(q) := \sigma_{(q_{true}-q)}/\mu(q_{true})$. We compared our method to the constrained version of the unregularized method proposed in [8], which is most closely related.

3.1   Software phantom data

We simulated 11679 uptake curves with a software phantom using the AIF measured by Parker et al. [7] and the Patlak model. Motivated by kidney data from the Haukeland clinic, we set the parameters for the two regions constantly to $p = 0.08$, $q = 0.25$ and $p = 0.01$, $q = 0.16$, respectively. To simulate the smooth structure within the kidney, the parameter maps were smoothed with a Gaussian

Table 1. Reconstruction results for software phantom data, 11,679 spatial locations, 16 time points. The relative errors and standard deviations of the parameter maps p and q obtained by the method of [8] and the new regularized method are summarized.

Unregularized model [8]	RE(p)	SD(p)	RE(q)	SD(q)
SNR = 7	0.1488	0.0990	0.1994	0.1307
SNR = 10	0.0969	0.0658	0.1024	0.0740
no noise	0.0361	0.0189	0.0132	0.0071
Regularized approach	RE(p)	SD(p)	RE(q)	SD(q)
SNR = 7	0.0667	0.0637	0.0770	0.0740
SNR = 10	0.0710	0.0478	0.0467	0.0477
no noise	0.6702	0.3393	0.4716	0.2507

filter. The result is displayed in Fig. 1. The uptake curves were generated in a time interval $[0\,\mathrm{s}, 40\,\mathrm{s}]$ at a time resolution of 0.1 s. Afterwards the MR measurements were simulated by taking only every 25th value, which corresponds to a measurement every 2.5 s. White Gaussian noise was added to the simulated uptake curves at various signal-to-noise ratios (SNRs). Given the mentioned parameters, stable reconstruction with a relative error less than 10% was possible up to a noise level of SNR = 7, distorting the uptake curves in the second region almost completely. Representative examples of these simulations are shown in Fig. 3.1. The regularization parameters were determined experimentally and were fixed at $\alpha_1 = 3.75, \alpha_2 = 1, \alpha_3 = 1$. In order to remove the dependency on scale, we renormalized the integral of the estimated AIF after the calculation to be the same as the integral of the AIF of the ground truth. Results are displayed

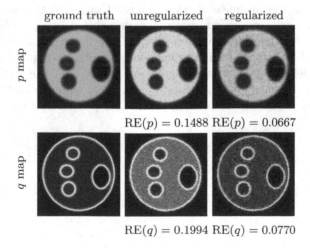

Fig. 1. Reconstruction of p and q maps by the unregularized method [8] compared to the new regularized method. Phantom data with SNR = 7.

in Fig. 1 and Tab. 1. The results for the regularized approach without noise are most likely problems of the employed optimization algorithm and are subject to current investigations.

3.2   Clinical data

One healthy human volunteer was scanned on a 1.5T MRI system (Siemens Avanto, Siemens, Erlangen, Germany) using a TWIST sequence after injection of 4ml MultiHance injected as a bolus at a rate of 3ml/s. A time sequence of 49 images with variable spacing between 2.5 s and 60 s was acquired. The DCE-MRI images were registered and contrast agent concentrations were calculated from the MRI data. Afterwards, the kidney medulla and the cortex were segmented. For details on the scan and the postprocessing pipeline [9]. We employed our new regularized method to calculate the 3D parameter maps for p and q as well as the AIF. The results are shown in Fig. 3. The results were normalized such that $I(r, A) = 1$. Due to the dependency of our model on scale, we confined to a visual evaluation. Clear to see is that the distribution of the amount of vascularization p is sharper as compared to the filtration parameters q. A cause for this can lie in the distinguished distribution of blood vessels. Given the regularization parameters, which were optimized for the 2D test case, no major visual differences between the old and the new method can be determined.

4   Discussion

We have proposed a new method to estimate DCE-MRI parameters as well as the AIF. A simulation shows that it is indeed possible to eliminate the dependency of the Patlak model on the AIF and reconstruct the parameter maps up to scale reliably, even in the presence of severe noise. Compared to the unregularized method [8], the relative error in noisy data is reduced by up to 55% for p and by 61% for q. Furthermore, our new method has the great advantage of being easily extendable to other compartment models, different regularization such as TV and time delay or smoothness assumptions on the AIF. Due to the underlying model, our method cannot yet estimate parameters uniquely and thus a proper scaling approach has still to be identified. This problem affects especially the

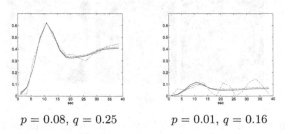

$p = 0.08, q = 0.25$ $p = 0.01, q = 0.16$

Fig. 2. Uptake curves and their reconstructions with our proposed method at SNR = 7.

unregularized method regularized method

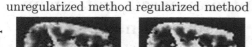

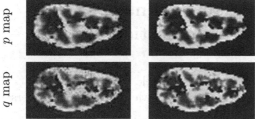

Fig. 3. 3D reconstruction of p and q from the left kidney by the unregularized and the regularized method for kidney data from Haukeland clinic. Slice 34 is shown, regularization parameters are $\alpha_1 = 3.75, \alpha_2 = 1, \alpha_3 = 1$.

evaluation on clinical data. Several options are subject to current investigation to overcome this problem: Prior knowledge of tissue parameters in specific body regions would certainly eliminate the problem. Another approach would be to establish estimates on properties of the AIF, such as its integral. Furthermore, for a more robust processing of clinical data, we are currently elaborating the parameter choice. In summary, we have proposed a new regularized method for reliable voxel-wise GFR estimation in DCE-MRI sequences of kidney data without the need of an auxiliary AIF.

References

1. National Kidney Foundation. K/DOQI clinical practice guidelines for chronic kidney disease. Am J Kidney Dis. 2002;39(2):1–266.
2. Hackstein N, Heckrodt J, Rau WS. Measurement of single-kidney glomerular filtration rate using a contrast-enhanced dynamic gradient-echo sequence and the Rutland-Patlak plot technique. J Magn Reson Imaging. 2003;18(6):714–25.
3. Sourbron SP, Michaely HJ, Reiser MF, et al. MRI-measurement of perfusion and glomerular filtration in the human kidney with a separable compartment model. Invest Radiol. 2007;43(1):40–8.
4. Sourbron SP, Buckley DL. Classic models for dynamic contrast-enhanced MRI. NMR Biomed. 2013;26(8):1004–27.
5. Patlak CSC, Blasberg RGR, Fenstermacher JDJ. Graphical evaluation of blood-to-brain transfer constants from multiple-time uptake data. J Cereb Blood Flow Metab. 1983;3(1):1–7.
6. Mendichovszky IA, Cutajar M, Gordon I. Reproducibility of the aortic input function (AIF) derived from dynamic contrast-enhanced magnetic resonance imaging (DCE-MRI) of the kidneys in a volunteer study. Eur J Radiol. 2009;71(3):576–81.
7. Parker GJM, Roberts C, Macdonald A, et al. Experimentally-derived functional form for a population-averaged high-temporal-resolution arterial input function for dynamic contrast-enhanced MRI. Magn Reson Med. 2006;56(5):993–1000.
8. Riabkov DY, Di Bella EVR. Estimation of kinetic parameters without input functions: analysis of three methods for multichannel blind identification. IEEE Trans Biomed Eng. 2002;49(11):1318–27.
9. Hodneland E, Kjørstad Å, Andersen E, et al. In vivo estimation of glomerular filtration in the kidney using DCE-MRI. Proc ISPA. 2011; p. 755–61.

Vermessung des Mitralapparats mit einem optisch getrackten Zeigeinstrument für die virtuelle Annuloplastie

Sandy Engelhardt[1], Bastian Graser[1], Raffaele De Simone[2],
Nobert Zimmermann[2], Matthias Karck[2], Hans-Peter Meinzer[1], Diana Nabers[1],
Ivo Wolf[1,3]

[1]Abteilung für Medizinische und Biologische Informatik, DKFZ Heidelberg
[2]Klinik für Herzchirurgie, Universitätsklinikum Heidelberg
[3]Institut für Medizinische Informatik, Hochschule Mannheim
sandy.engelhardt@dkfz-heidelberg.de

Kurzfassung. Bei einer OP-Indikation für Mitralklappeninsuffizienz ist die Beurteilung der Pathophysiologie ausschlaggebend, um eine geeignete chirurgische Technik auszuwählen. Eine dieser Techniken stellt das Einnähen eines Annuloplastie-Ringmodells dar, welches in verschiedenen Größen und Formen kommerziell erhältlich ist. Die intraoperative Ringselektion beschränkt sich bisher auf visuelle Begutachtung und auf einfache manuelle Messmethoden. Diese erlauben jedoch keine akkurate Messung der komplexen dreidimensionalen Anatomie der Mitralklappe. Wir schlagen eine neue intraoperativ durchführbare computerassistierte Messmethode vor. Mit Hilfe eines optisch getrackten Zeigeinstrumentes wird die Geometrie der Mitralklappe vermessen. Dabei werden 16 anatomische Landmarken auf dem Mitralapparat angefahren. In einer Studie wiederholten vier Herzchirurgen die Vermessungen jeweils drei mal an einem frisch exzidierten Schweineherz. Anschließend wurden 14 verschiedene Standard-Ringformen mit dem vermessenen Annulus verglichen unter Benutzung einer eigenen automatischen Analyse-Software. In 11 von 12 Fällen wurde der Carpentier-Edwards Physio-Ring als Ring mit der geringsten Abweichung vorgeschlagen. Dies zeigt, dass das Messverfahren eine stabile Ringselektion ermöglicht.

1 Einleitung

Das Konzept der Remodelierungsannuloplastie mit Einsatz von prothetischen Ringen wurde 1968 eingeführt und hat seither den Weg zu rekonstruktiver Klappenchirurgie geebnet [1]. Heute ist die Mitralklappenrekonstruktion eine weit verbreitete und angewandte chirurgische Alternative zum Einsatz von künstlichen Herzklappen. Bei der Rekonstruktion bleibt das natürliche Klappengewebe sowie der subvalvuläre Halteapparat erhalten. Das chirurgische Ergebnis ist in den meisten Fällen dem des Mitralklappenersatzes überlegen, was sich in einer geringeren Sterbe- und Reinterventionsrate widerspiegelt [2].

Transösophageale Echokardiographie (engl. Abkürzung: TEE) wird gewöhnlich als bildgebende Methode benutzt, um den funktionellen Zustand der Klappe vor und nach der Operation aufzuzeigen. Es bietet damit ein essentielles Werkzeug um den Schweregrad der Mitralklappeninsuffizienz perioperativ festzustellen. Im letzten Jahrzehnt sind Bildverarbeitungsalgorithmen entwickelt worden, welche die (semi-)automatische Analyse der TEEs ermöglichen [3, 4]. Dazu gehört die automatische Annuloplastie-Ringselektionen nach Segmentierung des patientenindividuellen Annulus wie Graser et al. [5] aufzeigten. Allerdings ist die TEE-Analyse oft auf den Annulus und die Segel beschränkt. Der subvalvuläre Apparat, bestehend aus den Chordae Tendineae und den Papillarmuskeln, sind auf dem Ultraschall nur schwer zu erkennen. Genau diese Strukturen können jedoch im Fall einer Ruptur einen Prolaps der Segel verursachen.

Aufgrund der Einschränkungen durch die Resultate der bildgebenden Verfahren sind die Chirurgen dazu gezwungen, fundamentale Entscheidungen intraoperativ zu treffen. Daher wird die tatsächliche Rekonstruktionsstrategie erst im Operationsraum ermittelt, unter der Erschwernis eines limitierten Zeitfensters durch den Anschluss der Herzlungenmaschine und der Aortenklemme.

Operative Maßnahmen an der Mitralklappe erfordern hohe Präzision und können deshalb nur vorgenommen werden, wenn sich das geöffnete Herz in einem kardioplegischen Zustand befindet. Damit einhergehend finden in diesem Zustand neben der Exploration der patientspezifischen Mitralklappenpathologie manuelle Messungen in-situ statt, die mit einem konventionellen Sizer-Instrument oder einem Kaliper durchgeführt werden. Ein Sizer ist eine Schablone in der Größe des prothetischen Rings, welcher von dem Chirurgen an den platzierten Kommissuralnähten ausgerichtet über die Klappe gehalten wird. Visuell wird dann entschieden, ob die Schablone zum Patientenannulus passt. Die Genauigkeit der Methode wird von Bothe et al. [6] kontrovers diskutiert, mit dem Hintergrund, dass die Wahl des passenden Ringmodells ein wesentlicher Faktor für die Güte des rekonstruktiven Ergebnisses ist.

Um den Chirurgen während dieser entscheidenden Phase zu unterstützen, schlagen wir eine neue präzise Methode vor, die eine Exploration der patientenindividuellen Klappengeometrie intraoperativ mit einem optischen Trackinggerät ermöglicht. Wichtige anatomische Punkte werden mit einem Zeigeinstrument genau lokalisiert. In einer vorherigen Studie [7] wurde die Machbarkeit und Reproduzierbarkeit der Methode untersucht und morphologisch wichtige Distanzen berechnet. Die Distanzen wurden mit einer mittleren Variabilität von 2.45 ± 0.75 mm zwischen den Experten aufgenommen. Die Abweichungen sind auf den Tremor sowie auf die verschiedenen Interpretationen der anatomischen Variationen zurückzuführen [7]. Ziel dieser Arbeit ist zu zeigen, dass trotz der Abweichungen zwischen den Experten mit dieser Messmethode eine stabile automatische Annuloplastie-Ringauswahl möglich ist.

2   Material und Methoden

Es wurden sechszehn anatomische Punkte in der linken atrioventrikulären Struktur, welche den Mitralapparat umfasst, definiert [7]. Insbesondere wurden Landmarken ausgesucht, die während der Klappenrekonstruktion von Bedeutung sind und beispielsweise bei einer virtuellen Annuloplastie behilflich sein können. Die Vermessungs-Software wurde als Plugin innerhalb des Open Source Software Toolkits Medical Imaging Interaction Toolkit(MITK) [8] realisiert. Dieser Prototyp beeinhaltet Vermessungsschemata, wie der Screenshot in Abb. 1 zeigt.

Die Positionen der Landmarken werden mit einem Zeigeinstrument angefahren, welches durch ein Infrarot-Stereokamerasystem Polaris Spectra (NDI, Ontario, Canada) lokalisiert wird. Das optische Tracking System zeichnet sich durch eine Genauigkeit von 0.35 mm im quadratischen Mittel sowie einer hohen Bandbreite aus [9]. Die Integration des NDI Systems erfolgte über MITK-IGT. Die Messungen wurden auf einem exzidierten pathologisch-unauffälligen Schweineherzen durchgeführt, welches in Abb. 2 gezeigt ist. Das Herz wurde in einer Röhre stabilisiert und durch zwei Holzstäbchen fixiert. Wie bei einer Annuloplastie üblich wurden rund um den Annulus Nähte zur Stabilisierung platziert. Der linke Ventrikel wurde mit Wasser gefüllt, um den systolischen Zustand der Mitralklappe als Ausgangspunkt für die Vermessungen anzunähren. Während der Messungen wurde der Füllungszustand nicht verändert. Vier Herzchirurgen

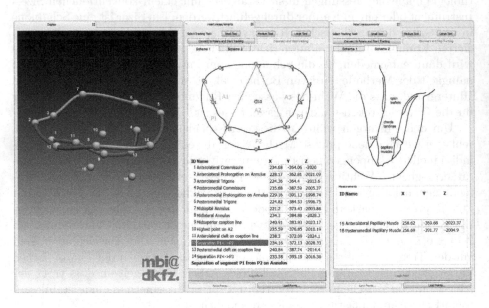

Abb. 1. Das MITK-Plugin Interface: Links ist eine 3D-Ansicht gegeben, welche die Relation der aufgenommenen Punkte zueinander aufzeigt. Das Vorgehen während des Messungen wird durch die Schemas auf der rechten Seite bestimmt (linkes Schema: Merkmale auf Segel und Mitralannulus, rechtes Schema: Spitze der Papillarmuskeln).

Abb. 2. (a) Fixiertes Schweineherz. Der linke Ventrikel ist mit Wasser gefüllt. (b) Messvorgang mit Zeigeinstrument. (c) Carpentier Physio Ring (grün in (d)). (d) Virtuelle Annuloplastie. Die schmalen Kurven stellen die interpolierten Annulusformen aus den drei Messversuchen von Experte 2 dar.

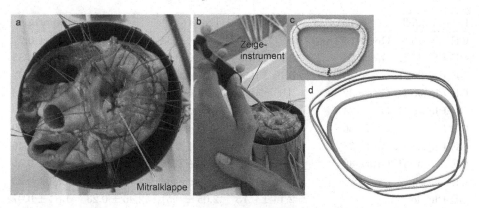

haben anschließend jeweils drei Messversuche an dem Schweineherz nach dem definierten Vermessungsschema (Abb. 1) durchgeführt.

In Bezug auf die Auswertung ist von Interesse, ob bei der automatischen Selektion eines kommerziell erhältlichen Annuloplastie-Rings bei allen Messversuchen der gleiche Vorschlag generiert wird. Eine Ringauswahl wird aufgrund der am wenigsten abweichenden Form zwischen Annulus und Annuloplastie-Ring generiert, da in diesem Fall die geringsten Zugkräften am Annulus erwartet werden [5]. Dafür wurde auf Basis der Punkte 2-3-7-6-5-14-8-12 (Abb. 1) die Form des Mitralannulus durch eine geschlossene Spline-Interpolation rekonstruiert. Eine Liste der 14 Ringmodelle ist in Tab. 1 aufgezeigt. Für eine konkrete Ringauswahl wird eine Fehlermetrik minimiert (Abb. 3): Der Ring wird auf den Abstand der projizierten Kommissurpunkte skaliert (Punkt 2 und 5); dann wird der Ursprung der Kurven errechnet und Ebenen senkrecht zur Annulusebene durch den Mittelpunkt in 10° Schritten mit den Kurven geschnitten. Ausgehend

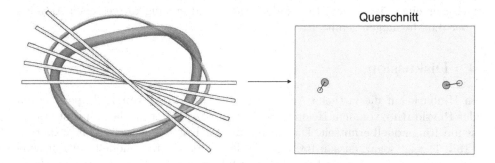

Abb. 3. Berechnung der Abweichung zwischen einem Ringmodell (grün) und dem Annulus (weiß). Im Querschnitt zeigt die gestrichelte Linie die Euklidische Distanz an.

Tabelle 1. Mittelwert und Standardabweichung der mittleren Abweichungen von Schweineherzannulus und einem kommerziell erhältlichen Annuloplastie-Ringmodell (CE = Carpentier-Edwards, CMA = Carpentier-McCarthy-Adams) bei dreimaliger Messung. *variiert je nach Größe in der Form.

Ring Modell	Experte 1	Experte 2	Experte 3	Experte 4
CE Physio II, Größe 26*	3.21 ± 0.33	2.57 ± 0.33	3.6 ± 0.21	2.88 ± 0.27
CE Physio II, Größe 28*	3.7 ± 0.37	2.91 ± 0.25	4.0 ± 0.24	3.25 ± 0.35
CE Physio II, Größe 30*	3.74 ± 0.39	2.98 ± 0.26	4.05 ± 0.22	3.31 ± 0.32
CE Physio II, Größe 32*	2.99 ± 0.25	2.36 ± 0.31	3.21 ± 0.18	2.63 ± 0.43
CE Physio II, Größe 34*	2.98 ± 0.29	2.33 ± 0.30	3.22 ± 0.19	2.63 ± 0.39
CE Physio II, Größe 36*	3.13 ± 0.23	2.41 ± 0.31	3.23 ± 0.24	2.59 ± 0.39
CE Physio II, Größe 38*	3.34 ± 0.37	2.57 ± 0.26	3.56 ± 0.18	2.97 ± 0.46
CE Physio II, Größe 40*	2.99 ± 0.31	2.32 ± 0.28	3.24 ± 0.17	2.68 ± 0.45
CE Classic	3.39 ± 0.08	3.30 ± 0.44	3.74 ± 0.28	2.83 ± 0.23
CE Physio	2.14 ± 0.15	2.05 ± 0.51	2.46 ± 0.23	1.84 ± 0.07
Edwards GeoForm	3.74 ± 0.36	3.52 ± 0.56	3.15 ± 0.43	2.62 ± 0.15
CMA IMR ETlogix	2.90 ± 0.09	2.86 ± 0.52	3.08 ± 0.27	2.35 ± 0.15
Edwards Myxo ETlogix	3.64 ± 0.42	2.86 ± 0.12	4.05 ± 0.25	3.21 ± 0.21
St. Jude Medical Rigid Saddle	3.69 ± 0.27	2.84 ± 0.35	3.73 ± 0.31	2.92 ± 0.31

von den Schnittpunkten wird der jeweilige Euklidische Abstand ermittelt und ein mittleres Fehlermaß über diese Distanzen berechnet.

3   Ergebnisse

In 11 von 12 Vermessungen wurde aufgrund der Minimierung der Fehlermetrik der gleiche Annuloplastie-Ring ausgewählt. Der erste Versuch von Experte 2 generierte einen Vorschlag für den Carpentier-Edwards Physio II-Ring, Größe 40. In den übrigen Versuchen kam die geringste Fehlermetrik bei dem Carpentier Physio-Ring zu Stande. Tab. 1 zeigt die Mittelwerte und Standardabweichung zwischen einem jeweiligen Ringmodell und dem dreimalig vermessenen Annulus über die Messungen gemittelt.

4   Diskussion

In Hinblick auf die virtuelle Annuloplastie wurde in 11 von 12 Experimenten der Physio Ring von dem Hersteller Edwards-Carpentier als das am besten passende Ringmodell ermittelt. Die Mittelung der Ergebnisse von einem Experten (Tab. 1) zeigt sogar, dass in 100% der Fälle das gleiche Ringmodell gewählt wurde. Für dieses Experiment kann geschlussfolgert werden, dass die Messmethode trotz kleinerer Ungenauigkeiten eine stabile Ringselektion ermöglicht. Die Akquise der Punkte dauerte 1-2 Minuten und konnte schneller fertig gestellt werden, je öfter die Messungen wiederholt wurden. Zudem hat sich das vorgeschlagene Vermessungsprotokoll als einprägsam erwiesen. Die Aufnahme dauert somit nicht wesentlich länger als die herkömmliche Sizing-Prozedur. Die zügige Durchführbarkeit deutet darauf hin, dass die Anwendung des neuen Messverfahrens in klinischer Routine potentiell möglich sein wird.

Abschließend bleibt zusammenzufassen, dass die in dieser Arbeit präsentierte Messmethode unseres Wissens nach das erste computerbasierte Verfahren ist, welches bei Mitralklappenrekonstruktionen durchgeführt werden kann. Wir haben darüber hinaus gezeigt, dass die inakkuraten konventionellen Sizingstrategien durch virtuelle Annuloplastie ersetzt werden können. Mithilfe der aufgenommenen Punkte können detailliertere Aussagen über die Annulusform gemacht werden; Bereiche mit hohen zu erwartenden Abweichungen vom selektierten Ring können erkannt werden und damit potentiell hohe Zugkräfte sichtbar gemacht werden. Zudem ist eine Erweiterbarkeit der Landmarkenanzahl jederzeit möglich. So ist eine Ringselektion, die auch die Größe der Mitralklappensegel mit einbezieht, realisierbar. In dem Schema (Abb. 1) ist bereits ersichtlich, das über die Annuluslandmarken hinaus weitere Punkte aufgenommen wurden, deren Information für die Ringselektion hinzugezogen werden sollen.

Danksagung. Diese Arbeit wurde im Rahmen des von der Deutschen Forschungsgemeinschaft geförderten SFB/TRR 125 Cognition-Guided Surgery (Projekt B01) erstellt.

Literaturverzeichnis

1. Carpentier A, Deloche A, Dauptain J, et al. A new reconstructive operation for correction of mitral and tricuspid insufficiency. J Thorac Cardiovasc Surg. 1971;61(1):1–13.
2. Taggart D, Wheatley D. Mitral valve surgery: to repair or replace? Brit Heart J. 1990;64(4):234–35.
3. Voigt I, Mansi T, Ionasec RI, et al. Robust physically-constrained modeling of the mitral valve and subvalvular apparatus. Proc MICCAI. 2011; p. 504–11.
4. Schneider RJ, Perrin DP, Vasilyev NV, et al. Mitral annulus segmentation from three-dimensional ultrasound. Proc ISBI. 2009; p. 779–82.
5. Graser B, Wald D, Al-Maisary S, et al. Using a shape prior for robust modeling of the mitral annulus on 4D ultrasound data. Int J Comp Assist Radiol and Surg. 2013; p. 1–10.
6. Bothe W, Miller DC, Doenst T. Sizing for mitral annuloplasty: where does science stop and voodoo begin? Ann Thorac Surg. 2013;95(4):1475–83.
7. Engelhardt S, De Simone R, Nabers D, et al. Intraoperative measurements on the mitral apparatus using optical tracking: a feasibility study. Proc SPIE. 2014;9036.
8. Nolden M, Zelzer S, Seitel A, et al. The medical imaging interaction toolkit: challenges and advances. Int J of Comput Assist Radiol and Surg. 2013;8:607–20.
9. Wiles AD, Thompson DG, Frantz DD. Accuracy assessment and interpretation for optical tracking systems. Proc SPIE. 2004;5367:421–32.

Wizard-Based Segmentation for Cochlear Implant Planning

Daniela Franz[1,2], Mathias Hofer[3], Matthias Pfeifle[4], Markus Pirlich[3],
Marc Stamminger[2], Thomas Wittenberg[1,2]

[1]Fraunhofer Institute for Integrated Circuits (IIS), Erlangen
[2]Computer Graphics Group, University of Erlangen-Nuremberg
[3]ENT Department, University Hospital of Leipzig
[4]Neurosurgical Department, University Hospital of Tübingen
daniela.franz@iis.fraunhofer.de

Abstract. The planning of a cochlear implantation requires careful segmentation of various structures within the middle and inner ear. Due to usability issues, many planning tools have not been integrated in the daily clinical routine yet. We propose an easy-to-use and intuitive wizard-based approach for the segmentation of structures of the ear. The wizard guides the user through the segmentation process, translating image processing into medical terminology. Semiautomatic corrections integrate the users medical expertise into the process so far. We have evaluated the wizard with a small user study including questionnaires and compared the segmentation result among different users.

1 Introduction

Many intervention planning tools have not yet been able to bridge the gap between high-end computer programs for image data segmentation and daily clinical expectations for intervention support. To address this problem, the well-known wizard interaction pattern [1] can be used to support, accelerate, and ease the interaction between clinical experts and a software tool. Such a wizard guides the user through a number of steps of a certain task. After each step, the user gets visual feedback about the result and can refine and undone them, until the desired result is achieved. The wizard interaction pattern can be used to translate technical image processing terms into problem-oriented medical terminology, thus closes the semantic gap between software and the medical expert. There already exist some examples of medical image processing wizards, such as wizards for filtering in AMIDE [2] or a wizard for neurosurgical planning including segmentation in [3]. In this contribution, we present a novel wizard for cochlear implant (CI) planning. The wizard guides medical experts without technical background through the steps necessary to segment different structures in the ear. Segmentation pipelines are encapsulated in an easy-to-use wizard, resulting in an efficient workflow for cochlear implant planning.

A CI is an electronic hearing aid, that is inserted into the cochlea. The operating field contains high-risk structures such as the facial nerve and the tympanic chord and is characterized by a limited intra-operative visibility. In CT-based CI planning, a combination of various anatomical structures provide detail and overview information of the ear and help the surgeon adjust his access strategy to the anatomy of a specific patient. Various approaches for the segmentation of the middle and inner ear have been proposed. E.g., in [4] a segmentation scheme has been suggested to segment various anatomical structures manually, based on thresholding, in [5] it is based on region growing. In [6] a complete CI planning including a segmentation of anatomical structures has been implemented. All these approaches do not integrate the users knowledge and experience with the data into the segmentation approach, while the proposed wizard-based approach is made by – and not for – image processing experts, but tailored to medical experts.

2   Materials and methods

We have developed a wizard-based interactive segmentation approach for CT-based CI planning, referred to as CI wizard.

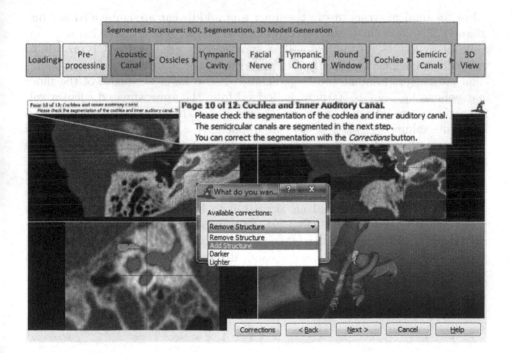

Fig. 1. CI wizard sequence (top) and CI wizard page for cochlea segmentation with 2D slice and 3D view, short instructions, and corrections (bottom).

Table 1. Methods in the segmentation pipelines for all anatomical structures in the order they are presented by the CI wizard. Abbreviations: (ROI) region of interest, (RG) region growing or thresholding, (MO) morphological filters, (DM) 2D/3D features, e.g. 2D area, 2D circularity, 2D/3D connectivity, (FV) vesselness filter, (DF) distance field, and (UI) user interaction, e.g. seed points.

Wiz. Step	Ear Structure	ROI	RG	MO	DM	FV	DF	UI	Prior Knowledge
1 (AC)	Acoustic Canal		x	x	x				Diameter, Shape
2 (OS)	Ossicles	x	x	x				x	Mean Volume
3 (TC)	Tympanic Cavity	x	x	x			x		Mean Volume
4 (NF)	Facial Nerve		x					x	Diameter
5 (NC)	Tympanic Chord		x					x	Diameter
6 (RW)	Round Window	x				x		x	Diameter, Shape
7 (CO)	Cochlea	x	x	x	x	x			Mean Volume
8 (SC)	Semicirc. Canals	x				x			Shape, Diameter

2.1 Segmentation pipelines

Most anatomical structures in the inner and middle ear are embedded in bony tissue. Therefore, inter-subject variations in shape, relative position and volume of structures are limited. This knowledge is used in the CI wizards to set ROIs for segmentation pipelines and restrict the search space for segmentation parameters (volume too large/small). E.g. a lower threshold of the inner ear volume $V_{\text{InnerEar}} > 500 \, \text{mm}^3$ is derived from the approximated cochlea volume $V_{\text{Cochlea}} \approx 106 \, \text{mm}^3$ (cone, $r = 4.5 \, \text{mm}$, $h = 5 \, \text{mm}$) and the approximated vestibule volume $V_{\text{Vestibule}} \approx 524 \, \text{mm}^3$ (sphere, $r = 5 \, \text{mm}$)[7]. One example of a segmentation sub-pipeline is depicted in Fig. 2 and describes the complete segmentation of the cochlea (Tab. 1, Step 7). Here, the ROI is computed beforehand and uses prior knowledge, such as the average length of the inner ear and its position medial to the round window [7]. The cochlear segmentation pipeline is based on thresholding and an algorithm to find a 2D connected region in axial direction in each slice (Fig. 2). The cochlear pipeline uses two criteria to determine if the cochlea has already be found. First, if the seed points for region selection are available and second, if the volume of the region selection

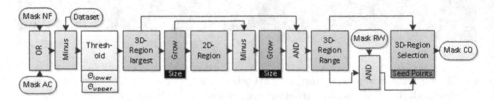

Fig. 2. Cochlea segmentation pipeline. The colors correspond to different methods: set operations (green), morphology (orange), connectivity (blue), thresholding (white). Structures abbreviations can be found in Tab. 1.

$V_{\text{InnerEar}} \geq 500\,\text{mm}^3$. While these criteria are not fulfilled, the upper and lower thresholds ($\Theta_{\text{lower/upper}}$, Fig. 2) are adjusted. The pipelines for the other structures have been designed similarly. An overview of the used methods in the sub-pipelines for all structures is given in Tab. 1 in the order they are presented in the wizard, which is mainly from lateral to medial.

2.2   User guidance with CI wizard

An image processing expert iteratively develops segmentation pipelines, describes its default values and a restricted parameter space for other parameters. In a segmentation pipeline three types of parameters can be distinguished (Fig. 2), that are all handled differently by the wizard (Fig. 1). Fixed parameters are constant for all data (Fig. 2, black). E.g. in the cochlear pipeline, the size of the grow filters is suitable for all data. Default parameters are constant for most of the data, but can manually be changed for interactive corrections (Fig. 2, gray). In the cochlear pipeline, e.g. the seed points for region selection are given by the round window. In some cases, the seed points have manually adjusted with "Add/Remove Structure". Normal parameters are chosen by the user. A default value is the basis for interactive corrections (Fig. 2, white). E.g. in the cochlear pipeline the thresholds $\Theta_{\text{lower/upper}}$ are manually adjusted with "grow/shrink"(Fig. 1). Whenever possible and for most anatomical structures the wizard shows automatic segmentation proposals, as for most users it is easier to adjust provided segmentation suggestions instead of creating new ones from scratch.

2.3   Initial user study

So far, two main features of the CI wizard (i.e., usability, segmentation quality) were interactively evaluated on four spiral CT datasets of one ear of adult patients with a mean pixel size of $0.24\,\text{mm}^2$ and a mean slice distance of $0.4\,\text{mm}$ in axial direction. Four users with different anatomical experience levels (technical student, medical student, ENT surgeon, experienced ENT surgeon) segmented all ear structures with the CI wizard and filled out a questions regarding the segmentation quality. The users quality ratings Q to the question "How well could you segment . . . ?" were translated into numerical values: "Very good" = 3, "With smaller errors" = 2, "With larger errors" = 1, and "Insufficiently" = 0. The mutual Jaccard index for the segmentations A and B ($J(A,B) = |A \cap B|/|A \cup B|$) was assessed. For more than two segmentations, the mean mutual Jaccard index J was computed to measure segmentation similarity.

3   Results

Mean runtime of the CI wizard on a standard PC was $t = 14\,\text{min}(\sigma = 6\,\text{min})$. On average the runtime was perceived appropriate by the users. A 3D result wizard view is shown in Fig. 3. On average user gave quality ratings of $Q =$

Fig. 3. 2D slices and 3D view of a CI planning result in intraoperative perspective.

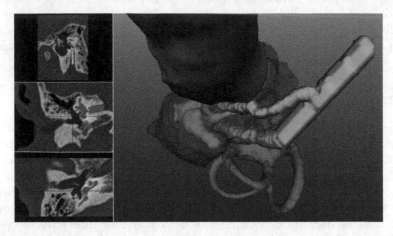

$2,17 (\sigma = 0,83)$, mean values per anatomical structure are depicted in Fig. 4 (left). Fig. 4 (right) shows the mean mutual Jaccard distance for all but the nerve segmentations, where no automatic segmentation proposal is available in the CI wizard. Fig. 5 depicts the segmentation variance for two different datasets and typical segmentation errors. The mean mutual Jaccard index J of the facial nerve (NF) was $J_{NF} = 0.29$ ($\sigma = 0.02$). The tympanic chord of the facial nerve (NC), easily detectable in only one dataset, was identified by three users, in all other datasets only by the most experienced user was able to identify the NC.

4   Discussion

In this study we presented the segmentation of the ear for CI planning for adult patients and evaluated it in a small user study with four users. On average the

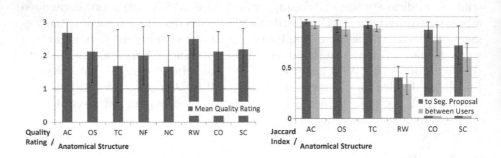

Fig. 4. Subjective mean segmentation quality ratings (left) and mean mutual Jaccard distance between users and in comparison to automatic segmentation proposals (right). The nerves NF and NC are excluded, because for them no automatic segmentation proposal exists.

Fig. 5. Segmentation variance for dataset 3 (right) and 1 (middle, left). The color coding refers to the number of users that have consistently classified a voxel. Arrows point out segmentation errors. Only one user was able to identify the tympanic chord (left). Two users segmented the oval instead of the round window (middle). Users choose different endpoints for the facial nerve (right).

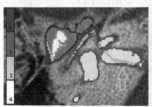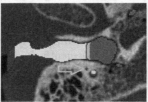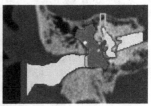

users were able to segment all structures, except nerves. A high mean quality rating and the structure specific quality ratings in Fig. 4 (left) indicate the users content with the segmentations. A lower quality rating of the tympanic cavity can be explained with the anatomically difficult separation of tympanic cavity and antrum. Also the tympanic chord is not clearly visible in all of the data, so the users often were not able to identify it (Fig. 5, middle). Although the average quality rating for the round window was high, segmentation similarity in Fig. 4 (right) is low. This is due to the fact, that in two cases users identified the oval instead of the round window (Fig. 5, right). This was not related to anatomical expertise of the users. We are currently continuing our study to obtain data from more user and cases.

A wizard-based segmentation can enhance the interaction between surgical planning tools and medical experts, which do not want to deal with image processing details, but to focus on the image data and the results of a segmentation with respect to the surgical planning process.

References

1. Tidwell J. Designing Interfaces. O'Reilly; 2007.
2. Loening A, Sanjiv G. AMIDE: A free software tool for multimodality medical image analysis. Int J Mol Imag. 2003; p. 131–7.
3. Ahmadi SA, Pisana F, DeMomi E, et al. User friendly graphical user interface for workflow management during navigated robotic-assisted keyhole neurosurgery. Proc CARS. 2010.
4. Rodt T, Ratiu P, Becker H, et al. 3D visualisation of the middle ear and adjacent structures using reconstructed multi-slice CT datasets, correlating 3D images and virtual endoscopy to the 2D cross-sectional images. Neuroradiol. 2002;44:783–90.
5. Todd C, Kirillov M, Tarabichi M, et al. A computer-based, interactive tool for semi-automatic extraction, visualization and pre-operative assessment of the inner ear. JCMIT. 2009.
6. Gerber N, Bell B, Gavaghan K, et al. Surgical planning tool for robotically assisted hearing aid implantation. Int J Comput Assist Radiol Surg. 2013;7(1):133–6.
7. Kirsch J. Taschenlehrbuch Anatomie. Thieme Georg Verlag; 2010.

Measurement of the Stratum Radiatum/Lacunosum-Moleculare (SRLM)

Steffen Oeltze[1], Hartmut Schütze[2], Anne Maaß[2], Emrah Düzel[2,3,4], Bernhard Preim[1]

[1]Department of Simulation and Graphics, University of Magdeburg
[2]Institute of Cognitive Neurology and Dementia Research, University of Magdeburg
[3]German Centre for Neurodegenerative Diseases (DZNE), Standort Magdeburg
[4]Institute of Cognitive Neuroscience, University College London, UK
stoeltze@isg.cs.uni-magdeburg.de

Abstract. Alzheimer disease (AD) at an early stage is characterized by a synaptic loss and atrophy in the apical layer of the CA1 part of the hippocampus, the stratum radiatum and stratum lacunosum-moleculare (SRLM). It was shown in vivo that patients with mild AD exhibit a reduced thickness of the SRLM. We propose a new approach to measure SRLM thickness in coronal brain sections. It is based on the interpolated contour of the manually segmented SRLM and its medial axis. We automatically compute the axis by combining Voronoi diagrams and methods from graph analysis. While existing measurement approaches require a mental segmentation of the SRLM and a repeated local estimate of its center, we obviate the latter. We evaluate our approach based on coronal $T2^*$-weighted 7 T MR images of 27 subjects.

1 Introduction

At an early stage, Alzheimer disease (AD) is characterized by episodic memory dysfunction. The hippocampus – a brain structure existing in both hemispheres and being part of the limbic system – plays a crucial role in consolidating episodic memory [1]. Postmortem studies found that synaptic loss and atrophy in the apical layer of the CA1 part of the hippocampus, the stratum radiatum and stratum lacunosum-moleculare (SRLM, Fig. 1(a)), coincide with earliest cognitive symptoms [2]. Kerchner et al. [3] showed that patients with mild AD exhibit a reduced SRLM thickness. Their analysis was based on coronal $T2^*$-weighted images from ultra-high field 7 T MRI. Only ultra-high field imaging provides an in-plane resolution ($< \approx 0.5$ mm) high enough to identify hippocampal subfields (Fig. 1(b)). Since normal SRLM thickness is about 1 mm, its width covers only a few pixels. Within each transection of the hippocampus, the SRLM is heavily quantized and borders to adjacent structures form a step-wise pattern. Since the CA1 apical neuropil is affected in early stages of AD, a correct measurement of SRLM thickness could serve as an objective imaging biomarker for AD pathology and moreover, contribute to judging the (e.g. protective) effects of physical or cognitive training in early AD patients as well as healthy older people.

Two approaches to measuring SRLM thickness have been published. A manual approach was presented by Kerchner et al. [3]. For each hemisphere in two consecutive slices, the user draws three lines extending over the local width of the SRLM. The approach is subjective, it is restricted to a subset of the slices that show the SRLM, and it poorly acknowledges the variance in thickness along the SRLM. Recently, Kerchner et al. [4] proposed a semi-automatic measurement. The user first draws in the medial axis of the SRLM in all slices. Orthogonal signal intensity profiles are then determined at equidistantly sampled points along a spline that is fit to the user-defined line. A single thickness value is computed per slice based on the average signal intensity change from the medical axis of the SRLM to the surrounding subfields. The approach is less subjective but sensitive to the user's definition of the medial axis. The definition requires a mental segmentation of the SRLM and a concurrent, repeated local estimate of its center. The latter is particularly tedious in regions of very small SRLM thickness (1-2 pixels). Furthermore, the measured local thickness depends on the signal intensity distribution of the surrounding subfields. SRLM sites being equally thick may result in different measurement values. This effect is mitigated by averaging the local intensity profiles but hampers a real local analysis.

The shape of the SRLM in coronal slices is similar to the shape of the corpus callosum (cc) in mid-sagittal slices (Fig. 1(a), cc in upper inset). An overview of approaches to measuring callosal thickness is part of [5]. Most approaches rely on the medial axis of the cc and determine thickness orthogonal to it. We propose a related SRLM measurement approach which is based on the interpolated contour of the manually segmented SRLM and the medial axis of this contour, i.e., of the SRLM. In contrast to [4], we automatically compute the axis. The contour increases the range of possible measurements, e.g., by area or curvature. Another advantage is the coherent local computation of SRLM thickness independent of the signal intensities of surrounding structures.

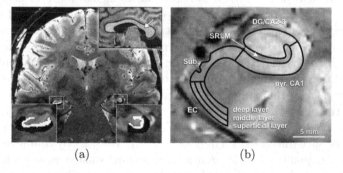

(a)   (b)

Fig. 1. (a) Coronal $T2^*$-weighted Magnetic Resonance image with overlaid ROIs of the stratum radiatum and stratum lacunosum-moleculare (SRLM, white) and pyramidal CA1 (black). The upper inset shows the corpus callosum (arrow). Its shape is similar to SRLM shape. (b) Schematic of the subfields in the hippocampal body.

2   Materials and methods

2.1   Study data and SRLM segmentation

The data were collected in an ultra-high field 7 T MRI study at the Institute of Cognitive Neurology and Dementia Research of the University of Magdeburg, Germany. The study combined a visual learning paradigm with high resolution functional measurements and very high resolution structural images for 14 subjects. A pre-study with 13 subjects was conducted. For both studies, healthy young people were recruited (age 25±2, 14 male). MRI data were acquired using a 7 T MRI system (Siemens, Erlangen, Germany) with a 32-channel head coil. The high resolution partial structural volume was acquired (T2*-weighted imaging, $TE = 18.5$ ms, $TR = 680$ ms, in-plane resolution 0.33 mm×0.33 mm, slice thickness 1.5 mm + 25% gap, 45 slices, FOV 212 mm×179 mm, matrix 640×540), with a slice alignment orthogonal to the hippocampal main axis. The pre-study was conducted with the same sequence and similar parameters.

The segmentation of hippocampal subfields was performed for each hemisphere using MRIcron (Chris Rorden, Version 4, April 2011). First, subfields in the hippocampal body were traced according to [6]. Next, the parahippocampal regions were delineated. Then, the hippocampal head was segmented into subregions according to [7]. The hippocampal tail was not delineated. Overall, the hippocampus was segmented into subiculum (Sub), CA1-stratum pyramidale (pyr. CA1), CA1-stratum radiatum/stratum lacunosum-moleculare (SRLM, Fig. 1(b)) and the remaining portion comprising CA2, CA3, and DG (DG/CA2-3). Only the SRLM part in the hippocampal body is used in the thickness evaluation.

2.2   SRLM measurement

Our measurement of the SRLM is based on its medial axis. A good survey of medial axis computation algorithms is part of [8]. The pixel-based medial axis generated by topological thinning or distance transform algorithms is too coarse since the width of the SRLM in some regions covers only 1-2 pixels. Surface sampling methods allow for a more fine-grained determination but require a representation of the objects boundary by a dense cloud of sample points. Our measurement algorithm starts by computing this point cloud.

Given the binary mask of the SRLM resulting from segmentation, we process this mask slice-by-slice (Fig. 2(a)). A 3D measurement is not feasible due to the considerable slice thickness (1.5 mm+25% gap). We start by computing a smooth contour of the quantized binary mask. A marching squares algorithm with linear interpolation provides an initial sharp-edged contour. The contour is enhanced via B-spline interpolation followed by a Laplacian smoothing with displacement adjustment to avoid shrinkage [9]. The smoothing parameters have been determined empirically: 10 smoothing passes with a factor of 0.1 and a window of 3 points. The final contour is resampled equidistantly with a sample point density that fulfills the requirements for an accurate medial axis computation [10].

The medial axis is derived from the Voronoi diagram of the sample points [10] (Fig. 2(b)). A Voronoi diagram divides the space into regions such that each seed (contour sample point) is contained in a separate region which comprises all points that are closer to this seed than to any other. The edges of the Voronoi diagram, which are completely contained within the SRLM contour, constitute its medial axis. They are determined based on point-in-polygon tests. The Voronoi approach is sensitive to noise in the contour. Slight deviations from a perfectly smooth curve cause short side branches originating from the medial axis (Fig. 2(b)). Hence, pruning is often carried out as a post-processing step [10].

We suggest an inverse strategy that separates the ideal medial axis MA_{ideal} from the noisy one MA_{noisy} (Fig. 2(c)). Due to the normally non-branching, tubular shape of the SRLM within a coronal slice, MA_{ideal} is a simple polyline extending from one end to the other. Its separation is based on the observation that MA_{ideal} corresponds to the longest of the shortest paths between any pair of terminal vertices of MA_{noisy}. We treat MA_{noisy} as an undirected, unweighted, acyclic graph. Each of the n vertices is a node and an edge exists between two nodes if they are connected by a line segment in MA_{noisy}. We describe the graph by its $n \times n$ symmetric adjacency matrix A, whose entries equal 1 if the two corresponding nodes are connected by an edge and 0 otherwise. Terminal vertices of MA_{noisy} are characterized by a single 1 in their corresponding row or column of A. For each pair of terminal vertices, we find the shortest in-between path, i.e., along MA_{noisy}, by Breadth-First Search on A. The longest of these shortest paths represents MA_{ideal}.

To measure SRLM thickness, we equidistantly resample MA_{ideal} according to a user-defined number of thickness measurements (Fig. 2(c)). At each sample point, we erect an orthogonal line. Its intersections with the lower and upper part of the SRLM's contour delimit the local thickness. If a line intersects the contour more than twice, the two intersections which are on either side of the line and closest to MA_{ideal} are chosen. The Euclidean distance between the intersection points corresponds to the local thickness of the SRLM.

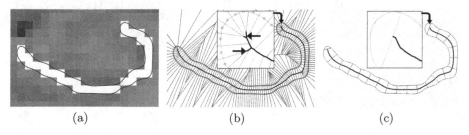

(a)   (b)   (c)

Fig. 2. Measurement approach. (a) Computation of the contour (black) of the SRLM mask (white). (b) Voronoi diagram (net-like structure) of the contour points (circles). The medial axis (thick polyline) is part of the diagram. The inset shows erroneous side branches. (c) Ideal medial axis and thickness measurements (thin, orthogonal lines).

3   Results

We have applied our measurement approach to data of 27 subjects. For each subject, the SRLM of the two hemispheres has been segmented in ≈10 slices resulting in 594 SRLM contours. The algorithm was set to equidistantly sample SRLM thickness at 20 locations along the medial axis. All medial axes and orthogonal lines defining local SRLM thickness were visually verified. Local thickness was correctly represented in > 95% of the orthogonal lines. Figure 3 shows typical examples for successful and failed representations, and illustrates the shape variety of the SRLM. In $(a - c)$, common shape variants and their reasonable measurements are displayed. The contours in $(d - f)$ represent increasing deviations from the typical SRLM shape leading to incorrect thickness measurements (thick lines). It can be seen that these errors occur mostly at sites of high bending or where one part of the contour bends significantly different than the opposite part. The branchings seen in $(g - h)$ result from uncertainty during segmentation which is due to similar signal intensities of blood vessels or surrounding structures. Although a reasonable medial axis can be computed, thickness measurements are disturbed by the second branch and it remains unclear which branch represents the SRLM. Instead of neglecting individual thickness measurements, we completely removed cases similar to $(d - h)$ from our analysis (22% of the contours were removed).

The SRLM thicknesses of all subjects had a mean of 0.95 mm ($\sigma = 0.17$ mm) and showed a very high correlation between both hemispheres ($r = 0.93, p < 0.01$), which suggests that an individual property of the subjects was indeed obtained. Kerchner et al. reported thickness values in the range $0.4 - 0.6$ mm [4]. The differences to our values are most likely due to their conservative estimate of where SRLM ends and where surrounding structures begin based on the signal intensities. While they choose the approximate middle of the unsure transition zone, we include the entire zone during segmentation.

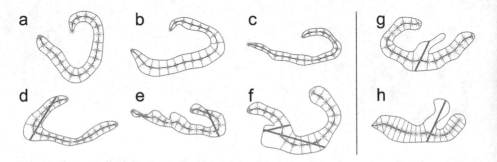

Fig. 3. Successful (a-c) and failed (d-h) evaluations of SRLM thickness. Thick lines represent unreasonable measurements due to strong local differences in the bending of the lower and upper SRLM contour parts (d-f) or due to a branching contour (g-h).

4 Discussion

Our method is largely dependent on the individual rater bias during pixel-wise delineation of the SRLM. However, if either a conservative or a slightly relaxed segmentation strategy is consistently chosen for all subjects of a study, the bias should be minimized. Hence, comparing a group of subjects with mild Alzheimer disease or mild cognitive impairment and a control group is feasible. We aim at correlating thickness and performance measures of recognition memory tests. Hereby, differences in thickness between groups and reproducible measurements are rather important than absolute real thickness values.

The reasons for erroneous thickness measurements (Fig. 3 d–f) have been also acknowledged by Herron et al. in measuring the corpus callosum (cc) [5]. However, their proposed solution involves a strict anatomically based definition of the cc's center. The computation of a similar center for the SRLM is hampered by its higher shape variability (Fig. 3). A promising solution in regions of high SRLM bending is based on electric field lines and was presented for measuring the cerebral cortex in 2D histological sections [11].

References

1. Milner B. The medial temporal-lobe amnesic syndrome. Psychiatr Clin North Am. 2015;28(3):599–611.
2. Thal DR, Holzer M, Rüb U, et al. Alzheimer-related τ-pathology in the perforant path target zone and in the hippocampal stratum oriens and radiatum correlates with onset and degree of dementia. Exp Neurol. 2000;163:98–110.
3. Kerchner GA, Hess CP, Hammond-Rosenbluth KE, et al. Hippocampal CA1 apical neuropil atrophy in mild alzheimer disease visualized with 7-T MRI. Neurology. 2010;75(15):1381–7.
4. Kerchner GA, Deutsch GK, Zeineh M, et al. Hippocampal CA1 apical neuropil atrophy and memory performance in alzheimer's disease. Neuroimage. 2012;63(1):194–202.
5. Herron TJ, Kang X, Woods DL. Automated measurement of the human corpus callosum using MRI. Front Neuroinformatics. 2012;6(25):1–15.
6. Mueller SG, Stables L, Du AT, et al. Measurement of hippocampal subfields and age-related changes with high resolution MRI at 4T. Neurobiology of Aging. 2007;28(5):719–26.
7. Wisse LEM, Gerritsen L, Zwanenburg JJM, et al. Subfields of the hippocampal formation at 7T MRI: in vivo volumetric assessment. Neuroimage. 2012;61(4):1043–9.
8. Foskey M, Lin MC, Manocha D. Efficient computation of a simplified medial axis. Proc SMA. 2003; p. 96–107.
9. Vollmer J, Mencl R, Müller H. Improved laplacian smoothing of noisy surface meshes. Comput Graph Forum. 1999;18(3):131–8.
10. Brandt JW, Algazi VR. Continuous skeleton computation by voronoi diagram. Comput Vis Image Underst. 1992;55(3):329–38.
11. Schmitt O, Böhme M. A robust transcortical profile scanner for generating 2-D traverses in histological sections of richly curved cortical courses. Neuroimage. 2002;16(4):1103–19.

Automatic Design of Realistic Multiple Sclerosis Lesion Phantoms

Jan Rexilius, Klaus Tönnies

Department of Simulation and Graphics, University of Magdeburg
`rexilius@isg.cs.uni-magdeburg.de`

Abstract. The segmentation and quantification of multiple sclerosis (MS) lesions is an important issue in medical image analysis. To reach clinical acceptance, a careful evaluation of each algorithm is required. Today, the standard approach is a comparison with results of patient data sets generated by domain experts. Unfortunately, the underlying ground truth is unknown in these data sets, and the results of expert analyses suffer from intra- and inter-rater variabilities. In this work, we present an automatic approach to develop digital MS lesion phantoms. The algorithm combines a statistical map of lesion positions with a lesion model extracted from actual patient data. A standard brain phantom is used as reference data set. Instead of creating one best phantom, our approach allows to parametrically generate a large range of different phantoms. This way, we can capture the variability of MS lesions encountered in practice without the need of manual interactions during the phantom design process. To evaluate our approach, a visual assessment is performed by a clinical expert. Furthermore, a published MS lesion segmentation algorithm is used to segment the phantom data. The results indicate the applicability of our approach.

1 Introduction

Magnetic resonance imaging (MRI) is widely used in clinical practice to study multiple sclerosis (MS). As part of standard diagnostics as well as for follow-up examinations and clinical trials, manual to fully automatic segmentation algorithms have been proposed to compute the total number of lesions and the lesion volume [1]. In order to reach clinical acceptance, and to understand the intrinsic characteristics of a method, dedicated evaluation strategies are required. During the last years, on-site competitions of several research teams during a conference have become popular, e.g., the Grand Challenge workshops at the MICCAI conference [2].

To evaluate an algorithm, most approaches compare the quality of a method with some kind of reference. Such a gold standard is presumed to contain the correct result (the ground truth) or be at least close to it. A common approach uses patient data and associated manual segmentations, which serve as a surrogate ground truth. However, a large data pool is required to account for major anatomical variations and pathologies. Furthermore, exact measurements of parameters such as the volume of an imaged organ are not possible with patient data sets.

Another way to establish a gold standard are physical or software phantoms [3, 4, 5], because the exact ground truth for the modeled parameters is available. However, building a phantom usually requires a large manual effort, and changing anatomical structures can be time-consuming and cost-intensive. Nevertheless, many data sets are required for an in-depth evaluation. A popular phantom in medical image analysis is the brain phantom introduced in [4] known as BrainWeb. It consists of ten tissue classes including gray matter, white matter, and cerebrospinal fluid extracted from a single volunteer. An extension with additional volunteer data sets and more structures such as blood vessels is proposed in [6].

In this paper, we propose an extension of the BrainWeb phantoms by an additional MS lesion class. Instead of developing a small amount of hand-crafted lesions, we present a fully automatic approach that allows to generate an arbitrary number of MS data sets. For each lesion object, different parameter models are available including shape, position, and volume. To ensure the quality of the resulting data sets, a qualitative assessment is performed by a clinical expert. Furthermore, results from a published segmentation algorithm are compared with measurements of the same method on our phantom data.

2   Materials and methods

In this section, we describe the steps that are used to develop MS lesion phantoms. An important aspect for our algorithm is a reasonable design of lesion parameters such as shape and position. Manually segmented lesions from actual patient data sets provide the basis for this task.

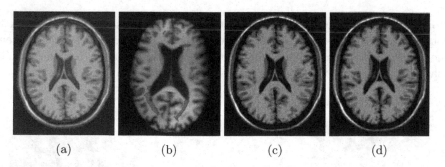

(a)   (b)   (c)   (d)

Fig. 1. Registration results. (a) Reference data. (b) Patient data after brain extraction with lesion mask overlay. (c) Reference data with patient data overlay (affine registration). (d) Reference data with patient data overlay (affine + B-spline registration).

2.1 Position map

In the first step of our algorithm, the spatial distribution of lesions is analyzed. We generate a statistical map of lesion positions by transforming a list of patient data sets into a common coordinate system. The BrainWeb data are used as reference.

The implemented registration process can be divided into three steps: First, the brain is separated from surrounding non-brain tissue of each patient data set based on an evolving deformable model [7]. This is a crucial pre-processing step, which helps to reduce the degrees of freedom during registration. In the next step, we perform a global affine registration. Since we observe a large inter-patient variability in the shapes of anatomical structures, the final step is a local nonrigid registration using a B-spline approach [8]. To generate the map of lesion positions, we apply the resulting transformations to the corresponding manual segmentation masks. An example of the registration results shown as overlay on the BrainWeb data is given in Fig. 1.

2.2 Lesion objects

After calculating reasonable lesion positions within the reference data set, we now focus on features of a single lesion.

Shape. The shape of a lesion is position-specific, e.g., due to anatomical constraints, and a single global model will not be sufficient. Therefore, the lesion shape is extracted from the segmentation mask that has been registered into the reference frame as described in the previous section. To account for manual segmentation errors, we update each shape by morphological filtering and smoothing operations. Additional patient data sets will be added to enhance the anatomical variability to our lesion models.

Volume. The volume is extracted from a given lesion segmentation mask by counting all segmented voxels. To model partial volume effects to some extent, the binary lesion mask is upsampled to a voxel size about 10 times smaller than the resolution of the reference data. This high-resolution data set is then

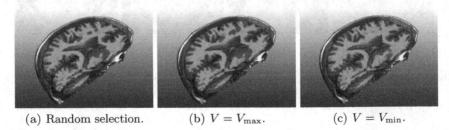

(a) Random selection.   (b) $V = V_{\max}$.   (c) $V = V_{\min}$.

Fig. 2. Visualization the effect of different lesion volumes $V \in [V_{\min}, V_{\max}]$.

downsampled again using trilinear interpolation. The resulting probability map defines the amount of partial volume at each voxel.

To add further variability, an individual volume range is defined for each lesion, depending on the original volume. The final lesion volume is then chosen randomly within this range so that the same lesion shape will have different volumes in different data sets. Fig. 2 shows the result of this approach for different lesions.

Gray value and noise. We assume homogeneous lesions with a constant intensity value as well as Gaussian noise. The noise standard deviation is set approximately equal to the noise of the reference data. The lesion gray values are computed from the ratio between mean white matter and lesion gray value, extracted from all patient data sets.

2.3   Lesion selection and placement

Given the position map and the lesion objects described above, we can now combine reference data and lesions to a single phantom data set. To enable an automatic object placement within the BrainWeb data, we randomly select positions from the map. The corresponding lesion objects with computed volume and gray values are then added to the data. Additionally, we account for inflammation that often appears around a lesion by smoothing the lesion probability map. The output of this step is a map with the amount of lesion tissue at each voxel plus the final phantom data set. Fig. 4 shows results of the MS lesion phantom generation process.

3   Results

Twenty patient data sets [2] with manually segmented lesions acquired on a 3T MRI scanner are used to calculate the position map and also form the basis of

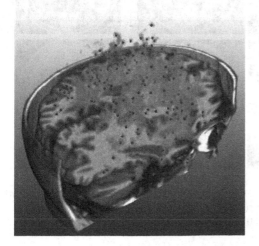

Fig. 3. Reference data with resulting statistical map of lesion positions and center of gravity of lesions (red points).

our lesion models. The data-acquisition protocol contains T1-, T2- and FLAIR-weighted images. The T1-weighted data are used for the initial brain extraction algorithm. After registration to the reference brain phantom, approximately 500 lesions are extracted. The lesion volumes range from 0.001 ml to 4.38 ml (mean = 0.25 ml). An illustration of the resulting position map and the center of gravity for each lesion is shown in Fig. 3.

Three lesion phantoms have been generated, each with 20 lesions. The total lesion loads (TTL) for the three data sets are 7.18 ml, 5.19 ml, and 8.39 ml. An example slice of each data set is shown in Fig. 4. To evaluate our phantoms, a domain expert was asked to assess the overall quality. A rating scale was used based on fuzzy terms (poor, low, average, high, very high). The expert rating for all data sets is "high".

Another evaluation that can increase the confidence in our approach is to apply an already published algorithm and compare the results with those from patient data. In this work, we use the segmentation algorithm proposed by

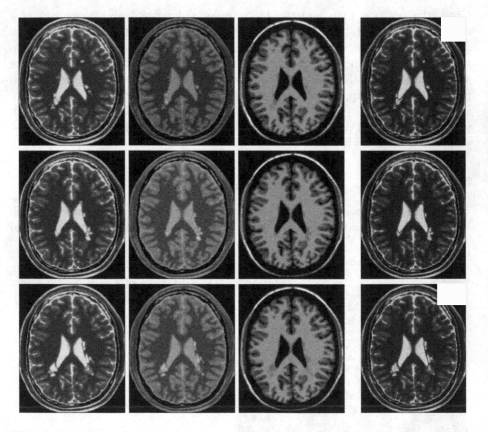

Fig. 4. Resulting phantom data sets. Column 1-3: T2-, PD-, T1-weighted data. Column 4: Phantoms with segmentation result overlay, red: algorithm result [9], yellow: phantom data using only voxel with ≥ 50% lesion probability.

Leemput et al. in [9]. The dice similarity coefficient $DSC = 2|A \cap B|/(|A|+|B|)$, ($A$ = Algorithm Result, B = Ground Truth) for the patient data sets given in the paper is $DSC = 0.45$. The same algorithm is now used to segment all phantom data set. An illustration of the results is given in Fig. 4 (right column). Since the segmentation algorithm computes a binary lesion mask, the phantom lesion load is calculated by counting all voxels with $\geq 50\%$ lesion probability. The computed similarity values $DSC = \{0.75, 0.71, 0.76\}$ are about 1.5 times higher compared to those reported by Leemput et al. Increasing the complexity of our lesion model could lead to results comparable to those given in literature. An in-depth analysis is required for a more thorough assessment.

4 Conclusion

The main objective in this work is to develop a novel approach that enables a fully automatic generation of MS lesion phantoms. An expert validation acknowledges the quality of these phantoms. A comparison of segmentation results from published work might indicate that the models used for our phantoms do not yet meet all relevant anatomical requirements. Nevertheless, we believe that our approach provides a sound basis that could serve as gold standard for the evaluation of segmentation and quantification algorithms. The resulting data will be made available publicly. Future work will focus on an extension of the lesion model. For example, to improve anatomical variability of the lesion shape, additional geometric deformations of the segmented data could be used.

References

1. Mortazavi D, Kouzani AZ, Soltanian-Zadeh H. Segmentation of multiple sclerosis lesions in MR images: a review. Neuroradiology. 2012;54(4):299–320.
2. Styner M, Lee J, Chin B, et al. 3D segmentation in the clinic: a grand challenge II: MS lesion segmentation. Proc MICCAI. 2008; p. 1–6.
3. Tofts PS, Barker GJ, Filippi M, et al. An oblique cylinder contrast-adjusted (OCCA) phantom to measure the accuracy of MRI brain lesion volume estimation schemes in multiple sclerosis. Magn Reson Imaging. 1997;15:183–92.
4. Collins D, Zijdenbos A, Kollokian V, et al. Design and construction of a realistic digital brain phantom. IEEE Trans Med Imaging. 1998;17(5):463–8.
5. Rexilius J, Hahn HK, et al. Evaluation of accuracy in MS lesion volumetry using realistic lesion phantoms. Acad Radiol. 2005;12:17–24.
6. Aubert-Broche B, Evans AC, Collins DL. A new improved version of the realistic digital brain phantom. Neuroimage. 2006;32(1):138–45.
7. Smith S. Fast robust automated brain extraction. Hum Brain Mapp. 2002;17(3):143–55.
8. Klein S, Staring M, Murphy K, et al. Elastix: a toolbox for intensity based medical image registration. IEEE Trans Med Imaging. 2010;29(1):196–205.
9. Leemput KV, Maes F, Vandermeulen D, et al. Automated segmentation of multiple sclerosis lesions by model outlier detection. IEEE Trans Med Imaging. 2001;20(8):677–88.

Illustrative Visualization of Endoscopic Views

Kai Lawonn, Patrick Saalfeld, Bernhard Preim

Department for Simulation and Graphics, OvG University Magdeburg
lawonn@isg.cs.uni-magdeburg.de

Abstract. This paper deals with the application of illustrative line renderings on endoscopic views. We examine different line drawing concepts and assess the ability to represent interior branches as well as specific anatomic features. Furthermore, we conduct a qualitative evaluation to rate the results of different illustrative visualization methods. We evaluate how well branches are depicted according to a shaded object and which of the technique is rated as the most expressive. We use different anatomical surfaces which were derived from clinical image data. Moreover, we identify the limitations of the illustrative visualization and derive requirements for the application.

1 Introduction

Virtual endoscopy is utilized for the examination of air-filled or fluid-filled structures, such as colon, blood vessels, kidney, bladder, larynx, paranasal sinus, and so forth to present endoluminal views. While real endoscopy involves anesthesia and is involved with some risk, virtual endoscopy may partially replace this procedure and increase patient safety. Virtual endoscopy is restricted to intensity data from CT and MRI instead of the full-color information in real endoscopy. Despite this problem, pathologies are detected in modern virtual endoscopy systems with a high sensitivity. Mostly, the virtual endoscopy is used for screening colorectal cancer or bronchogenic carcinoma. The virtual endoscopy surface models can be reconstructed by clinical image data such as CT data. Often, the endoscopy is used for examination and for detection of polyps, tumors, calcified plaques, and stenosis. Especially for lectures for the doctors-to-be it is interesting to illustrate polyps, tumors, or plaques as known from anatomical atlases. There, only essential information are depicted while unnecessary ones are avoided to prevent visual clutter. Therefore, illustrative visualization has a high potential in medical applications such as surgery planning [1] and intra-operative visualizations [2]. In this paper, we focus on illustrative surface renderings. We introduce different line drawing concepts and employ them to endoscopic views. This idea is motivated by its high potential to depict interesting objects in normal shading and illustrate surrounding non-essential context objects with line drawing techniques or vice versa. Line drawing techniques attempt to convey the surface by drawing several lines. Here, we distinguish between feature lines and hatching. While feature lines try to depict only salient regions by separate lines, hatching uses a bunch of lines to illustrate the object. First, we show that current feature line methods are not able to illustrate the endoscopic view let alone to convey a spatial impression, whereas hatching methods are able to depict the spatiality. Here, we focus on the hatching method by Praun et al. [3] and Zander et al. [4]. Furthermore, we use the ConFIS method by Lawonn et al. [5], which can be seen as a hybrid between feature line and hatching. We give an overview about the presented methods in Section 2. The contribution of this paper is to examine the application of line drawing techniques to endoscopic views. We present feature line methods and hatching techniques. We show that feature lines are not appropriate for endoscopic views. Furthermore, we introduce hatching methods. Moreover, we conduct a qualitative evaluation to assess the proficiency of these methods in order to gain a spatial impression of endoscopic views in comparison to surface shading.

2   Material and methods

This section gives an explanation about the underlying surface data sets as well as a brief overview about the line drawing techniques that we want to evaluate.

2.1   Endoscopic data

We use clinical image data such as CT or MRA to acquire the anatomical information as well as the surface model. We reconstruct the surface mesh by applying a simple thresholding segmentation followed by a connected component analysis. The resulting segmentation mask is used to construct the surface by a marching cubes algorithm. Afterwards, the mesh quality is improved by a combination of edge collapses, edge flips, smoothing, and remeshing.

2.2   Methods

First, we present some feature line methods and explain the key idea.

Feature lines There are several feature line techniques: ridges and valleys [6], suggestive contours [7], apparent ridges [8], and photic extremum lines [9]. These methods are explained in more detail in [10]. Ridges and valleys are defined as the loci of points where the principle curvatures reaches an extremum in the principle curvature direction. As ridges and valleys are not view-dependent, suggestive contours attempt to resolve this issue. Suggestive contours extend the normal definition of the contour. These lines are defined as the set of points where the diffuse lighting reaches a minimum in the direction of the projected view vector. Unfortunately, objects without concave regions have no suggestive contours. In contrast, apparent ridges are a view-dependent approach that tries to depict also features which are missed by suggestive contours. Apparent ridges extend the definition of ridges and valleys by using a view-dependent approach. It defines view-dependent curvatures as well as view-dependent principle curvature directions. Hence, apparent ridges are also defined as the set of points where these curvature assumes an extremum in these directions. Last, photic extremum lines are the loci of points where the variation of illumination in its gradient direction is a local maximum. Figure 1 illustrates that these methods are not appropriate for endoscopic views. In [10] this result was also confirmed at the trachea model.

Hatching We consider three different techniques: the method by Praun et al. [3], Zander et al. [4], and Lawonn et al. [5]. All three methods use an underlying curvature direction field. For this, we build a curvature field according to Rusinkiewicz [11]. He approximates the second fundamental tensor by linear differences of the vertex normals and least square methods. Afterwards, the determination of the eigenvalues and eigenvectors of the second fundamental tensor yields the curvatures and the principle curvature direction. Praun et al. introduced real-time hatching. They generate line-art tonal art maps for different shading levels. Afterwards, lapped textures are applied to map the line-art textures onto the surface. Thereby, the textures are mapped randomly onto the surface and missing facets are processed by querying a list of non-covered facets. Then, those textures are used which correspond to the underlying shading. Zander et al. employ high-quality hatching, a geometry-based method. They do not use textures, but streamlines. These streamlines are generated on the entire surface and propagated along the principle curvature directions. The shading of each streamline part corresponds to the underlying surface shading. Lawonn et al. developed ConFIS. This method seeds only streamlines at relevant regions determined by the mean curvature and its gradient. They define a contour margin and feature regions. These regions are relevant for streamlines. The streamlines are traced along the principle curvature directions. Seeding streamlines at certain regions yields a faster approach than a generation on the entire surface.

2.3 Evaluation

We performed a qualitative evaluation of the three line drawing techniques to rate the ability for assessing the spatial impression. For the evaluation, four sur-

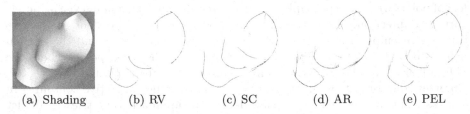

(a) Shading   (b) RV   (c) SC   (d) AR   (e) PEL

Fig. 1. Endoscopic view rendered with simple shading (a), ridges and valleys (RV) (b), suggestive contours (SC) (c), apparant ridges (AR) (d), and photic extremum lines (PEL) (e).

Table 1. The left table shows which method was rated as most effective for the four data sets (left column). The participants could also vote for two techniques (maximum is seven). The right table shows how many participants counted the right number of branches.

	Real-time	High-quality	ConFIS		Real-time	High-quality	ConFIS
1	4	0	6	1	5	5	7
2	2	0	6	2	5	7	7
3	5	0	2	3	7	7	7
4	1	0	7	4	6	6	6

face models were chosen. The evaluation was conducted with seven researchers who are familiar with medical visualizations. We generated the illustrations and showed the results in different order. The sequence of the data sets was the same. The ordering of the line drawing techniques changed. First, we showed the researchers different results and asked them if they are able to perceive branches and other features from the resulting pictures. After all illustrative pictures were shown, we presented the normal shaded image. Then, we asked if they would have expected this model. Afterwards, we showed all results to compare between the different methods. Here, we wanted to figure out if some features were misinterpreted or missed. In comparison of all line drawing methods with the shaded model, the participants should rate which technique is more appropriate to capture salient regions as well as the spatiality and which limitations they noticed. During the evaluation, we noted the spoken comments by the participants.

3 Results

In Figure 2 the shaded models are shown. For each model the results of the different hatching methods are depicted. The results of our evaluation are summarized in Table 1. We assessed two findings. First, which technique was rated as most expressive and second which method delivers a good result for perceiving the right number of branches. The spoken comments of the participants were mostly the same. The real-time hatching (RT) gives a good spatial impression, whereas the high-quality hatching (HQ) is insufficient for a 3D impression. The ConFIS is also able to deliver a spatial impression and tries to depict salient regions. Especially for the third model, the cut-off between the two branches was illustrated appropriately. In contrast, the HQ could not depict it well. Furthermore, the participants liked the consistent drawing of the ConFIS method. Whenever a branch is depicted, the lines wrap around the outgoing structure. The RT technique is able to illustrate the model according to the light intensity. Therefore, the result is very close according to the shaded image. Two participants realized some distortions of the RT method as this is a texture projection method. We implemented the method but used another parameterization technique. Nevertheless, they mentioned that these artifacts were not distracting to focus on the object branches. One participant thought of an improvement of HQ and ConFIS by attenuating the lines according to the distance to gain better depth cues. In summary, the ConFIS technique was rated as the most expressive technique and gives the best impression for branches.

4   Discussion

The result of our evaluation can be summarized such that all methods are able to illustrate the underlying surface model. The RT method uses the underlying shading to create an illustrative visualization result which is close to the shaded image. The HQ technique generates streamlines on the whole surface and shades them according to the underlying illumination. In comparison to their method, the ConFIS technique used a different method. Here, this method depicts the spatiality by illustrating the contour margin as well as curvature-based features. Therefore, if the user demands a salient representation with a spatial impression, we recommend the ConFIS method. For a full visualization of the object and using an alternative to diffuse lightning, we would recommend the RT method. As the method by Praun et al. uses a projection of the texture onto the surface, it is sensitive to surface noise and the results depend strongly on the local parameterization. To avoid distortions, the mapped texture should be small to prevent a covering of a large high frequent surface. This implies a longer preprocessing time for determining the lapped textures and a result which is close to

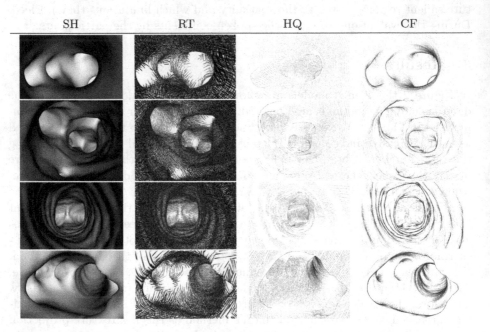

Fig. 2. Endoscopic view illustrated in simple shading (SH), real-time hatching (RT), high-quality hatching (HQ), and ConFIS (CF).

normal shading. HQ and ConFIS depend on the underlying curvature field. The presented curvature field by Rusinkiewicz is robust against surface noise. Here, we notice that the ConFIS method is faster than the high-quality hatching. This is explainable by the fact that ConFIS draws only streamlines at salient regions and therefore less streamlines than the high-quality hatching. Surprisingly, all methods were able to illustrate noised surface well. This can be seen from the second data set of our evaluation. Regarding our evaluation, we can state that hatching methods are able to offer an alternative to normal shading. They can be used for context-aware medical illustrations in endoscopic views as well as learning illustrations for textbooks.

References

1. Tietjen C, Isenberg T, Preim B. Combining silhouettes, surface, and volume rendering for surgery education and planning. Proc IEEE EuroVis. 2005; p. 303–10.
2. Ritter F, Hansen C, Preim B, et al. Real-zime illustration of vascular structures for surgery. Proc IEEE. 2006;12:877–84.
3. Praun E, Hoppe H, Webb M, et al. Real-time hatching. Proc ACM. 2001; p. 581–6.
4. Zander J, Isenberg T, Schlechtweg S, et al. High quality hatching. Comput Graph Forum. 2004;23(3):421–30.
5. Lawonn K, Mönch T, Preim B. Streamlines for illustrative real-time rendering. Comput Graph Forum. 2013;33(3):321–30.
6. Interrante V, Fuchs H, Pizer S. Enhancing transparent skin surfaces with ridge and valley lines. Proc IEEE. 1995; p. 52–9.
7. DeCarlo D, Finkelstein A, Rusinkiewicz S, et al. Suggestive contours for conveying shape. Proc SIGGRAPH. 2003;22(3):848–55.
8. Judd T, Durand F, Adelson EH. Apparent ridges for line drawing. Proc SIGGRAPH. 2007;26(3):19.
9. Xie X, He Y, Tian F, et al. An effective illustrative visualization framework based on photic Extremum Lines (PELs). IEEE Trans Vis Comput Graph. 2007;13:1328–35.
10. Lawonn K, Gasteiger R, Preim B. Qualitative evaluation of feature lines on anatomical surfaces. Proc BVM. 2013; p. 187–92.
11. Rusinkiewicz S. Estimating curvatures and their derivatives on triangle meshes. Symp 3D Data Process Vis Transmis. 2004; p. 486–93.

Investigating Contrast Settlement Using Virtual Angiography

Jürgen Endres[1], Thomas Redel[2], Markus Kowarschik[2], Joachim Hornegger[1,3]

[1] Pattern Recognition Lab, Friedrich-Alexander-Universität Erlangen-Nürnberg
[2] Siemens AG, Healthcare Sector, Forchheim
[3] Erlangen Graduate School in Advanced Optical Technologies (SAOT), Erlangen
juergen.endres@cs.fau.de

Abstract. Hemodynamic parameters based on the temporal behavior of contrast agent flow in cerebral aneurysms represent important indicators of the effectiveness of deployed micro devices. These measurements are also interesting for the assessment of virtual treatment planning strategies such as virtual device implantation combined with CFD simulations of blood flow and subsequently generated synthetic angiograms (virtual angiography). Due to settlement effects, contrast agent residence time may increase. As of today, virtual angiography does not explicitly model these effects such that differences between real and virtual angiograms are existent. Hence, we present an approach to examine this contrast agent settlement in virtual angiograms by adding a gravitational effect on simulated contrast agent. The model is evaluated on several cases with different characteristics by generating virtual angiograms with and without the proposed gravity model and comparisons against acquired, real angiograms. Primarily with regards to wash-out behavior and residence time, virtual angiograms including a gravity component show a significantly improved concordance with acquired angiograms.

1 Introduction

A recent method for intracranial aneurysm treatment is flow diversion [1], where fine-meshed stents, called flow diverters (FD), are inserted into the parent artery to reduce the flow inside the aneurysm and to recover the original blood flow.

To assess the efficacy of a flow-diverting device, 2D digital subtraction angiographic (DSA) sequences are acquired after the treatment and compared against 2D DSA sequences before treatment. To quantitatively evaluate the differences, time-intensity curves (TICs) of the injected contrast agent inside the aneurysm are often considered. Characteristic differences between the curves of DSA sequences may finally allow evaluating the efficacy of the implanted device [2].

In this context, an observation is the stagnation of contrast agent/blood mixture within the aneurysm, especially observable for large and giant ones. According to [3], this effect is presumably attributed to density differences between contrast agent/blood mixture and pure blood, leading to a descent of the mixture due to the influence of gravity. On the other hand, a settlement of contrast agent in a mixture with blood could not be reproduced in ex-vitro experiments since density differences are usually only small [4], leading to the assumption this effect is also originating from specific flow patterns inside the aneurysm.

Computational fluid dynamics (CFD) is a recent technique to investigate hemodynamic parameters such as flow velocity and pressure within the aneurysm using numerical methods [5]. Combined with virtual device implantation, this method can be used in order to simulate the treatment outcome of alternative interventional procedures. A first evaluation approach of these CFD results may be based on virtual angiography [6, 7] by comparing them against real, acquired 2D DSA scenes. Including advection and diffusion into virtual angiography calculations, the results fail to show or explain the extended contrast residence time and contrast settling inside the aneurysm.

To examine this effect in our virtual angiography model, we exert a gravity-based velocity vector on virtually injected contrast agent, which leads to an observable stagnation inside the aneurysms.

2   Materials and methods

2.1   Clinical data

In this study, seven data sets were used (Tab. 1). Each data set consists of a 3D rotational angiogram (3D RA) providing spatial information of the vasculature, as well as a 2D DSA sequence which provides dynamic flow information. For three data sets, both pre and post stenting 2D angiograms were available. The data sets contain cases with large/giant aneurysms (Pat1, Pat2) as well as small/medium-sized aneurysms (Pat3, Pat4).

2.2   Virtual angiography considering gravitational effect

In order to introduce the settling effect into virtual angiogram generation, we extend the workflow as presented in [7]. Based on a particle representation of contrast agent, an algorithm consisting of alternating advection and diffusion steps models the propagation of contrast agent through the vasculature. In order to model the settling effect, the workflow is extended by a third component, as depicted in Fig. 1. This gravitational step processes each individual particle, where $\rho_i(t)$ denotes the position of the particle i at time t, δt denotes the (fixed) time step for the repeated process and v_g describes a constant velocity vector pointing towards the center of earth. This velocity vector is deduced from the gravitational force and can be considered as constant since all particles share the same mass and are processed using the same fixed time step δt. That means, contrast agent (an ensemble of individual particles) gets a constant, downward drift during propagation within the vessels. We additionally include a constraint, which intends to overcome the limitations of using dimensionless particles. Due to that property, contrast agent (i.e., particles) may agglomerate as a thin layer

Table 1. Overview of clinical data sets. FD denotes flow diverter.

Dataset	DSA duration	DSA [fps]	Flow diverter	Contrast settlement
Pat1	12.5 s	30	×	✓
Pat1 w/ FD	12.3 s	30	✓	✓
Pat2	11.8 s	4	×	×
Pat2 w/ FD	11.8 s	4	×	✓
Pat3	6.7 s	30	×	×
Pat4	3.7 s	15	×	×
Pat4 w/ FD	8.0 s	15	✓	✓

at the bottom part of the aneurysm. However, by introducing a partitioning V_p of the vasculature into (cubic) subvolumes and restricting the number of particles per volume by a saturation constant C, particles will stack up resulting in a volumetric bulk rather than a flat plane. Hence there are two parameters for controlling the gravity process; v_g as the velocity vector and C as the particle threshold for subvolumes. This constraint is used for the gravity step only

$$\rho_i(t+1) = \begin{cases} \rho_i(t) + \delta t \cdot v_g \ , \text{ if } \quad V_p(\rho_i(t) + \delta t \cdot v_g) < C \\ \rho_i(t) \qquad , \text{ else} \end{cases} \tag{1}$$

2.3 Experiments

Patient-specific virtual angiograms were generated using both the conventional workflow [7] as well as the proposed workflow including gravity. That means, virtual angiograms were generated such that they best match the corresponding 2D DSA sequence for that data set in terms of vessel geometry, inflow velocities, injection bolus, etc. at the position which corresponds to the inlet boundary of the CFD simulation. Subsequently, comparisons between real and virtual angiograms (w/ and w/o gravity) are examined using both qualitative as well as quantitative parameters as described in [2] (Tab. 2 and 3). For the partitioning

Fig. 1. Extended virtual angiography algorithm.

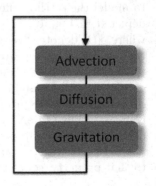

Table 2. Measured quantities for data set Pat1. Full width at half maximum (FWHM) is given in seconds [s], average inflow (avgIF) and average outflow (avgOF) are given in change of gray-level values per second [I/s]. The values in brackets behind the measured data denote the differences between the measurements from the corresponding virtual angiogram and the measurements from the real data set. In the last column, the improvement (given in percentage points) is given when switching from virtual angiograms without gravity to virtual angiograms with gravity.

Dataset Pat1		Real DSA	Virtual DSA w/o grav		Virtual DSA w/ grav		Improvement (% points)
Proximal	FWHM	1.28	1.27	(-0.8%)	1.24	(-3.1%)	-2.3
	AvgIF	211	242	(14.7%)	240	(13.7%)	1.0
	AvgOF	220	202	(-8.2%)	228	(3.6%)	4.6
Distal	FWHM	2.45	1.42	(-42.0%)	1.42	(-42.0%)	0.0
	AvgIF	88	83	(-5.7%)	87	(-1.1%)	4.6
	AvgOF	33	91	(175.8%)	93	(181.8%)	-6.0
Aneurysm	FWHM	2.90	2.20	(-24.1%)	2.78	(-4.1%)	20.0
	AvgIF	89	84	(-5.6%)	80	(-10.1%)	-4.5
	AvgOF	13	27	(107.7%)	14	(7.7%)	100.0

V_p, the CFD output data grid is used, where single voxels represent the subvolumes. Parameters v_g (gravity vector) and C (saturation variable for subvolumes) are heuristically determined for one data set using comparisons with real DSA series and transferred to all other data sets. For the following experiments, $|v_g|$ = 0.1 m/s, and $C = 8 \cdot 10^2$ (for a total amount of $8 \cdot 10^5$ particles) is used.

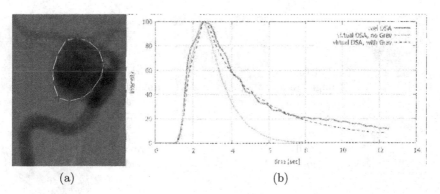

(a)   (b)

Fig. 2. (b) shows the TICs for the acquired angiogram (data set Pat1) as well as for both virtual angiograms (w/ and w/o gravity), calculated for the region of interest covering the complete aneurysm dome (a).

3   Results

In Tab. 2, we present the quantitative measurements of the virtual angiograms for data set Pat1 and compared the results against measurements of the acquired angiogram. The quantities are calculated according to [2], whereas the differences between real and virtual angiograms are expressed as deviation from the real angiogram. To point out the influence of the gravitational effect, the improvement from virtual angiograms without gravity model to virtual angiograms with gravity model is calculated (given in percentage points, see last column of Tab. 2). Tab. 3 lists these improvements for all data sets.

For illustration purposes, real and virtual angiograms both without and with gravitational effect are shown in Fig. 3 for data set Pat1, as well as the corresponding time intensity curves for the region of interest covering the aneurysm dome, Fig. 2 (b).

4   Discussion

By adding the presented gravity model, we achieved significant improvements when comparing CFD-based virtual angiograms with acquired angiograms where contrast settlement is observable in real angiograms (Pat1, Pat1 w/ FD, Pat2 w/ FD, Pat4 w/ FD). The quantities particularly improve for the measurements covering the complete aneurysm dome. Measurements proximal and distal to the aneurysm are not significantly affected by the gravity component, as expected from real angiograms. More important, in cases where no intense contrast settlement is visible in real angiograms (Pat3, Pat4), no significant changes are observable between virtual angiograms with and without gravity component.

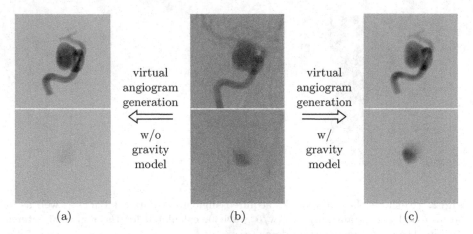

(a)   (b)   (c)

Fig. 3. (b) shows images of the acquired angiogram of a giant aneurysm from AP view. The upper part of the image shows the contrast agent distribution at time t = 2.3 s, the lower part at time t = 6.2 s. (a) shows the respective virtual angiogram without gravitational effect, (c) including the gravitational effect.

Table 3. Improvement in percent of virtual angiograms with and without gravity.

		Pat1	Pat1 w/FD	Pat2	Pat2 w/FD	Pat3	Pat4	Pat4 w/FD
Proximal	FWHM	-2.3	-4.5	2.0	-1.0	0.0	2.3	4.0
	AvgIF	1.0	-2.0	7.2	1.2	10.7	6.0	-9.4
	AvgOF	4.6	-3.6	-5.2	-14.5	-10.5	31.2	7.6
Distal	FWHM	0.0	-3.5	-12.6	-3.9	1.5	-6.7	0.7
	AvgIF	4.6	-9.3	-10.2	4.3	3.0	-5.1	-0.4
	AvgOF	-6.0	11.6	5.4	-13.4	5.6	9.6	-5.6
Aneurysm	FWHM	20.0	56.0	2.6	2.0	1.4	0.7	12.0
	AvgIF	-4.5	7.4	-10.8	-1.1	2.2	-5.0	-4.9
	AvgOF	100.0	166.7	0.0	560	9.6	18.6	31.3

In this study, we model contrast settlement using a gravity model for virtual angiograms that suggests the gravity contributes to the contrast settlement. For further understanding, especially on the contribution of specific flow patterns and their interaction with gravity, additional experiments with an increased number of cases are needed. Future work may also discuss exisiting limitiations of our study; i.e., segmentation accuracy, flow and mixing behaviour of blood and contrast agent, as well as flow changes due to the injection process. More in-depth analysis may further be accomplished using multi-phase CFD approaches.

Acknowledgement. We thank Prof. Dörfler and his team, Dept of Neuroradiology, University Erlangen-Nuremberg, for discussions and data providing.

References

1. Byrne JV, Szikora I. Flow diverters in the management of intracranial aneurysms: a review. EJMINT Orig Artic. 2012;1225000057:1–22.
2. Struffert T, Ott S, Kowarschik M, et al. Measurement of quantifiable parameters by time-density curves in the elastase-induced aneurysm model: first results in the comparison of a flow diverter and a conventional aneurysm stent. Eur Radiol. 2013;23(2):521–7.
3. Wang ZJ, Hoffmann KR, Wang Z, et al. Contrast settling in cerebral aneurysm angiography. Phys Med Biol. 2005;50(13):3171–81.
4. Lieber BB, Sadasivan C, Hao Q, et al. The mixability of angiographic contrast with arterial blood. Med Phys. 2009;36(11):5064–78.
5. Larrabide I, Aguilar ML, Morales HG, et al. Intra-aneurysmal pressure and flow changes induced by flow diverters: relation to aneurysm size and shape. Am J Neuroradiol. 2013;34(4):816–22.
6. Ford MD, Stuhne GR, Nikolov HN, et al. Virtual angiography for visualization and validation of computational models of aneurysm hemodynamics. IEEE Trans Med Imaging. 2005;24(12):1586–92.
7. Endres J, Kowarschik M, Redel T, et al. A workflow for patient-individualized virtual angiogram generation based on CFD simulation. Comput Math Methods Med. 2012;2012(306765):1–24.

Neuartige Röntgensimulation für ein ERCP-Trainingsphantom

M. Vietz[1], V. Aurich[1], K.-E. Grund[2]

[1]Institut für Informatik, Heinrich-Heine-Universität Düsseldorf
[2]Experimentelle Chirurgische Endoskopie, Eberhard-Karls-Universität Tübingen
vietz-bvm2014@acs.uni-duesseldorf.de

Kurzfassung. Die Endoskopisch Retrograde Cholangio- Pankreatiko-graphie (ERCP) bedarf als komplexer endoskopisch/radiologischer Eingriff im Gallengangsystem eines intensiven Trainings von Arzt und Assistenz. In der Experimentellen Endoskopie des Universitätsklinikums Tübingen wurde für das Training speziell dieses Einsatzes ein realistisches Hands-On-Trainingsphantom entwickelt, das bisher über eine virtuelle Röntgensimulation verfügt, mit der die Lage einfacher endoskopischer Instrumente innerhalb des Gallengangsystems dargestellt werden kann. Für ein effektives uneingeschränktes Training aller diagnostischen, therapeutischen und interventionellen Eingriffe bei der ERCP reicht die bisherige Röntgensimulation jedoch noch nicht aus; in diesem Beitrag stellen wir ein neuartiges Verfahren vor, mit dem deutlich detailliertere und realistischere Röntgenbilder auch von komplexen Instrumenten erzeugt werden können. Damit wird erstmals ein effektives und realitätsnahes ERCP-Training ohne Strahlenbelastung möglich.

1 Problemstellung

Die Endoskopisch Retrograde Cholangio-Pankreatikographie (ERCP) ist ein minimalinvasives endoskopisch/radiologisches Verfahren, das Diagnostik und Interventionen in den Gallenwegen und im Pankreasgangsystem ermöglicht. Die ERCP gehört zu den sehr komplexen endoskopischen Eingriffen und erfordert deshalb viel Training und große Erfahrung, um Komplikationen zu vermeiden.

Aktuell wurde für das Training dieser anspruchsvollen Eingriffe in der Experimentellen Endoskopie des Universitätsklinikums Tübingen ein ERCP-Phantom, der sog. Tübinger Biliphant entwickelt, der die Nachteile bisheriger Trainingssimulatoren vermeidet [1, 2, 3]. Es besteht aus realitätsnahen Nachbildungen des menschlichen oberen Gastrointestinaltrakts mit integriertem biliopankreatischem System. Es können Läsionen und Pathologika (Engstellen, Tumore, Steine etc.) als Module eingebracht werden. Alle Komponenten entsprechen einer korrekten humanen Anatomie und bestehen aus speziellen Materialien, die hygienisch unbedenklich sind, kein Tiermaterial enthalten und in Optik und Haptik weitgehend menschlichem Gewebe entsprechen. Insbesondere die Papille kann, genau wie beim Patienten, hochfrequenzchirurgisch geschnitten werden.

Ein entscheidender Punkt ist die Notwendigkeit, alle ERCP-Interventionen unter Röntgendurchleuchtung auszuführen, was eine Strahlenbelastung für Trainees und Tutoren bedeutet. Im Tübinger Biliphanten sind alle Organe und Module mit definierter Röntgendichte ausgeführt, sodass er sich wie ein menschlicher Patient mittels eines üblichen C-Bogens durchleuchten lässt.

Die daraus resultierende hohe Strahlenbelastung ist aber vor allem für weibliche Teilnehmer nicht vertretbar. Neuere Studien [4] zeigen, dass selbst bei Nutzung aller Strahlenschutzmaßnahmen insbesondere die Strahlendosis für die Augenlinse in der Praxis kaum unter dem von der Internationalen Strahlenschutzkommission IRCP empfohlenen Grenzwert gehalten werden kann. Trainingssituationen, die naturgemäß eine um ein Mehrfaches längere Durchleuchtungszeit als eine Intervention am Patienten erfordern, überschreiten somit alle Grenzwerte der Strahlenexposition in nicht tolerabler Weise.

2 Methoden

Zur Lösung des Problems der hohen Strahlenbelastung wurde in das Gesamtsystem eine virtuelle Röntgensimulation implementiert. Diese umfasst zwei Berechnungsschritte: Zunächst wird der „Hintergrund", der alle statischen Bereiche des simulierten Röntgenbildes beinhaltet, berechnet und anschließend das Instrument geometrisch korrekt als "Vordergrund" eingeblendet. Die Erzeugung des Röntgenbildes wird mittels 3D-Rendering unter Verwendung von OpenGL vorgenommen. Dies hat den Vorteil, dass sich das virtuelle Röntgenbild wie ein reales Röntgenbild innerhalb gewisser Grenzen um alle Achsen rotieren, verschieben, etc. lässt.

2.1 Berechnung des Hintergrundbildes

Für die Berechnung des Hintergrundes wird ein CT-Volumendatensatz des Biliphanten mittels klassischem Raycasting gerendert. Die Intensitäten aller Voxel auf einem Sehstrahl werden dabei aufintegriert. Anschließend wird ausgehend von diesem Integral analog zur physikalischen Erzeugung eines realen Röntgenbildes nach dem Lambert-Beer'schen Gesetz

$$I = I_0 * \exp\left(-\int \mu(x)dx\right)$$

der Intensitätswert für diesen Sehstrahl ermittelt. Hierbei ist $\mu(x)$ der sog. lineare Abschwächungskoeffizient, der die „Röntgendichte" des durchleuchteten Materials am Ort x beschreibt. Dieser lässt sich relativ direkt aus dem CT-Datensatz ableiten.

2.2 Bisherige Berechnung des Instrumentabbildes

Für die Berechnung des Abbilds des Instruments existiert neben dem hier vorgestellten, neuen Verfahren bereits eine einfachere Version [2]. Mit diesem einfacheren Verfahren kann ein virtuelles Röntgenbild eines linienhaften Instruments, wie z.B. eines Führungsdrahts oder eines Papillotoms, erzeugt werden. Das Hintergrundbild wird auf ähnliche Weise berechnet. Für Anfänger ist dies durchaus ausreichend, da diese zunächst die Navigation im Gallengangsystem erlernen müssen, wofür sich das einfache Verfahren gut eignet. Die eingesetzte Sensorik ist aber z.B. nicht dazu in der Lage, ein in Schlaufen liegendes Instrument detailgetreu wiederzugeben. Auch können damit aufwändigere Instrumente, wie z.B. Ballons zur Gefäßdilatation, Zangen zur Steinextraktion oder sog. Dormia-Körbchen, nicht dargestellt werden, was für fortgeschrittene Anwender aber unerlässlich ist. Dies wird erst mit dem neuartigen Verfahren ermöglicht, das im Folgenden beschrieben werden wird.

2.3 Neuartige Berechnung des Instrumentabbildes

Die Grundidee des Verfahrens beruht auf der einfachen Überlegung, dass sich die Bilderzeugung eines realen Röntgenbildes z.B. durch einen C-Bogen in vielen wesentlichen Eigenschaften kaum von der Erzeugung eines Schattenbildes durch eine optische Kamera unterscheidet: Sowohl Röntgengerät als auch optische Kamera liefern eine Projektion des aufgenommenen dreidimensionalen Objekts auf eine zweidimensionale Bildebene.

In der Standardausstattung sind die nachgebildeten Gallengänge intransparent. Für die verbesserte Röntgensimulation wurden diese dahingehend modifiziert, dass wichtige Stellen des Gangsystems, wie z.B. Verzweigungen oder Engstellen (Stenosen), transparent für sichtbares Licht sind. Anschließend wurde eine optische Kamera eingebaut. Diese Kamera wurde so montiert, dass sie ein Bild von diesen wichtigen Stellen liefert. Auf der Rückseite der transparenten Gallengangsegmente befindet sich eine flächenhafte Lichtquelle, sodass eine gleichmäßige Beleuchtung von der Rückseite her stattfindet.

Wird nun ein Instrument, z.B. eine Zange, in den Gallengang eingeführt, so wird es aufgrund der Beleuchtung von der Rückseite im Bild der Kamera als Schattenriss sichtbar. Dieser Schattenriss bildet die Grundlage für die weiteren Verarbeitungsschritte hin zum fertig simulierten Röntgenbild.

2.4 Verarbeitungsschritte

Die Instrumente, von denen ein Röntgenbild simuliert werden soll, haben durchaus sehr unterschiedliche Gestalt. Ein Dilatationsballon wirft, sofern er mit Kontrastmittel gefüllt wurde, einen großflächigen Schatten, während ein Dormia-Körbchen oder gar ein Metallstent eine sehr filigrane, komplexe Struktur besitzen. Einen Bildverarbeitungsalgorithmus zu entwickeln, der im Kamerabild in jeder Situation genau das gewünschte Instrument segmentiert, erweist sich deswegen als schwierig. Ein gänzlich anderer Ansatz, der aus der Subtraktionsangiographie bekannt ist, erweist sich als einfacher. Hierbei wird vor Beginn des simulierten Eingriffs zunächst ein Bild B_r der Kamera als Referenzbild aufgenommen. Anschließend wird bei allen später aufgenommenen Bildern die Differenz $B_d(x,y) := B_a(x,y) - B_r(x,y)$ zwischen dem aktuellen Bild und dem Referenzbild berechnet. Im Idealfall hat das Differenzbild in allen Pixeln, die nicht zum

Instrument gehören, den Wert 0, während dort, wo sich das Instrument befindet, sehr große Grauwerte vorkommen.

2.5 Berechnung des Gesamtbildes

Nachdem das Hintergrundbild berechnet wurde, wird das segmentierte Instrument anschließend geometrisch korrekt mittels Alpha-Blending über dieses Hintergrundbild gelegt. Dazu wird das Differenzbild B_d als Textur auf eine Ebene abgebildet, die so in das Volumen eingepasst wird, dass ihre Lage der Lage der realen Kameraebene innerhalb des Phantoms entspricht. Diese Einpassung wird anhand von Markern vorgenommen, die sowohl in den Volumendatensatz als auch in das Phantom eingebracht wurden und im Bild der Kamera leicht gefunden werden können. Abhängig von der Anatomie des Phantoms kommen 8 - 16 Marker zum Einsatz, die direkt am Gallengangsystem befestigt sind. Beim Rendern der Ebene wird der Texturwert in jedem Punkt der Ebene als Alphawert interpretiert, der die Transparenz der Ebene in diesem Punkt definiert. Die Ebene selber ist komplett schwarz. Auf diese Weise wird die eingeblendete Ebene an den Stellen, wo in B_d eine große Differenz gespeichert ist, sehr dunkel, während sie dort, wo keine oder kaum Differenzen vorhanden sind, nahezu transparent ist. In Abschnitt 3 sind einige Beispielbilder zu sehen.

2.6 Korrektur bei elastischen Deformationen

Ein Problem, welches bei der Berechnung von Differenzbildern immer wieder auftritt, besteht darin, dass sowohl die Kamera als auch die gesamte Anordnung der aufgenommenen Szene absolut starr sein müssen, damit es bei der Differenzbildung nicht zu unerwünschten Artefakten kommt. Die Position der Kamera im Phantom kann zwar relativ gut fixiert werden, jedoch ist das Gallengangsystem bis zu einem gewissen Grad elastisch. Aus diesem Grund verbietet sich die naive Erzeugung des Differenzbildes, wie sie in Abschnitt 2.4 beschrieben wurde, in der Praxis.

Der gewählte Lösungsansatz besteht darin, dass vor der Berechnung des Differenzbildes B_d eine Korrektur des aktuellen Bildes B_a vorgenommen wird, die etwaige Deformationen korrigiert. Das Differenzbild berechnet sich danach durch $B_d(x, y) := B_a(x', y') - B_r(x, y)$, wobei $(x', y') := (x, y) + T(x, y)$ die korrigierte Position ist, an der im Bild B_a zugegriffen werden muss. Hierbei ist T ein diskretes Vektorfeld $\mathbb{Z}^2 \to \mathbb{Z}^2$, welches für jedes Pixel in B_a die Verzerrungskorrektur beschreibt.

Die Marker, die in Abschnitt 2.5 erwähnt wurden, dienen nicht nur der Einpassung der Kameraebene ins Volumen, sondern können darüber hinaus dazu eingesetzt werden, das Korrekturfeld T durch Interpolation der Markerpositionen zu berechnen. Für die Interpolation werden die Marker zunächst einmalig im Referenzbild B_r und anschließend in jedem neuen Bild B_a detektiert. Wird die Menge der Markerpunkte als Eckpunkte eines Polygonzugs aufgefasst, reduziert sich das Interpolationsproblem auf die Aufgabe, ein Polygon P_1 auf ein (ähnliches) anderes Polygon P_2 abzubilden. Für diese Interpolationsaufgabe eignet sich die Verwendung Verallgemeinerter Baryzentrischer Koordinaten als Gewichte. Für den vorliegenden Beitrag wurden Mean Value Coordinates [5] verwendet.

3   Ergebnisse

Folgende Abbildungen geben einen Eindruck über die erzeugten virtuellen Röntgenbilder. Als Vergleichsbild soll Abb. 1(a) dienen, die ein echtes Röntgenbild eines Sondierungsdrahts zeigt. Abb. 1(e) und Abb. 1(f) zeigen einen Vergleich eines korrigierten mit einem nicht korrigierten Differenzbild. Zur besseren Sichtbarkeit wurden die Grauwerte invertiert und die Artefakte grün markiert. Man sieht sehr schön, dass die Artefakte durch die Korrektur praktisch vollständig vermieden werden können.

Die Berechnung des Hintergrundbilds findet komplett in der GPU des Rechners statt, sodass diese sehr schnell vonstatten geht. Das Instrumentabbild wird von der CPU des Rechners berechnet; es zeigt sich jedoch, dass ein handelsüblicher Intel I5-Prozessor mit 2,6 Ghz eine Bildrate von mindestens 10 Bildern pro Sekunde erreicht. Die Simulation des Röntgenbilds ist also echtzeitfähig.

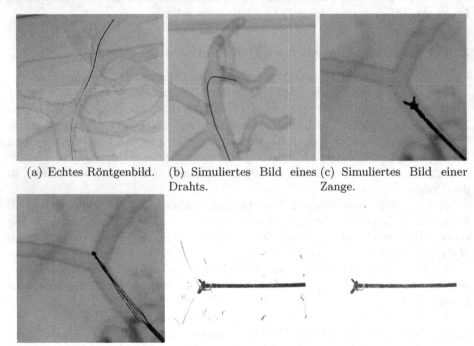

(a) Echtes Röntgenbild.   (b) Simuliertes Bild eines (c) Simuliertes Bild einer
                          Drahts.   Zange.

(d) Simuliertes Bild eines (e) Nicht korrigiertes Diffe- (f) Korrigiertes Differenz-
Dormia-Körbchens.   renzbild. Es sind deutliche bild. Keine Artefakte.
                           Artefakte vorhanden (grün
                           markiert).

Abb. 1. Erzeugung virtueller Röntgenbilder.

4 Diskussion

Die ERCP gehört zu den schwierigsten endoskopischen Prozeduren. Das Risiko für schwere Komplikationen ist relativ hoch, deshalb ist ein intensives Training von Arzt und Assistenz unumgänglich. Mit dem Tübinger Biliphanten steht ein leistungsfähiges Trainingskonzept zur Verfügung, das jedoch bisher unter der unvermeidbaren Röntgenbelastung bei der ERCP leidet. Mit der Integration der Röntgensimulation der ersten und ganz besonders der zweiten Version konnte dieses Problem weitestgehend gelöst werden, sodass nun nahezu alle üblichen Eingriffe ohne jede Strahlenbelastung beliebig oft wiederholbar und vor allem reproduzierbar trainiert werden können.

Der Biliphant wurde inzwischen in über 15 Trainingskursen erfolgreich eingesetzt. Die herkömmliche Röntgensimulation ist dabei sowohl von Experten als auch von Trainingsteilnehmern durchweg positiv aufgenommen worden. Mit der Integration der verbesserten Röntgensimulation mittels optischer Erkennung können nahezu alle Eingriffe in gewohnter Weise radiologisch dargestellt und kontrolliert werden. Die Einführung von Instrumenten in die Gangsysteme und die Manipulationen dort werden kontinuierlich realitätsgetreu in Echtzeit dargestellt (Abb. 1(b) - Abb. 1(d)). Auch schwierige Interventionen lassen sich in jeder Phase radiologisch verfolgen; dabei wird jedoch jede Strahlenbelastung vermieden. Für die verbesserte Simulation stehen bisher nur wenige Erfahrungswerte und Bewertungen zur Verfügung, die jedoch hoch positiv sind, sodass dieser Ansatz für die Zukunft sehr vielversprechend ist.

Literaturverzeichnis

1. Grund K, Ingenpaß R, Durst F, et al. Neuartiges Hands-on-Phantom für das realistische Training der gesamten diagnostischen und therapeutischen ERCP. Endo heute. 2012; p. 14–7.
2. Vietz M, Özmen D, Grund K, et al. Neuartige virtuelle Simulation des Röntgenbildes und der Endoskop-Position für das phantomgestützte Hands-on-Training ohne Strahlenbelastung. Endo heute. 2013;26:17.
3. Grund K, Ingenpaß R, Schweizer U, et al. Neues ERCP-Trainings-Modell für alle diagnostischen und therapeutischen Eingriffe. Z Gastroenterol. 2012; p. 4–5.
4. Galster M, Guhl C, Uder M, et al. Exposition der Augenlinse des Untersuchers und Effizienz der Strahlenschutzmittel bei fluoroskopischen Interventionen. Rofo. 2013; p. 474–81.
5. Joshi P, Meyer M, DeRose T, et al. Harmonic coordinates for character articulation. ACM Trans Graph. 2007;26(3). Available from: http://doi.acm.org/10.1145/1276377.1276466.

Identifikation und Simulation intraoperativer Fehlerquellen bei einer orthopädischen Umstellungsosteotomie

Sebastian Kallus[1], Christoph Auer[1], Urs Eisenmann[1], Sebastian Wolf[2],
Jürgen Korber[2], Thomas Dreher[2], Hartmut Dickhaus[1]

[1]Institut für Medizinische Biometrie und Informatik, Universität Heidelberg
[2]Orthopädische Klinik, Universitätsklinikum Heidelberg
sebastian.kallus@med.uni-heidelberg.de

Kurzfassung. Umstellungsosteotomien sind in der orthopädischen Chirurgie von großer Bedeutung und stellen häufig die einzige Möglichkeit dar pathologische Fehlstellungen des Bewegungsapparates zu korrigieren. Der Therapieerfolg bleibt in einigen Fällen trotz genauer Planungsdaten deutlich hinter den Erwartungen zurück. Die seit Jahren beobachtete Streuung der Therapieergebnisse im Follow-Up ist bisher nicht erklärbar. Kliniker sehen als wahrscheinlichste Ursache Unsicherheiten beim operativen Eingriff. Mit Hilfe eines hier entwickelten Simulationsmodells wurde das Fehlerpotential bei einem solchen OP-Verfahren erstmalig quantitativ erschlossen. Auswertungsergebnisse belegen, dass die feststellbare Streuung durch methodische Probleme bei der OP-Durchführung und -Kontrolle erklärt werden kann und entschlüsseln die Beiträge einzelner Fehlerquellen zur Gesamtabweichung. Hiermit wurden neue Erkenntnisse gewonnen, wie sich die korrekte Planungsumsetzung bei der OP-Durchführung sicherstellen lässt.

1 Einleitung

Bei Patienten mit ausgeprägten Gangstörungen, aufgrund knöcherner Fehlstellungen der Beine, werden häufig chirurgische Eingriffe vorgenommen, um den physiologischen Gang wiederherzustellen. Spezialisierte orthopädische Zentren können komplexe Gangstörungen, wie sie z.B. bei frühkindlicher Hirnschädigung vorliegen, durch eine instrumentelle 3D-Ganganalyse genau quantifizieren. Die hier häufig festgestellte Innen- oder Außenrotation der Beine wird durch eine femorale Derotationsosteotomie (FDO) um den zuvor in der Planung berechneten Korrekturwinkel kompensiert. [1] Dazu wird der Oberschenkelknochen durchtrennt und das knienahe Segment rotiert. Mit einer winkelstabilen Osteosyntheseplatte werden beide Segmente anschließend fixiert (Abb. 1). Durch einen Stellungsvergleich der vorher eingebrachten Kirschnerdrähte (K-Drähte) wird mit Hilfe eines analogen Winkelmessers der intraoperativ umgesetzte Korrekturwinkel ermittelt. [2]

Trotz technisch aufwendig ermittelter Planungsdaten und sorgfältiger operativer Umsetzung des Korrekturwinkels bleibt der Therapieerfolg häufig hinter den Erwartungen zurück. So ist bei der postoperativen Funktionsanalyse nach 12 Monaten eine hohe interindividuelle Streuung von ± 10 Winkelgraden zu beobachten. [3] Abweichungen in dieser Größenordnung können für den einzelnen Patienten eine erneute Operation oder eine bleibende Behinderung der Gehfähigkeit bedeuten.

Die Ursachen sind bisher nicht eindeutig geklärt. Das größte Fehlerpotential wird jedoch von erfahrenen Chirurgen in der Operationsdurchführung selbst vermutet. Mit dem hier entwickelten Computermodell wird erstmalig der Ansatz verfolgt potentielle intraoperative Fehlereinflüsse, die das Therapieergebnis einer FDO beeinflussen können, zu simulieren und quantitativ zu charakterisieren. Hiermit sollen Erkenntnisse darüber gewonnen werden, ob und wie sich die Qualität der OP-Intervention verbessern lässt.

2 Material und Methoden

2.1 Identifikation intraoperativer Fehlerquellen bei einer FDO

Mit der Unterstützung chirurgischer Experten der Orthopädie Heidelberg konnten während klinischer OP-Besuche sowie mittels Analysen von Planungs- und OP-Daten (Kinematik, Röntgenbilder, etc.) mehrere potentielle Fehlerquellen bei der OP-Durchführung aufgedeckt werden (Tab. 1). Bereits der Planungstransfer in den OP ist nicht exakt möglich, da der Eingriff auf der anatomischen Knochenachse vollzogen werden muss, die sich von der funktionalen Planungsachse aus der 3D-Ganganalyse unterscheidet (Abb. 2).

Auch gelingt es den Chirurgen nicht immer den Oberschenkelknochen exakt senkrecht zu durchtrennen, sodass die tatsächliche Korrekturachse in der Praxis noch stärker von der funktionalen Planungsachse abweichen kann. Analysen intraoperativer Kontroll-Röntgenbilder zeigen hier Abweichungen von bis zu $20°$.

2.2 Virtuelles FDO-Modell

Modelldefinition. Um den Einfluss der identifizierten Fehlerquellen auf das OP-Ergebnis quantitativ zu untersuchen, wurde ein Computermodell für femorale Derotationsosteotomien (FDOs) entworfen und in Matlab implementiert. Mit

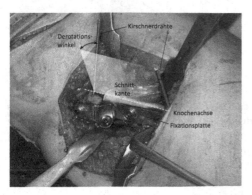

Abb. 1. Operationsbereich FDO. Es sind die Kirschnerdrähte und die Fixierungsplatte sichtbar. Der Korrekturwinkel, die Schnittkante und die anatomische Knochenachse sind schematisch eingezeichnet. (Quelle: Orthopädie Heidelberg).

Tabelle 1. Zusammenfassung der vermuteten Fehlerquellen einer FDO.

Nr.	Potentielle intraop. Fehlerquellen	Bereich max. Abweichung
1	Planungs- vs. anatom. Knochenachse	$6 \pm 2°$
2	Schiefe Schnittebene/Korrekturachse	$\leq 20°$
3	K-Drähte (Winkeloffset)	$[-5°, \ldots, +5°]$
4	Ableseposition Winkelmesser	20-40 cm zu distalem K-Draht vom Knie; max. 20 cm re./li. bzw. ober-/unterhalb vom Kniegelenkszentrum
5	Plattenverschraubung	-

Hilfe eines präparierten FDO-Knochenphantoms wurde die Geometrie eines genormten Femurs (mittlere Größenverhältnisse bei einem gesunden Erwachsenen) mit einem elektromagnetischen Trackingsystem (NDI Aurora) abgetastet und vermessen. Im Knochenphantom weicht die Lage der funktionalen Planungsachse von der anatomischen Knochenachse um 6, 5° ab. Die Schnittebene befindet sich ca. 8 cm vom Kniegelenkzentrum entfernt. Die geometrischen Zusammenhänge und modellierten Aspekte der FDO werden in Abb. 2 erklärt.

FDO-Durchführung. Zur virtuellen Durchführung einer FDO können im Modell Lage und Winkel der Schnittebene variabel definiert und die daraus resultierende Korrekturachse berechnet werden.

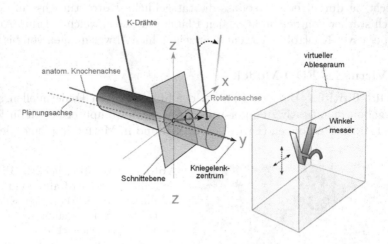

Abb. 2. Schematische Darstellung des virtuellen FDO-Modells. Das Modell besteht aus folgenden Parametern: funktionale Planungsachse, anatomische Knochenachse, initiale Stellung der K-Drähte, Lage der Schnittebene, Geometrie des Knochenquerschnitts, Knochen-Teilsegmente (proximal und distal) sowie aus dem Rotationszentrum und der entstehenden Korrekturachse.

Nach Einstellung des beabsichtigten Korrekturwinkels werden die Knochensegmente neu ausgerichtet, sodass die Osteosyntheseplatte direkt an den angrenzenden Schnittkanten beider Knochensegmente fixiert werden kann. Die operative Drehachse wird dabei verschoben. Betrag und Richtung der Verschiebung ergeben sich aus der unsymmetrischen Form der gegeneinander rotierten Schnittkanten des distalen und proximalen Segmentes.

Neben den auftretenden Verschiebeeffekten lässt sich der virtuell eingestellte Drehwinkel mit den wirksamen Winkelkomponenten auf der Knochenlängsachse und der funktionalen Verbindungsachse vergleichen. Bei der Simulation des manuell abgelesenen Korrekturwinkels kann der Winkelmesser im virtuell defierten Ableseraum frei verschoben werden (Abb. 2). Über die Positionsangabe des Winkelmessers wird gleichzeitig die Projektionsrichtung vorgegeben, entlang derer sich der abgelesene Korrekturwinkel errechnet.

Fehlersimulation der FDO. Mit dem hier entwickelten Modell lassen sich FDOs für beliebig geplante Korrekturwinkel virtuell durchführen, indem die intraoperativ ermittelten Störgrößen (Schnittfläche in Lage und Winkel, manuelle Ablesung, ...) frei parametrisierbar sind.

Zur Ermittlung signifikanter Unterschiede zwischen OP-Planung und OP-Umsetzung wurde mit Hilfe eines entwickelten Generators der virtuelle Fehler-Parameterraum in den klinisch relevanten Definitionsgrenzen (Tab. 1) vollständig durchsucht. Die daraus resultierenden Ergebnisdatensätze (> 169781 Parameterkombinationen) wurden nach Größe der Rotationsabweichungen und Verschiebungen hin ausgewählt.

Durch geeignete Fehlerplots und Dimensionsreduktion der multidimensionalen Daten konnten einige Zusammenhänge zwischen bestimmten Parameterkombinationen und hohen Ergebnisabweichungen ermittelt werden.

3 Ergebnisse

3.1 Rotationseffekte

Die Simulationsergebnisse zeigen, dass bei der femoralen Deroationsosteotomie mehrere geometrische Zusammenhänge berücksichtigt werden müssen, um den geplanten Korrekturwinkel intraoperativ korrekt abzubilden. Dabei haben die initiale Stellung der K-Drähte, die richtige Ableserichtung mit dem Goniometer und der gewählte Planungswinkel den größten Einfluss auf ein korrektes Gelingen (Tab. 2).

Findet die Ablesung nicht exakt auf der Planungsachse statt, so wird der korrigierte Winkel über die Stellung der K-Drähte auf Grund auftretender Parallaxenfehler falsch eingeschätzt. Liest der Chirurg den tatsächlichen Drehwinkel mit Hilfe des Goniometers beispielsweise weit oberhalb bzw. unterhalb des Kniegelenkzentrums ab, so kann dieser um bis zu 8.4° überschätzt werden. Hingegen besteht bei einer seitlichen Ablesung die Gefahr, den Korrekturwinkel um bis zu

Tabelle 2. Risikofaktoren, die die korrekte Rotationsumsetzung negativ beeinflussen.

Fehlerquelle	Auswirkung auf Rotationsumsetzung
Ablesung mit Goniometer	$[-7.2°,\ldots, +8.4°]$
Planungswinkel	Je größer der Planungswinkel, desto größer das Fehler-potential bei der manuellen Ablesung.
Initiale Stellung der KDs	$[-5°,\ldots, +5°]$
Schnittebene	Nebeneffekt (s.o.)
Planungs- vs. Knochenachse	$< 1°$

$7.2°$ zu unterschätzen (Abb. 3). Berücksichtigt man darüber hinaus ein mögliches Offset der K-Drähte ($\pm5°$), so sind damit Rotationsabweichungen von bis zu $13.4°$ durch das Modell erklärbar.

Aus einer schiefen Schnittebene resultiert nicht zwangsläufig ein Rotationsfehler. Dennoch birgt dieser Aspekt unerwünschte Nebeneffekte. So muss in diesen Fällen das distale Segment ungünstiger Weise um einen größeren Winkel rotiert werden als es bei einem senkrechten Schnitt der Fall wäre, sodass der geplante Effekt erreicht wird. In Extremfällen wäre ein Winkelzuschlag von bis zu $8.1°$ notwendig.

Die Plattenfixierung verursachte unter den Modellannahmen keine Rotationsfehler.

3.2   Verschiebeeffekte

Auftretende Verschiebeeffekte werden maßgeblich von der Schnittebene und dem Planungswinkel beeinflusst. Beide Faktoren korrelieren miteinander: Je größer der Planungswinkel und je schräger die Schnittebene, desto stärker wird der Kniemittelpunkt aus seiner ursprünglichen Position herausgedreht (Abb. 4). In den Simulationsfällen konnte eine maximale Verschiebung des Kniemittelpunktes um $2.9\,\mathrm{cm}$ beobachtet werden.

Dahingegen hatte die Plattenfixierung unter diesen Modellannahmen mit konstant ≤ 3 mm nur einen geringfügigen Einfluss auf die Verschiebung.

4   Diskussion

Die Simulationsergebnisse zeigen, dass die OP-Durchführung großen Spielraum für Optimierungen im Planungstransfer und in der Umsetzungsgenauigkeit bietet. Durch das hier entwickelte Modell lassen sich Unter- bzw. Überkorrekturen von $-13.4°$ bis zu $+12.2°$ sowie ungewollte Verschiebungen des Kniemittelpunktes von über 2.5 cm erklären. Die in der Praxis vorkommenden hohen Streuungen von ca. $\pm10°$ lassen sich durch die Simulationsergebnisse gut nachvollziehen. [3]

Da die möglichen Fehlerquellen an einem Normknochenmodell untersucht wurden, sind individuelle Abweichungen natürlich möglich. Ebenfalls ist zu beachten, dass eine mathematisch korrekte Umsetzung des Korrekturwinkels nicht einem idealen Therapieergebnis entsprechen muss. So sind kompensierende Effekte, die während des zwölfmonatigen Heilungsprozesses eine Rolle spielen (z.B. durch Reorganisation der Motorik), mit diesem Modell nicht erklärbar.

Um die Durchführungsqualität der FDO zu verbessern, bietet sich für dieses OP-Szenario die Entwicklung eines computerassistierten OP-Systems (CAS) an. Durch eingebrachte Sensoren an den einzelnen Femursegmenten lässt sich mit Hilfe eines Trackingsystems die relative Lageänderung der Knochensegmente über die Sensorstellung quantitativ erfassen. Gelingt es, die anatomische Knochenachse und die Schnittkante zu rekonstruieren, kann der eingestellte Korrekturwinkel in Echtzeit genau berechnet werden. Mit einem solchen CAS könnten die Fehlerquellen unabhängig vom geplanten Drehwinkel ausgeschlossen bzw. stark reduziert werden.

Literaturverzeichnis

1. Dreher T, Wolf S, Braatz F, et al. Internal rotation gait in spastic diplegia - critical considerations for the femoral derotation osteotomy. Operat Orthop Traumatol. 2003;15(4):387–401.
2. Wagner M. The Supracondylar Femur Osteotomy for the Correction of a Genu Valgum. Gait Posture. 2007;26(1):25–31.
3. Kay RM, et al. Comparison of proximal and distal rotational femoral osteotomy in children with cerebral palsy. J Pediatr Orthop. 2003;23(2):150–4.

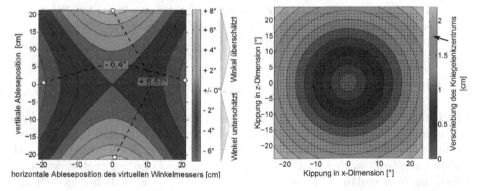

Abb. 3. Ablesefehler mit einem Goniometer bei 30° Rotation. Gemessen in 20 cm Entfernung zum Kniemittelpunkt. Horizontale Achse kodiert Ableseposition des Goniometers, wenn der Winkel seitlich vom Knie abgelesen wird. Vertikale Achse steht für Ablesung unter- bzw. oberhalb des Knies. Farbskala kodiert Ablesefehler.

Abb. 4. Verschiebeeffekte des Kniemittelpunktes, die durch schräge Schnittebenen bei einer 30° Winkelkorrektur entstehen. Horizontale Achse kodiert Kippung der Schnittebenen in einer Dimension. Vertikale Achse kodiert Kippungen in einer zweiten Dimension. Farbskala kodiert die Verschiebung des Kniemittelpunktes.

Nicht-lineare Zeitnormierung im Langzeit-EKG

Generierung einheitlicher Pseudo-Bilddaten aus Multikanal-Ableitungen

Malte Sartor[1], Stephan Jonas[1], Tobias Wartzek[2], Steffen Leonhardt[2],
Christoph Wanner[3], Nikolaus Marx[4], Thomas M. Deserno[1]

[1] Institut für Medizinische Informatik, Uniklinik RWTH Aachen
[2] Lehrstuhl für Medizinische Informationstechnik, RWTH Aachen
[3] Medizinische Klinik I, Universitätsklinikum Würzburg
[4] Klinik für Kardiologie, Pneumologie, Angiologie und Internistische Intensivmedizin,
Uniklinik RWTH Aachen

sjonas@mi.rwth-aachen.de

Kurzfassung. Die zeitliche Normierung von EKG-Signalen gewinnt mit automatischen Analyseverfahren an Bedeutung. Bisher wird jedoch zumeist nur eine lineare Normierung durchgeführt, welche bei wechselnden Herzfrequenzen auf Grund der Streckung oder Stauchung von Zyklus-Segmenten kein zufriedenstellendes Ergebnis erzielen kann. Daher stellen wir hier ein neues Verfahren basierend auf mathematischem Matching vor, welches eine nicht-lineare Anpassung von EKG-Signalen auf einen Referenz-Zyklus ermöglicht. Das vorgestellte Modell ist zudem auf allen in der Koronalebene aufgenommenen EKG-Kanälen einsetzbar und erzielt im Vergleich zu einem Referenzsignal einen durchschnittlichen RMSE von 0.19 mV. Durch die Normalisierung kann eine Bild- oder Volumen-Repräsentation der einzelnen EKG-Zyklen erstellt werden. Diese ist insbesondere für automatische Algorithmen zum Clustering und zum Textur-Vergleich der Zyklen wichtig.

1 Einleitung

Mit Elektrokardiographie (EKG) bezeichnet man die Aufzeichnung der elektrischen Impulse der Herzaktivität in verschiedenen Richtungen. Die bekannte Darstellung des EKG-Zyklus (Abb. 1(a)) beschreibt in der Regel Kanal I oder II, welcher von links nach rechts bzw. diagonal von rechts oben nach links unten durch das Herz verläuft. In der Regel werden sechs bis zwölf Richtungen (Kanäle) abgeleitet, die Richtungen der Ableitungen werden durch den Cabrerakreis (Abb. 2(a)) beschrieben.

Neuartige EKG-Geräte ermöglichen die Aufnahme von 12-Kanal-EKGs mit hoher zeitlicher Auflösung über einen langen Zeitraum. Dies wird in Zukunft einen Paradigmenwechsel bei der Betrachtung von EKG-Daten mit sich ziehen. Beispielsweise werden in klinischen Studien 12-Kanal EKG-Daten mit 1000 Hz über sieben Tage erhoben. Dies entspricht etwa 8 GB unkomprimierte Daten oder einem Papier-EKG von ca. 15 km Länge. Diese Datenmengen sind unmöglich manuell auszuwerten. Anders als bei bisherigen Verfahren, die einzelne Ereignisse in Langzeit-EKGs detektieren [1], soll die Gesamtheit der Daten in neuen Analyseverfahren betrachtet werden. Hierfür wird eine zeitliche Normierung benötigt, die Variationen auf Grund der Änderung der Herzfrequenz eliminiert.

Die einzelnen Segmente des EKG-Zyklus haben beschränkte Längen. Sie verschieben und strecken sich je nach Herzrate individuell [2]. Daher ist eine lineare Zeitnormierung nicht möglich (Abb. 1(b)). Thematisch ähnliche Arbeiten beschäftigen sich mit Personenidentifikation [3] oder der Simulation und Synthese von EKG-Daten [4]. Arbeiten zur nicht-linearen EKG-Normierung oder zum Matching vieler Zyklen sind uns derzeit nicht bekannt.

Wir beschreiben eine Methode zur mathematischen Modellierung der Kanäle, die in der Coronalebene ableiten. Das mathematische Modell wird verwendet, um eine nicht-lineare Anpassung auf einen Referenz-Zyklus vorzunehmen.

2 Material und Methoden

Zur Erstellung des mathematischen Modells wurde mit Hilfe des Summationsvektors der Frontralprojektion einer Herzerregung [5] die Approximationsformel nach Alwal et al. [6] erweitert, um die EKG-Kanäle I, II, III, aVL, aVR und aVF, die in der coronalen Ebene liegen, zu modellieren. Ausgehend von einem Ruhepol beschreibt der Summationsvektor die Richtung, in der die Spannung im Herzen während des EKG-Zyklus verläuft.

2.1 EKG-Daten Erhebung

Die zum Vergleich herangezogenen EKG-Daten wurden mit einem Vorseriengerät des Schiller medilog FD12+ (Schiller Medizintechnik GmbH, Feldkirchen) erhoben. Alle Daten wurden im 12-Kanal Modus mit 1000 Hz abgetastet. Von zwei Personen wurde ein Belastungs-EKG erstellt, bei dem auf einem Ergometer die Belastung und somit die Herzrate kontinuierlich gesteigert wurde. Weiterhin wurde mit einer der beiden Personen ein EKG ohne weitere Belastung angefertigt. Diese Daten wurden mittels des hier vorgestellten Verfahrens modelliert.

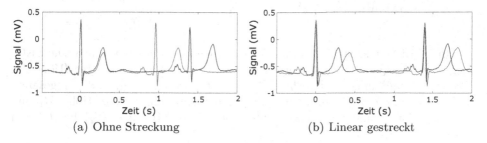

(a) Ohne Streckung   (b) Linear gestreckt

Abb. 1. Referenz- (rot) und Test-Zyklus (blau) unterschiedlicher Länge.

2.2   Filterung des EKG

Aufgrund von Signal-Rauschen und Schwankungen der Basisspannung durch Atmung und andere Einflüsse müssen die Zyklen vor der Anpassung an ein Modell gefiltert werden. Hierzu wurden ein Gaußscher Bandpass entworfen, welcher durch den Tiefpassanteil das Rauschen reduziert und durch den Hochpassanteil die auftretenden Gleichanteilschwankungen entfernt. Der Hochpassanteil wurde als $1 - TP_H$ ausgelegt. Die Filterparametrierungen wurden experimentell auf $\sigma_{TP_T} = 55.6\,\text{ms}$ und $\sigma_{TP_H} = 12.625\,\text{ms}$ festgelegt.

2.3   Modellbildung

Die Approximationsformel für ein EKG-Signal lautet nach Alwal et al. [6]

$$
\begin{aligned}
\text{ECG}(t) = M_P e^{-(\frac{t-\tau_P}{\sqrt{2}W_P})^2} + M_{Q_1} e^{-(\frac{t-\tau_{Q_1}}{\sqrt{2}W_{Q_1}})^2} + M_{Q_2} e^{-(\frac{t-\tau_{Q_2}}{\sqrt{2}W_{Q_2}})^2} + \\
M_S e^{-(\frac{t-\tau_S}{\sqrt{2}W_S})^2} + M_T e^{-(\frac{t-\tau_T}{\sqrt{2}W_T})^2} + \frac{d}{dt} M_R e^{-(\frac{t-\tau_R}{\sqrt{2}W_R})^2}
\end{aligned} \tag{1}
$$

Hierbei beschreibt M_P die Höhe, τ_P die Position und W_P die Breite der P-Welle. Dasselbe gilt für die anderen Zyklen-Elemente Q_1, Q_2, S und T, sowie für den Ableitungsterm der R-Welle. Dieses Modell wurde auf sechs Ableitungen erweitert. Hierzu wurden die Exponentialterme in (1) durch einen abschnittsweisen Term ersetzt, um Wellen, bei denen der Anstieg und Abfall unterschiedliche Zeiten dauern, genauer zu modellieren. Ein weiterer Anteil wurde hinzugefügt, um alle Elemente des EKG-Zyklus durch einen eigenen Term zu beschreiben

$$
\text{ECG}'(t) = \sum_{i \in P,Q,R,S,T} g(t, M_i, \tau_i, W_{1_i}, W_{2_i})
$$

$$
+ \frac{d}{dt} h(t, M_{1_{QRS}}, M_{2_{QRS}}, \tau_{QRS}, W_{1_{QRS}}, W_{2_{QRS}})
$$

$$
\text{mit}\ \ g(t, M_i, \tau_i, W_{1_i}, W_{2_i}) =
\begin{cases}
M_i e^{-(\frac{t-\tau_i}{\sqrt{2}W_{1_i}})^2} & \text{für } t - \tau_i < 0 \\
M_i e^{-(\frac{t-\tau_i}{\sqrt{2}W_{2_i}})^2} & \text{für } t - \tau_i >= 0
\end{cases} \tag{2}
$$

$$
\text{und}\ h(t, M_{1_i}, M_{2_i}, \tau_i, W_{1_i}, W_{2_i}) =
\begin{cases}
M_{1_i} e^{-(\frac{t-\tau_i}{\sqrt{2}W_{1_i}})^2} & \text{für } t - \tau_i < 0 \\
M_{2_i} e^{-(\frac{t-\tau_i}{\sqrt{2}W_{2_i}})^2} & \text{für } t - \tau_i >= 0
\end{cases}
$$

In (2) ist kein separates Modell für jeden Kanal mehr erforderlich. Die EKG-Segmente P, Q, R, S und T werden jeweils durch vier Parameter (Höhe M, Position τ und linke und rechte Komponente W_1 und W_2) und der gesamte QRS-Komplex durch fünf weitere Parameter (linke und rechte Höhe M_1 und M_2, Position τ und linke und rechte Komponente W_1 und W_2) beschrieben (Abb. 2(b)).

Die Positionen der einzelnen Segmente sind eindeutig aus τ abzulesen. Mit diesem Modell ist der Summationsvektor aus allen Richtungen näherungsweise abbildbar. Daraus ergibt sich eine Approximationsformel für die Kanäle I, II, III, aVL, aVR, und aVF. Das Modell kann zu einem Summationsvektor der Herzerregung umgerechnet werden. Mit Hilfe des Cabrerakreises können die Anteile der jeweiligen Ableitungen zu den Richtungen berechnet werden.

2.4 Anpassung des Modells

Die einzelnen Ableitungen der tatsächlichen EKG Zyklen wurden mittels des Levenberg-Marquardt-Algorithmus (LMA) an das Modell angepasst. Hierbei werden aus dem Zyklus zunächst die Positionen und Höhen der einzelnen Komponenten mittels lokaler Hoch- und Tiefpunktsuche ermittelt, mit denen dann der LMA initialisiert wird. Anschließend werden die 25 Parameter aus (2) iterativ an die Kurve angepasst. Das Residuum wird als Differenz des mathematischen Modells und des Zyklus berechnet. Dieses Verfahren wird für alle Ableitungen der Frontalprojektion einzeln durchgeführt.

2.5 Summationsvektors aus Rekonstruktion und Modellierung

Aus den Ableitungen kann ein Summationsvektor gebildet werden. Hierzu werden die Richtungsanteile der Ableitungen anhand des Cabrerakreises berechnet und aufsummiert. Anschließend werden diese in einem zweidimensionalen Plot aufgezeichnet (Abb. 4(a)). Aus diesem Plot ergibt sich eine nicht von der Zykluslänge abhängige zweidimensionale Repräsentation der Herzerregung.

2.6 Normalisierung der Zykluszeit

Als weiteres Verfahren zur vergleichbaren zweidimensionalen Darstellung von Zyklen unterschiedlicher Länge wird die Länge des Signals zunächst mit Hilfe des mathematischen Modells normalisiert.

Hierzu werden die zeitlichen Faktoren τ_i und W_i des zu normierenden Zyklus durch die eines Zyklus in Normlänge N ersetzt. Anschließend wird das Residuum

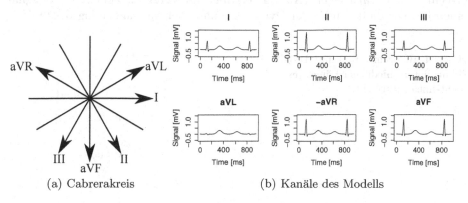

(a) Cabrerakreis   (b) Kanäle des Modells

Abb. 2. Cabrerakreis und Kanäle des Modells mit konstruierten Parametern.

Abb. 3. Mögliche 2D-Darstellungen des Signals als Summationsvektorplot (links) und als Grauwertplot der normierten Kanäle und Residualfunktion über acht Zyklen (rechts).

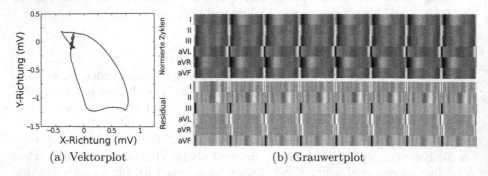

(a) Vektorplot   (b) Grauwertplot

abschnittsweise linear skaliert. Die Abschnittsgrenzen markieren die Zeitpunkte $\tau_P, \tau_Q, \tau_R, \tau_S$ und τ_T. Das skalierte Residuum wird zum berechneten Modell addiert. Dieses ergibt den normalisierten Zyklus.

2.7 Generierung von 2D Daten aus normierten Zyklen

Aus den so gewonnenen normierten Zyklen werden Pseudobilder generiert. Hierzu werden die Werte der 6 Kanäle als Grauwerte in jeweils eine Spalte geschrieben. Dies ergibt ein Abbild des Zyklus normierter Größe, das mit Verfahren der Bildanalyse ausgewertet werden kann (Abb. 4(b)). Dasselbe Verfahren wird zur Generierung eines Residuumplots auf den nicht durch das Modell erklärbaren Anteil des Signals angewandt.

3 Ergebnisse

Die Modellparamerter für die betrachteten Daten wurden berechnet. Die damit errechneten Normierungen (Abb. 4) ergaben im Vergleich zum Referenzsignal einen RMSE von 0.19 mV. Der Dynamikumfang der Messungen lag bei 1 mV.

Abb. 4. Referenz- (rot) und Test-Zyklus (blau) unterschiedlicher Länge aus Abb. 1 nicht-linear gestreckt.

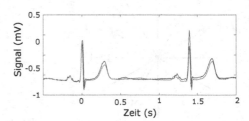

4 Diskussion

In dieser Arbeit haben wir eine mathematische Modellierung der EKG-Kanäle I, II, III, aVL, aVR und aVF vorgestellt. Das Modell kann verwendet werden, um eine nicht-lineare Anpassung eines Zyklus an eine Referenz zu gewährleisten, was für weiterführende Verarbeitungen wichtig ist. Gleichzeitig kann dieses Modell zur Segmentierung verwendet werden, da die Positionen der einzelnen EKG-Segmente vom Modell berechnet werden. Hiermit lassen sich Standard-EKG-Messwerte wie z.B. die QT-Zeit automatisch in den ca. 600.000 Zyklen einer Langzeitableitung über 7 Tage berechnen und statistisch auswerten. Dieser Paradigmenwechsel in der EKG-Analyse verspricht neue Erkenntnisse in der Kardiologie.

Weitere Schritte werden daher eine Erweiterung des Modells auf alle zwölf Kanäle beinhalten und eine 3D-Darstellung des Erregungsvektors sowie eine Modellierung von pathologischen Zyklen ermöglichen. Eine Outlier-Detektierung im Parameterraum wird das Modell zusätzlich verbessern. So könnten die Parameter, welche die Positionen der einzelnen EKG-Segmente beschreiben, leicht auf Plausibilität getestet werden.

Die hier vorgestellte Methode kann auch verwendet werden, um die EKG-Daten als Volumina zu visualisieren. Dazu werden die Zyklen als Bilder mit gleicher Größe dargestellt, deren Textur einfach analysiert oder verglichen werden kann. Die Residualfunktion des Matchings, also der Teil des Signals, der nicht durch das Modell erklärt werden kann, wird als potentiell pathologisch betrachtet und ist – als Bild dargestellt – mit Pattern-Matching-Methoden weiter verarbeitbar.

Danksagung. Diese Arbeit wurde durch die European Foundation for the Study of Diabetes (EFSD) und Boehringer Ingelheim im Bereich „Mechanisms Relating Renal Dysfunction to Cardiovascular Disease in Type 2 Diabetes" (Kennzeichen HT6J2012) gefördert.

Literaturverzeichnis

1. Waseem K, Javed A, Ramzan R, et al. Using evolutionary algorithms for ECG arrhythmia detection and classification. Proc IEEE ICNC. 2011;4:2386–2390.
2. Reed MJ, Robertson CE, Addison PS. Heart rate variability measurements and the prediction of ventricular arrhythmias. QJM. 2005 Jan;98(2):87–95.
3. Tawfik MM, Selim H, Kamal T. Human identification using time normalized QT signal and the QRS complex of the ECG. Proc CSNDSP. 2010; p. 755-9.
4. Sovilj S, Magjarevic R, Lovell NH, et al. A simplified 3D model of whole heart electrical activity and 12-lead ECG generation. Comput Math Meth Med. 2013;2013:134208.
5. Schmidt RF, Lang F. Physiologie des Menschen mit Pathophysiologie. Heidelberg: Springer-Medizin-Verlag; 2010.
6. Awal A, Mostafa SS, Ahmad M. Simplified mathematical model for generating ECG signal and fitting the model using nonlinear least square technique. Proc ICME. 2011; p. RT–011.

Fusion of X-Ray and Video for an Intraoperative Navigation System for PCNL Procedures

Arthur Teimourian[1], Michael Müller[1], Dogu Teber[2], Martin Wagner[3], Hans-Peter Meinzer[1]

[1]Division of Medical and Biological Informatics, DKFZ Heidelberg
[2]Department of Urology, Heidelberg University Hospital
[3]Department of Surgery, Heidelberg University Hospital
a.teimourian@dkfz-heidelberg.de

Abstract. Percutaneous nephrolithotomy (PCNL) is the most commonly used procedure to remove large stones from the human kidney. To improve the speed and safety of PCNL, researchers have been developing an intraoperative navigation system which employs a marker-based registration technique to superimpose CT images on the video stream of a tablet computer. In this paper, we present our work on the fusion of intraoperative X-ray and video aimed at improving the existing system. For the fusion, we used automatic marker-detection algorithms and then processed the data by using thin-plate spline transformation and landmark warping. The evaluation of the technique was performed by testing it on a silicone phantom. The results of the evaluation are very promising, showing a mean geometrical error of 0.9 mm. The aggregated runtime of our algorithms is 0.086 ms, which gives the fusion real-time capability. The fusion enables the detection of organ deformations by the surgeon. Possible future work could include the development of a registration framework to automatically detect organ deformations. Furthermore, algorithms for needle detection in fluoroscopic images would greatly improve intraoperative navigation. The location of the needle could then be superimposed on the tablet screen.

1 Introduction

Renal lithiasis can be extremely painful; indeed kidney stones are one of the sources of the most severe pain a human being can experience [1]. For the removal of kidney stones, there are various possible procedures. For large and complex kidney stones percutaneous nephrolithotomy (PCNL) is the treatment of choice. A needle-shaped instrument is inserted through a small incision in the skin and is navigated to the renal collecting system [2]. Once reached, the kidney stone is crushed to pieces using ultrasound techniques. To perform such a procedure, physicians usually employ images generated by pre-procedural computed tomography (CT) and intraoperative X-ray (fluoroscopy). They use CT images to locate the kidney stone and to estimate its size. This means that CT data is used to plan the procedure, while fluoroscopy gives surgeons a real-time component, e.g. by showing the current position of the needle. To improve the speed and safety of PCNL, researchers have been developing an intraoperative navigation system, which employs a marker-based registration technique to superimpose CT images on the video stream of a tablet computer [3]. This work builds on the existing system. A drawback of the existing approach is that it does not yet take account of real-time fluoroscopic data. This matter can be solved by incorporating the fusion of fluoroscopy and video which is presented in this work. Intraoperative navigation systems already exist, but they lack the ability to use real-time data such as fluoroscopy provides [4], or they use it as the main modality for registration which decreases user-friendliness and increases radiation [5, 6]. In our approach we only use fluoroscopic images which would have been generated anyway to gain additional information for the fusion. Integrating the fusion of fluoroscopy and video would have several advantages. For example, real-time fluoroscopic images would enable us to detect possible real-time organ deformations, thus obviating the problem caused by CT data normally being assembled days before the procedure.

2   Materials and methods

The existing system is made up of several components. A tablet computer is used to both record the procedure and display the results of the algorithms (Sec. 2.1). In the following sections we briefly introduce some important parts of the existing system and then the X-ray and video fusion.

2.1   Existing algorithms

The existing system utilizes both pre-operative CT and video data to assist surgeons during surgery. Cross-shaped markers are used to match these two modalities. The video images recorded by the tablet computer are streamed to a mobile server via Wi-Fi. The server runs algorithms to match the position of the markers in the CT dataset with the markers detected in the video stream. By sending the results back to the tablet, the server provides the data necessary to allow the surgeon to see the patient's internal structures (Fig. 2).

2.2   Fluoroscopy and video fusion

The fusion of fluoroscopic images with the video stream of the tablet computer brings numerous benefits (Sec. 1). The fusion's workflow proceeds in four steps (Fig. 3). First of all the images have to be preprocessed for the subsequent stages. This preliminary step consists of cropping and resizing the data to improve comparability. After preprocessing the images in this way, marker-detection algorithms are run on both the video and the fluoroscopic data. The output provides the thin-plate spline (TPS) algorithm with marker coordinates. TPS is a 2D analog of the cubic spline in one dimension. It is the solution of the biharmonic equation. Given a set of marker coordinates for the fluoroscopic

Fig. 1. Fluoroscopic image of the phantom with cross-shaped markers, artifical renal collecting system and additional structures.

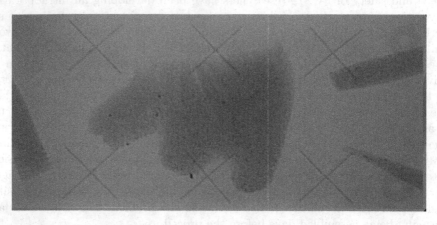

image, a weighted combination of thin-plate splines centered at each data point gives the interpolation function that passes through the points while minimizing the bending energy. The bending energy function is defined as the 2D integral of the squares of the second derivatives [7]. Most importantly, TPS is constrained not to move at grid points. Thus TPS matches the marker coordinates of the fluoroscopic image with the marker coordinates of the video image. This creates a shift vector field, which can be used to warp the fluoroscopic image appropriately (landmark warping). The warped fluoroscopic image is then superimposed on the video image.

2.3   Evaluation

The evaluation had two main objectives. The first and most important was to determine how much geometrical error there might be after all the necessary

Fig. 2.   Enhanced reality view of a patient's internal structures.

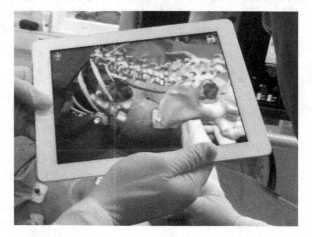

steps shown in Fig. 3 had been processed. The second was the measurement of the technique's runtime. Since the system is to be used under real conditions, the fusion has to have real-time capability. To perform the evaluation, we built a phantom out of pourable soft silicone (manufacturer: www.nedform.com, Fig. 4). The dimensions of the phantom were $24 \times 10 \times 4$ cm. We placed a model of a renal collecting system as well as three additional random structures inside the phantom to simulate a real setup for PCNL. The renal collecting system and the additional structures were soaked with a contrast agent and colored with black silicone dye. We used six cross-markers and two dot-markers impervious to X-rays. The diameter was 3.2 cm for a cross-marker and 0.4 cm for a dot-marker. All six cross-markers were located around the renal collecting system (region of interest). Fluoroscopic images were generated (Fig. 1) and fused with the video images. To determine the geometrical error accurately, we used video images from different angles between the system and the X-ray source (Fig. 4). These angles were classified as either steep (approx. 0°), regular (approx. 45°) or flat (approx. 60°). Of the six cross-markers five were used to track the phantom, while one cross-marker and the two dot-markers were used to determine the euclidean error. The locations of the markers were verified manually to eliminate possible error caused by the marker-detection algorithm. To quantify the geometrical error, we estimated the error shown in the registered image (Fig. 5). Since the geometrical error was assumed to approximate to the markers' size we expected that the geometrical characteristics close to one marker would correspond to the geometry of the marker itself. On account of our use of marker-based registration, we assumed that outside the region of interest and for flat angles accuracy would diminish. Furthermore, as this is a projected 3D error estimation on the surface of the phantom, we expect a greater 3D error inside the phantom.

3   Results

We used 27 different video images to perform the evaluation. The images were selected manually, care being taken that they were distributed equally amongst steep, regular and flat angles (Fig. 5). The results of the evaluation show that the mean euclidean error after registration of the fusion is approximately 0.9 mm (Tab. 1).

The aggregated runtime of the algorithms is 0.086 ms, which means that the fusion has real-time capability. The runtime was measured on a test server with

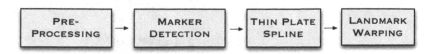

Fig. 3. Workflow of fluoroscopy and video fusion.

Table 1. Evaluation results depend on the angle between system and X-ray source.

Angle (System / X-ray Source)	Steep (ca. 0°)	Regular (ca. 45°)	Flat (ca. 60°)
Euclidian Error	0.4 ± 0.2 mm	0.8 ± 0.2 mm	1.6 ± 0.3 mm

an Intel i7-3930K processor and 32 gigabytes of main memory. The results also show diminishing accuracy outside the region of interest.

4   Discussion

In this paper, we have introduced a framework for fusing X-rays with video in an intraoperative navigation system. Experiments on a silicone phantom show promising results regarding both accuracy and runtime of the algorithms. Within the region of interest, the approximated accuracy of the framework is very good for regular and steep angles. As expected, the accuracy worsens outside the region of interest as well as in the case of flat angles. Since the markers are usually placed around the region of interest, this does not impede the use of the fusion. Furthermore, the tablet is not normally held at a flat angle. For the evaluation, we verified the location of the markers manually. It is to be expected that the geometrical error of this system using automatic marker-detection algorithms will be greater than that described in section 3. The fusion presented in this paper enables the detection of organ deformations by the surgeon. For our method no additional setup is necessary. This makes this system easy to use. The runtime on our test system (sec. 3) proved to be well below the real-time capability boundary. Future work should focus on using the findings presented in this paper to exploit the full potential of what fluoroscopy integration can contribute to an intraoperative navigation system. Integrating fluoroscopy would

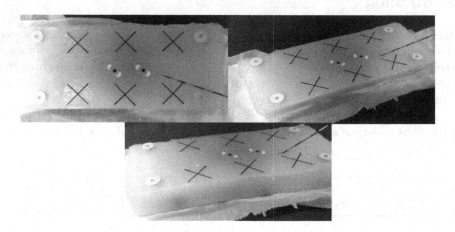

Fig. 4. View of the phantom from a steep (top left), regular (top right) and flat (bottom) angle, with the angles being approximately 0°, 45° and 60° respectively.

Fig. 5. Result of the superimposition for a steep angle. The numbered markers are used for the registration, while the unnumbered cross- and dot-markers serve as evaluation markers. The red markers are located in the fluoroscopic image. The black markers are situated in the video image. The 2D offset between red and black markers is the geometrical error of the fusion.

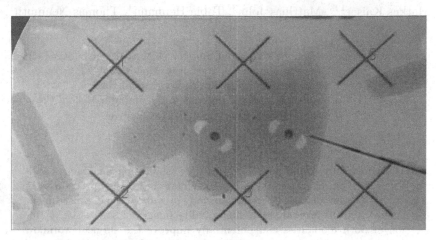

enable 2D-3D registration between CT and fluoroscopic images. As a result, possible organ deformations could be recognized automatically. Moreover, by detecting a needle in fluoroscopic images, we could show its position on the screen of the tablet for an even better navigational approach.

References

1. Gücük A, Kemahlı E, Üyetürk U, et al. Routine flexible nephroscopy for percutaneous nephrolithotomy in renal stones with low density: a prospective randomized study. J Urol. 2013.
2. Michel MS, Trojan L, Rassweiler JJ. Complications in percutaneous nephrolithotomy. Eur Urol. 2007;51(4):899–906.
3. Rassweiler JJ, Müller M, Fangerau M, et al. iPad-assisted percutaneous access to the kidney using marker-based navigation: initial clinical experience. Eur Urol. 2012;61(3):628–31.
4. Valenti DA, Boucher LM, Artho G, et al. Minioptical navigation system for CT-guided percutaneous liver procedures. Adv Comput Tomogr. 2013;2(3):77–82.
5. Egli A, Kleinszig G, John A, et al. Pose estimation quality assessment for intraoperative image guidance systems. Proc SPIE. 2013;8671:40–9.
6. Chen X, Wang L, Fallavollita P, et al. Error analysis of the X-ray projection geometry of camera-augmented mobile C-arm. Proc SPIE. 2012;8316:60–8.
7. Bookstein FL. Principal warps: thin-plate splines and the decomposition of deformations. IEEE Trans Pattern Anal Mach Intell. 1989;11(6):567–85.

Comparison of Optimizers for 2D/3D Registration for Fusion of Ultrasound and X-Ray

Markus Kaiser[123], Matthias John[3], Tobia Heimann[4], Thomas Neumuth[1],
Georg Rose[2]

[1]Innovation Center Computer Assisted Surgery (ICCAS), Universität Leipzig
[2]Otto von Guericke Universität, Magdeburg
[3]Siemens AG, Healthcare Sector, Forchheim
[4]Siemens AG, Corporate Technology, Imaging and Computer Vision, Erlangen
markus.kaiser@medizin.uni-leipzig.de

Abstract. Ultrasound and X-ray are two facilitating imaging modalities in the field of transcatheter-based minimally invasive procedures in structural heart disease. X-ray fluoroscopy provides excellent instrument imaging and ultrasound shows high-quality images of soft tissue. A fusion of both modalities can potentially improve the surgical workflow and the catheter navigation. A current approach shows the fusion of X-ray fluoroscopy with trans-esophageal echo (TEE) with the help of 2D/3D registration. An ultrasound probe model is registered to X-ray images which inherently provides a registration of ultrasound images to X-ray. In this paper, we evaluate the accuracy and the performance of four optimizing algorithms (Powell, Nelder-Mead, BFGS, CMA-ES) while registering digitally reconstructed radiographs (DRR) of the model to X-ray images. The DRRs were generated by mesh-rendering, not by ray casting. The optimizers show significant differences in accuracy and runtime.

1 Introduction

The number of procedures from open-heart surgery in the field of structural heart disease that are now performed minimally invasive and catheter-based is constantly increasing. Examples are trans-catheter aortic valve implantation or trans-catheter mitral valve repair. The drivers for this general tendency are the availability of advanced intra-procedural imaging and new catheter developments. Usually, these procedures are performed under C-arm fluoroscopic X-ray and trans-esophageal echo (TEE) guidance [1]. Commonly, these modalities are used independently during the intervention. An image fusion of both systems could lead to a better image understanding and potentially allow new kinds of procedures.

Gao et al. [2] introduced an approach for the fusion of ultrasound with fluoroscopic X-ray with the help of purely image based 2D/3D registration. A TEE probe is located in the X-ray image and the 3D position of the TEE probe relatively to the X-ray detector is derived. This inherently provides a registration of the ultrasound image to the X-ray image. To estimate the 3D position, artificial X-ray images (digitally reconstructed radiographs (DRRs)) of a model of the TEE probe are registered to the X-ray image via a 2D/3D registration algorithm. An approach to speed up the DRR generation, which is the most time consuming part of the 2D/3D registration, was presented in [3]. Here, a triangular mesh of the TEE model was rendered in a way, that it can be used instead of the normal ray-casted DRR image (Fig. 2 a,b) which is much faster. The authors of the paper did not employ their approach in a complete automatic 2D/3D registration process. Therefore, we adopted the presented technique and evaluated it within an automatic 2D/3D registration with different optimization algorithms.

2   Materials and methods

2D/3D registration can be described as an iterative process where DRRs, based on a 3D image of the object, are compared with the help of a similarity measure SM to the original X-ray image I_0. An optimizer determines new rigid transformation parameters $S = \{t_x, t_y, t_z, \theta_{\mathrm{yaw}}, \theta_{\mathrm{pitch}}, \theta_{\mathrm{roll}}\}$ until the similarity measure converges and results in the final parameters S'

$$S' = \mathrm{argmax} SM(I_0, DRR(\mathrm{Model}_{\mathrm{TEE}}, S)) \qquad (1)$$

The parameters are visualized in Fig. 2c. In general, one must differentiate between in-plane (t_x, t_z, θ_{yaw}) and out-of-plane parameters (t_y, θ_{pitch}, θ_{roll}). In-plane parameters are parallel to the image plane and causing a larger pixel shift in the projection than out-of-plane parameters. Therefore, it is easier to estimate in-plane than out-of-plane parameters.

Because a new DRR must be computed for every cost function evaluation, it is one of the main tasks of an optimizer to reduce this number of evaluations.

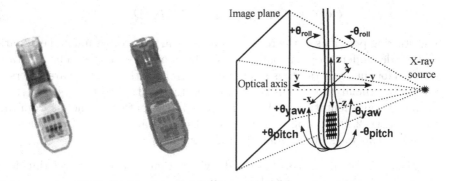

(a) Ray casting DRR (b) Mesh based DRR   (c) TEE probe rigid parameters

Fig. 1. Example of a conventional ray casted DRR and a mesh rendered DRR, together with a visualization of the six rigid parameters of the TEE probe.

Therefore, the optimizer strongly affects the speed of the 2D/3D registration system.

2.1 Optimizers

The six rigid parameters have no linear relationship. Therefore, a non-linear optimization problem must be solved. We employed the following four different optimizers with the ability to solve such a problem and compared them by accuracy and performance. All four optimizers have been used successfully for 2D/3D registration before.

1. Powell's method [4], which is a local optimizer and used successfully in similar registrations problems [2].
2. Nelder-Mead (or downhill simplex) method [5], belongs to the class of hill climbing techniques. It works without derivatives.
3. BFGS (Broyden-Fletcher-Goldfarb-Shanno algorithm) [6], is a Quasi-Newton method which uses derivatives.
4. CMA-ES (Covariance Matrix Adaptation Evolution Strategy) [7], is an evolutionary optimizer which approximates the normal distribution of sample points in a search space. It shows good ability for global optimization.

2.2 Optimizing strategy

The DRRs of the TEE probe were generated via the rendering of triangular meshes which was presented in [3]. The used similarity measure was the gradient correlation (GC) which is sensitive to high contrast structures e.g. a TEE probe.

For each optimizer, we used the same experimental setup. The C-arm's rotation offset between two images was always 90°. This has the advantage that the out-of-plane parameters of one image plane are becoming the in-plane parameters of the other plane and vice versa. The similarity measure GC was calculated and averaged over both imaging planes

$$GC = (GC(I_A, DRR_A) + GC(I_B, DRR_B))/2 \qquad (2)$$

The starting positions of the registrations were always rough manual estimations of the independent in-plane parameters in both biplane images. The 3D starting position for the registration is a combination from both in-plane parameters sets. The most crucial and extensive part is the registration of the roll (θ_{roll}). Due to the typical orientation of the TEE probe in the patient, which is from top to bottom (Fig. 2.2), the roll is still an out-of-plane parameter in both planes. We examined two ways of handling the roll parameter.

1. Manual estimation: this has the drawback that it takes a longer time for the user to determine an initial approximation.
2. Automatic registration: assuming that the other five rigid parameters are initialized very close, one can think about a line search over the whole roll parameter space. Unfortunately, the TEE probe is not a perfect cylindric

object. Therefore, it is not possible to do a line-search of the roll from ±180°, because the shape of the probe is changing too much (Fig. 2.2). A re-registration of the in-plane parameters becomes necessary.

While the registration strategy for the first approach is straight forward, the second one is more complex. Here we started several new registrations from the initial parameters, but each from a new roll angle. The offset between each step was 22.5°. From these multiple registrations, we picked the registration with the best value of the similarity measure.

3 Evaluation

The testing datasets for the optimizer evaluation contained over 42 different biplane scenes. The data was acquired during clinical interventions. We exclusively used projection images from C-arm CT rotational scans. The TEE probe was not moved during the acquisition. That gave us the ability to extract multiple biplane scenes, as well as to establish a suitable ground truth via manual registration with images from multiple viewing directions. All operations were carried out on a mobile computer with 2.2 GHz Intel CPU (8 cores) and a NVIDIA QUADRO 1000M graphics card.

We summarized the registration results for the first approach in Tab. 1. We measured the rate of registration success for each rigid parameter. The boundaries for a successful registration were defined as follows: 1.5 mm for t_x, t_y, t_z, 2° for θ_{pitch} and θ_{yaw} and for the out-of-plane parameter θ_{roll} 4°. One can see, that the CMA-ES outperforms the other employed optimization algorithms, but is also the slowest. Powell's method and BFGS are showing almost the same performance while the Nelder-Mead is worst.

Tab. 2 summarizes the results for the second approach. Powell's method is showing a good performance on the roll parameter, as well as CMA-ES which is slightly better for the rest of the parameters. BFGS and Nelder-Mead do

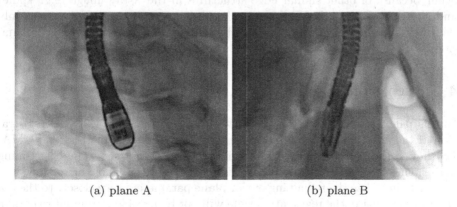

(a) plane A   (b) plane B

Fig. 2. Example of a biplane dataset for registration.

Table 1. Percentage of successful registrations per optimizer with manual roll initialization.

Optimizer	t_x	t_y	t_z	θ_{pitch}	θ_{yaw}	θ_{roll}	time [s]
Powell	84	74	71	82	82	68	2.97
Nelder-Mead	53	50	42	32	29	58	1.42
BFGS	87	76	79	76	74	63	2.89
CMA-ES	95	89	87	92	95	87	5.63

Table 2. Percentage of successful registrations per optimizer with automatic roll registration.

Optimizer	t_x	t_y	t_z	θ_{pitch}	θ_{yaw}	θ_{roll}	time [s]
Powell	87	81	82	84	82	71 | 79	32.8
Nelder-Mead	55	50	42	29	29	16 | 39	13.1
BFGS	89	87	79	74	66	26 | 63	23.7
CMA-ES	92	89	87	92	92	66 | 89	43.2

not show a good accuracy. Unfortunately, the two best optimizers are also the slowest. The second column of θ_{roll} shows the registration success if we increase the boundary to 10°. That means that in general, CMA-ES has a better ability of estimating the parameters than the other optimizers.

The results for the roll parameter are summarized in Fig. 3. The roll indicates a successful registration, because we observed that if one of the other parameters is not registered well, the roll registration will definitely fail. But if all other parameters are good, it is not sure that the roll is correct.

Failures of the overall registration process are commonly due to the inaccurate registration of the in-plane parameters. If the parameters t_x, t_z, θ_{yaw} are inaccurate, it is impossible that the out-of-plane parameters are registered properly. Because of the chosen similarity measure, errors in in-plane registration occur because of other similar edge structures in the X-ray image (e.g. spine) and along the TEE probe. Failures in the parameters θ_{roll}, θ_{pitch} are commonly because of visual symmetries of the probe between different roll/pitch combinations.

4   Discussion

In this paper we evaluated four optimization algorithms for a 2D/3D registration of the a TEE probe to biplane X-ray images. Powell's method and CMA-ES showed the best accuracy. Unfortunately, they do not show the best timing performance. To dramatically reduce the runtime of the whole algorithm, it is crucial to initialize the remaining out-of-plane parameters very closely to the optimum. Otherwise, the registration time will not be feasible during intervention. This can probably achieved with algorithms like proposed in [8]. Another possi-

Fig. 3. Rates of successful registrations for the roll parameter (θ_{roll}).

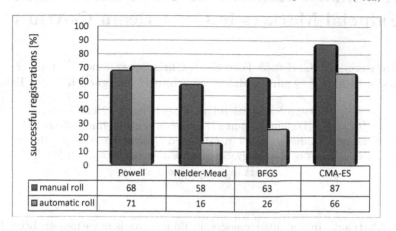

	Powell	Nelder-Mead	BFGS	CMA-ES
■ manual roll	68	58	63	87
■ automatic roll	71	16	26	66

ble improvement could be the combination of different optimization algorithms to gather a benefit of the different advantages, for example a rough estimation with CMA-ES combined with a Powell local search.

Acknowledgement. This work was funded by Siemens AG, Healthcare Sector. The authors want to thank the Heart Center Leipzig for the image data. The presented concepts and informations are based on research and are not commercially available.

References

1. Feldman T, Wasserman HS, Herrmann HC, et al. Percutaneous mitral valve repair using the edge-to-edge technique six-month results of the everest phase I clinical trial. J Am Coll Cardiol. 2005;46(11):2134–40.
2. Gao G, Penney G, Ma Y, et al. Registration of 3D trans-esophageal echocardiography to X-ray fluoroscopy using image-based probe tracking. Med Image Anal. 2012;16(1):38–49.
3. Kaiser M, John M, Borsdorf A, et al. Significant acceleration of 2D-3D registration-based fusion of ultrasound and X-ray images by mesh-based DRR rendering. Proc SPIE. 2013;8671:867111–6.
4. Brent RP. Algorithms for Minimization Without Derivatives. Courier Dover Publications; 1973.
5. Nelder JA, Mead R. A simplex method for function minimization. Comput J. 1965;7(4):308–13.
6. Flannery BP, Press WH, Teukolsky SA, et al. Numerical Recipes in C. Cambridge University Press; 1992.
7. Hansen N. The CMA evolution strategy: a comparing review. Towards New Evol Comput. 2006;192:75–102.
8. Mountney P, Ionasec R, Kaiser M, et al. Ultrasound and fluoroscopic images fusion by autonomous ultrasound probe detection. Proc MICCAI. 2012;7511:544–51.

Automatic Removal of Externally Attached Fiducial Markers in Cone Beam C-Arm CT

Martin Berger[1,2], Christoph Forman[1,3], Chris Schwemmer[1,3], Jang H. Choi[4], Kerstin Müller[1,3], Andreas Maier[1], Joachim Hornegger[1], Rebecca Fahrig[4]

[1]Pattern Recognition Lab, FAU Erlangen-Nürnberg
[2]Research Training Group 1773 "Heterogeneous Image Systems"
[3]Erlangen Graduate School in Advanced Optical Technologies (SAOT)
[4]Department of Radiology, Stanford University, Stanford, CA, USA
martin.berger@cs.fau.de

Abstract. In computed tomography fiducial markers are frequently used to obtain accurate point correspondences for further processing. These markers typically cause metal artefacts, decreasing image quality of the subsequent reconstruction and are therefore often removed from the projection data. The placement of such markers is usually done on a surface, separating two materials, e.g. skin and air. Hence, a correct restoration of the occluded area is difficult. In this work six state-of-the-art interpolation techniques for the removal of high-density fiducial markers from cone-beam CT projection data are compared. We conducted a qualitative and quantitative evaluation for the removal of such markers and the ability to reconstruct the adjoining edge. Results indicate that an iterative spectral deconvolution is best suited for this application, showing promising results in terms of edge, as well as noise restoration.

1 Introduction

A crucial step in medical image registration is to find accurate point correspondences, which can be clearly detected in all acquired images. In computed tomography (CT) fiducial markers, represented by small metallic beads, are often the method of choice. An advantage of fiducials is that they are well recognisable in the 2D projection images. However, after having exploited the markers' spatial information, it is often necessary to remove them prior to further processing. One reason for this is that metallic markers typically lead to increased streaking artefacts in the reconstructed domain, substantially decreasing image quality. The position of the markers might also be used to provide ground truth information for further, marker-free processing methods [1].

Marker removal recovers missing data in the areas occluded by the object, using the known, surrounding pixel values. In CT reconstruction, various methods have been proposed to remove high-density objects from projection data. A simple but often adequate approach is to linearly interpolate the missing regions based on a specified neighbourhood. Additionally, spline-based techniques have been proposed [1]. In contrast to spatial interpolation, an iterative spectral deconvolution approach has been introduced in [2], showing promising results on radiographic data. In [3], a concept has been proposed that also incorporates the hidden structural information underneath high-density objects.

Despite the multitude of available methods, little attention has been paid to the locational properties of the defects. Fiducial markers are usually attached externally at a distinct edge between two materials, e.g. skin and air. Accurately recovering this edge poses an additional challenge to the removal algorithm as many of them assume only low-frequency changes in a defect's neighbourhood. In this work we compare the performance of six different algorithms for marker removal with a special focus on their ability to restore material edges.

2   Materials and methods

2.1   Automatic marker detection

For marker detection we used a fully automatic pipeline based on the fast radial symmetry transform (FRST) [4]. Identifying corresponding markers over all projection images helps to reduce false positive detections. We solve this problem by an initial detection of the 3D marker positions. The algorithm works as follows:

1. Apply the FRST to all projection images $f_j(\boldsymbol{x})$, with $\boldsymbol{x} \in \mathbb{R}^2$ and $j \in [1, P]$.
2. Backproject a blurred version of the FRST outcome to 3D, yielding distinct blobs for each marker.
3. Binarise the blobs using the maximum entropy method [5] and apply a 3D connected component analysis. The components' centroids then represent the 3D reference positions of each marker, denoted as $\boldsymbol{v}_i \in \mathbb{R}^3$ with $i \in [1, B]$. The number of markers B is given by the number of components.
4. Given the projection matrices $\boldsymbol{P}_j$, forward project the 3D reference points onto each projection image yielding the 2D reference points $\overline{\boldsymbol{u}}_{ij} = \boldsymbol{P}_j \boldsymbol{v}_i$, where j and i denote the j-th projection and i-th marker.
5. Extract a set of 2D candidate points $\boldsymbol{u}_{ij}$ for each projection image from the initial FRST result, using a heuristically determined threshold and a 2D connected-components analysis.
6. Assign the candidate points to the closest 2D reference points, essentially solving the correspondence problem.

For a better accuracy, the 3D marker positions can be updated by the newly assigned candidate points and a method described in [6]. Thus, the algorithm can be applied iteratively by repeating step 4) to 6) with the updated 3D positions.

2.2   Marker removal

As input for the marker removal we had the estimated 2D marker positions $\boldsymbol{u}_{ij}$, which were then used to extract a binary defect mask

$$w_j(\boldsymbol{x}) = \begin{cases} 0 & \text{if } \|(\boldsymbol{x} - \boldsymbol{u}_{ij})\|_2 < r, \ \forall i \in [1, B] \\ 1 & \text{otherwise} \end{cases} \tag{1}$$

where r is derived from the marker size and determines the invalid area and $\|.\|_2$ denotes the L2-norm. The removal was done separately for each marker using a square region centred at the marker's position. Let us define the set

$$\Omega_{ij} = \{x \mid \|x - u_{ij}\|_\infty < N/2\} \tag{2}$$

that includes all pixel locations that are part of the square region, where N is the region's side length and $\|.\|_\infty$ the infinity norm. Hence, the inputs for a removal method are given by $f_j(x_\Omega)$ and $w_j(x_\Omega)$, for all $x_\Omega \in \Omega_{ij}$. Let us further define a subset of Ω_{ij} that contains all positions that are marked as defect, i.e.

$$\Gamma_{ij} = \{x \mid x \in \Omega_{ij} \wedge w_j(x) = 0\} \tag{3}$$

Then the marker removal is described by estimating the missing data values at positions Γ_{ij} given the known data points at positions $(\Omega_{ij} \setminus \Gamma_{ij})$.

Six different interpolation techniques are compared. First we used a linear interpolation (LinInt) approach. Further we applied cubic B-splines (BSpl), estimated for each row and column separately [1]. The interpolation at the missing position x_Γ is then computed by the mean of the corresponding row and column spline. We also used the more general thin-plate smoothing spline (TPSpl). Here a 2D surface is fitted to the valid pixels and evaluated at the missing positions. Normalised convolution (NConv) was applied as introduced in [7], which is a Gaussian low-pass filter, normalised by incorporating information from the given defect mask. We also applied the Subtract-and-Shift (SaS) method [3], which aims to recover remaining high-frequency structure from the occluded areas. Finally, the spectral defect interpolation (SpecInt) as proposed in [2] is applied. This method estimates the missing information by an iterative approach in the frequency domain, minimising the mean squared difference between the estimated and observed image over all positions in $(\Omega_{ij} \setminus \Gamma_{ij})$.

2.3   Data and experiments

We had access to a C-arm CT scan of a left knee, containing 8 fiducial tantalum markers with 1 mm diameter, attached at distinct positions at the height of the patella. The data was acquired on an Axiom Artis dTA (Siemens AG, Forchheim, Germany), with a detector resolution of 1240×960 pixels, a pixel size of $0.308 \times 0.308\,\text{mm}^2$ and an angular resolution of 496 projections acquired over a range of $200°$. Further we generated synthetic phantom projections, using the same geometry as for the real scan. The phantom consists of three encapsulated cylinders representing a simple model of tissue, bone and bone marrow. The cylinders have radii of 80 mm, 35 mm and 31.5 mm and their attenuation coefficients are set to water, bone and bone marrow, respectively. Eight metallic beads with 1 mm diameter are attached in a helical trajectory around the outer cylinder such that they overlap the cylinder's surface by 0.1 mm. We also created marker free reference projections, to obtain ground truth data.

Each removal method was applied to all 8 markers over 496 projections yielding a total of 3968 interpolation steps per dataset and algorithm. Afterwards,

Table 1. Quantitative results for each marker removal method based on the synthetic dataset. The evaluated edge separates water ($0\,\mathrm{HU}$) and air ($-1024\,\mathrm{HU}$). "None" equals the reconstruction without marker removal.

	None	LinInt	BSpl	TPSpl	NConv	SaS	SpecInt
RMSE [HU]	30.12	13.84	9.26	9.91	19.50	14.62	8.08
σ_{RMSE} [HU]	4.36	4.84	4.27	4.35	6.46	4.33	3.31

$256 \times 256 \times 256$ cubes were reconstructed centred at the bead positions, with a spacing of $0.125 \times 0.125 \times 0.125\,\mathrm{mm}^3$. We also reconstructed the non-corrected projections and the marker-less projections in the case of the synthetic data. For a quantitative comparison the root mean squared error (RMSE) between marker-free and interpolated reconstructions and its standard deviation over the different markers (σ_{rmse}) were computed. The methods' parameters, e.g. the window width N, have been manually adjusted on the synthetic data.

3   Results

The quantitative results are shown in Tab. 1. Spectral interpolation performed best with an RMSE of $8.08\,\mathrm{HU}$ and a standard deviation of $3.31\,\mathrm{HU}$. The spline-based approaches performed similarly well, followed by the linear interpolation and Subtract-and-Shift. The normalised convolution showed a substantially worse performance and also the highest standard deviation.

Fig. 1 depicts $16 \times 16\,\mathrm{mm}^2$ regions centred around each marker. The ground truth surface of the cylinder is overlayed as a dashed yellow line. Spectral interpolation shows the best result, almost perfectly recovering the cylinder's edge. The spline-based approaches show similar results with a slightly more blurred edge. Increased blurring can be seen with linear interpolation and SaS, where the latter could not remove the marker completely. Normalised convolution produced streaking artefacts and could not sufficiently restore the missing information. In Fig. 2 we show the results for the C-arm CT acquisitions, where Fig. 2a gives an overview of the full reconstruction. A considerable amount of noise was present which ideally would be restored in the defective area. The spectral interpolation approach performed best, yielding a distinct edge profile and also restoring the noise level. Compared to the synthetic data, the B-spline approach produced noticeable streaking artefacts, whereas the thin-plate-splines showed increased blurring making the outcome comparable to a linear interpolation. The SaS was not able to remove the marker completely, yet the edge was well restored and the noise level retained. The normalised convolution showed similar artefacts as for the simulated data and performed worst.

4   Discussion

The results show that the spectral interpolation approach accurately restores edges as well as noise properties. An important parameter for this algorithm is

Fig. 1. Bead removal results for the synthetic dataset. The images show a $16 \times 16\,\mathrm{mm}^2$ region centred around the marker. The display window was [-922, 51] HU.

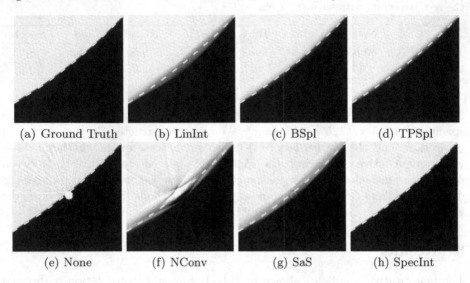

(a) Ground Truth   (b) LinInt   (c) BSpl   (d) TPSpl

(e) None   (f) NConv   (g) SaS   (h) SpecInt

the location and width of the support region. In our data the markers' size was constant and their positions known, which might be one reason for the good performance. The spline-based approaches did not retain the high performance seen from the synthetic data when applied to the real data. The B-Spline approach

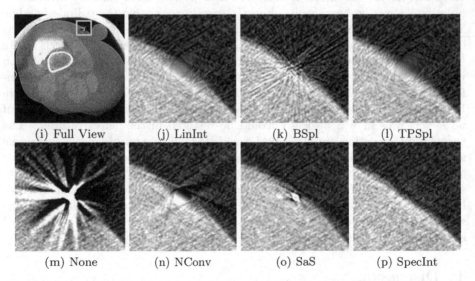

(i) Full View   (j) LinInt   (k) BSpl   (l) TPSpl

(m) None   (n) NConv   (o) SaS   (p) SpecInt

Fig. 2. Bead removal results for the real dataset. Fig. a) shows the full reconstruction. Fig. b) to h) show the method comparison focused on the marked rectangular region.

showed increased streaking artefacts which might be due to the increased noise level of the real data. This seems reasonable as values are determined by information based on the line and column only, not involving any other neighbourhood. The thin-plate-spline shows an increased smoothing effect on real data, which might be due to an additional increase in the regularisation parameter needed to cope with the noise level. Simple linear interpolation robustly removes markers but tends to smooth the adjoining edge. By definition the SaS method aims to retain high-frequency information, which is then aligned with the surrounding intensities [3]. The method was not able to remove the markers completely, which we think is due to the high frequency implied by the small markers itself. No sufficient performance was obtained when using the normalised convolution which does not seem to be suitable for marker removal on surfaces.

We compared six techniques for the removal of high-density fiducial markers from cone-beam CT projection data. The placement of the markers is typically done on a distinct surface, which makes a correct restoration of the 3D reconstruction more difficult. This study shows a qualitative and quantitative comparison for the removal of such markers and the ability to reconstruct the adjoining material edge. The results show that the spectral interpolation approach is best suited for our application, showing promising results in terms of edge, as well as noise restoration. Evaluation on arbitrarly shaped markers as well as data with patient-motion will be the subject of future work.

Acknowledgement. The authors gratefully acknowledge funding of the Research Training Group 1773 "Heterogeneous Image Systems" and the Erlangen Graduate School in Advanced Optical Technologies (SAOT) by the German Research Foundation (DFG).

References

1. Mitrovic U, Spiclin Z, Likar B, et al. 3D-2D registration of cerebral angiograms: a method and evaluation on clinical images. IEEE Trans Med Imaging. 2013;32(8):1550–63.
2. Aach T, Metzler VH. Defect interpolation in digital radiography: how object-oriented transform coding helps. Proc SPIE. 2001;4322:824–35.
3. Schwemmer C, Prümmer M, Daum V, et al. High-density object removal from projection images using low-frequency-based object masking. Proc BVM. 2010; p. 365–9.
4. Loy G, Zelinsky A. Fast radial symmetry for detecting points of interest. IEEE Trans Pattern Anal Mach Intell. 2003;25(8):959–73.
5. Kapur J, Sahoo PK, Wong A. A new method for gray-level picture thresholding using the entropy of the histogram. Computer Vis Graph Image Process. 1985;29(3):273–85.
6. Marchant TE, Amer AM, Moore CJ. Measurement of inter and intra fraction organ motion in radiotherapy using cone beam CT projection images. Phys Med Biol. 2008;53(4):1087.
7. Knutsson H, Westin CF. Normalized and differential convolution: methods for interpolation and filtering of incomplete and uncertain data. Proc Computer Vis Pattern Recognit. 1993; p. 515–23.

Kalman Filter-Based Head Tracking for Cranial Radiation Therapy with Low-Cost Range-Imaging Cameras

Jan Graßhoff, Ralf Bruder, Achim Schweikard, Floris Ernst

Institute for Robotics and Cognitive Systems, University of Lübeck
grasshof@informatik.uni-luebeck.de

Abstract. To allow for highly accurate localisation in stereotactic radiation therapy, patients are typically immobilised, equipped with optical markers or observed by stereoscopic X-ray imaging cameras. These methods decrease patient comfort and cause additional exposition to ionizing radiation. Consequently, there is a growing demand for contact-free approaches to compensate for patient motion. In this paper we present a first prototype for tracking head motion during radiation therapy using 3D range cameras. We propose a combination of global and local registration methods. We apply a Kalman movement model to observe head motions. The system's capabilities are analysed using a conventional Kinect-like camera which is mainly known as a low-cost consumer electronics device. Our tests show that the proposed setup has the potential of determining head positions with submillimeter accuracy in real-time. However, the use of low-cost cameras turns out to be problematic as they consistently cause substantial systematic errors in measuring depths.

1 Introduction

The success of cranial radiation therapy strongly depends on the possibilities to prevent or detect undesirable movements as it is crucial to irradiate the treated tissue with submillimeter accuracy. Therefore methods have to be found to match targets on the patient's diagnostic images (CT, MRT) with the actual location on the treatment couch. Today's state of the art is to immobilize the patient through frames. Invasive frames are rigidly fixed to the patient's skull and allow high accurate positioning below 0.8 mm [1]. Especially rigid frames are highly uncomfortable and lead to long preparation times as each frame has to be individually adapted. Besides, current systems are not capable of correcting possible errors continuously. Contact-free and non-ionizing approaches gain attractiveness. Purely optical devices have the potential to detect head-movements accurately with a high frequency and reduce patient setup times.

Nowadays a new generation of consumer electronics interfaces uses optical sensors to react to gestures and head movements in real-time. These systems show a high stability but forego millimeter accuracy as needed in medical applications. Nevertheless, Cerviño et al. demonstrated the feasibility of contact-free

Fig. 1. Overall architecture of the head tracker.

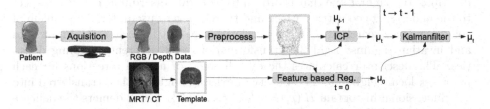

cranial radiosurgeries [2]. Wiersma et al. showed, that 3D surface imaging has the potential for submillimeter level tracking [3]. In this paper, we present a prototype capable of accurate head tracking at high frequencies with 3D cameras, in particular low-cost range-imaging cameras. We explore the possibilities to reduce the uncertainty of registration algorithms through a Kalman movement model. Our setup (Fig. 1) detects a specific surface within a 3D point cloud captured by a range-imaging camera and determines its rigid transformation over time. For that a previously taken head-template is globally characterized through Fast Point Feature Histograms (FPFH) feature-descriptors and thereby matched into the scene. Then the distance between the template points and the camera points is iteratively locally minimized through an Iterative Closest Point (ICP) algorithm. The detected movement is finally observed by a linear Kalman filter.

2   Materials and methods

2.1   Feature-based registration

To initialize our tracking software, the initial head position within the 3D scene has to be detected. The ICP algorithm is not suitable for this task as it may converge to local minima and doesn't take global surface properties into account. The feature-based alignment addresses the global registration problem.

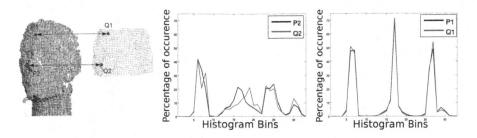

Fig. 2. Example of FPFH-descriptor with 33 bins for template (red) and camera data (black).

Among the huge amount of available 3D feature descriptors, the FPFH-descriptor, is the first one that is proven to be highly discriminative with respect to the underlying geometric surface and therefore very useful for the problem of correspondence search [4]. FPFH is relatively robust against noisy input data and invariant against rigid 3D transformations and different sampling densities. The descriptor calculates the overall trend of normal directions for each point's p_i local neighbors. The variety of existing angles is then transferred into a n-dimensional histogram $H(p_i) = \{h^1, h^2, \ldots, h^n\}$. Fig. 2 depicts the delicate sensitivity of FPFH towards different regions of the human face. The problem of determining the best registration solution can have a high computational complexity because of the enormous number of possible correspondences between similar points. Therefore the randomized SAC-IA [4] method (SAmple Consensus Initial Alignment) was used to find decent solutions for the correspondence problem in reasonable time.

2.2   Iterative closest point (ICP) algorithm

ICP is the most popular registration algorithm for point sets or surfaces when an initial estimate of the relative orientation exists. For our setup, a conventional point-to-point ICP with closest-point matching is used. The nearest neighbor search is accelerated using a k-d tree. Our setup uses the initial template position as determined by the feature-based registration as a starting point for ICP and then iteratively takes the last convergence point as a starting point in new camera data.

In medical applications we don't expect rapid head movements, hence the difference between two considered camera point clouds will be small. Therefore the registration problem turns from a global one as addressed in subsection 2.1 into a local one. Assuming small movements within two frames, the pairing of nearest neighbors will likely return pairs that actually correspond geometrically. Our experiments with different initial template positions and angles showed that the head template usually converges within 35 iterations, even with high offsets (Fig. 3).

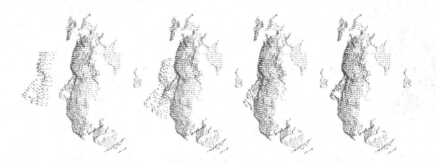

Fig. 3. Convergence of ICP for iteration 1, 2, 5 and 35 (from left to right).

2.3   Kalman filter

The Kalman Filter is a well-proven method to observe dynamic systems based on noisy measurements. Particularly movements of rigid objects can be exactly modeled by Kalman filters as they follow the physical laws of motion. The filter is initialized with the data determined by the feature-based registration and updated iteratively using the ICP results. Our linear Kalman model includes the head's position and RPY-orientation and their first derivatives

$$\mu = \left(X^{\mathrm{T}}, V^{\mathrm{T}} \right)^{\mathrm{T}} = \left(x, y, z, \mathrm{roll}, \mathrm{pitch}, \mathrm{yaw}, v_x, v_y, v_z, v_{\mathrm{roll}}, v_{\mathrm{pitch}}, v_{\mathrm{yaw}} \right)^{\mathrm{T}}$$

As a start, we chose a linear model. The linear state transition equations are derived as

$$X_t = X_{t-1} + V_{t-1} \Delta t + \alpha$$
$$V_t = V_{t-1} + \beta$$

The process noise (α, β) is assumed to be normally distributed: $(\alpha, \beta) \sim \mathcal{N}(0, Q)$. The covariance matrix Q was chosen to be diagonal. Let Z_t be the location and orientation vector as measured by the registration algorithms. Then the obversation model is given through

$$Z_t = X_t + \gamma$$

with $\gamma \sim \mathcal{N}(0, R)$ representing the uncertainty in our measurements. R is as well a diagonal matrix. The elements of Q and R were determined empirically. By balancing the elements of Q and R, the confidence in either the measurements or the process model can be adjusted. Higher certainty in the process model decreases the systems noise while higher certainty in observations increases the reactivity of the system.

3   Results

The systems's capabilities were tested using an "Asus Xtion Pro Live" low-cost Kinect-like camera.

3.1   Runtime and robustness

Different settings for the feature-based registration have been tested. At a point density of 8 mm for both the template's and the camera's points the algorithm finds a valid head position in 300 SAC-IA iterations with a probability of more than 99%. The runtime for a C++ implementation on a 2.93 GHz Intel Core i7 is less than 0.4 seconds. The highest stability for ICP was achieved with a slightly higher point density for the camera data. At a resolution of 7 mm for the template and 4 mm for the Kinect, the ICP converges in 30 ms. Including all other calculation steps, a tracking rate of 16 FPS was achieved.

Table 1. Standard deviation (SD) and trackable movements.

	x-axis	y-axis	z-axis	roll	pitch	yaw
Trackable velocity at 16 FPS	0.48 m/s	0.16 m/s	0.16 m/s	80°/s	40°/s	40°/s
SD of Kalman-filtered values	0.071 mm	0.19 mm	0.20 mm	0.21°	0.073°	0.12°
SD reduction through Kalman	17.4 %	9.5 %	12.4 %	9.7 %	25.5 %	16.0 %

The robustness of the prototype was measured by tracking robotized movements at different velocities. The highest processable velocities are 0.48 m/s and 0.16 m/s for x- and y-, z-axis, respectively (Tab. 1).

3.2 Accuracy

The basic setup for this measurement was a human head phantom made of styrofoam, which was mounted to an industrial robot (Adept Viper s850), serving as a ground truth and the mentioned Asus camera. To estimate the system's noise, the standard deviation of the Kalman-filtered values was calculated (Tab. 1).

To measure the intrinsic accuracy of our prototype, the robot was moved to 40 positions on each axis by increments of 2 mm. Each position was tracked for 20 seconds and the measured values were averaged. The error of the averaged distances to the first measurement is depicted in Fig. 4. To estimate the quality of our system, the RMS error was computed (Tab. 2). The measured values show a significant systematic error of 2.7% on the x-axis (depth). This aberration was reproducible. We suppose that the Asus camera as a consumer electronics device is not calibrated accurately enough to measure depths consistently. Provided that systematic errors in Kinect measurements can be calibrated, the RMS error decreases (Tab. 2). To estimate the effect of a decent calibration, each camera axis was corrected with a best-fit line.

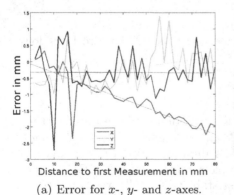

(a) Error for x-, y- and z-axes.

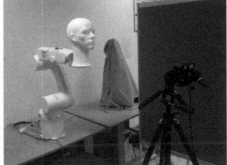

(b) Experimental setup.

Fig. 4. Estimation of tracking errors.

Table 2. RMS-error for measured distances.

	x-axis	y-axis	z-axis
RMS-Error	1.34 mm	0.62 mm	0.71 mm
RMS with calibration	0.34 mm	0.52 mm	0.63 mm

4 Discussion

In this paper we presented a first prototype for tracking head motion with a Kalman movement model. The proposed setup might be applied for head-tracking during radiation therapy. We showed that a combination of a feature-based global registration algorithm and an Iterative Closest Point optimizer is stable and reliable. The ICP showed great robustness in tracking movements of about 0.16 m/s. at 16 FPS. The expected movements on a treatment coach are many times lower, thus our prototype is robust enough to observe normal patient motion. The Kalman filter decreased uncertainties in measurements substantially and is thus an appropriate method for noise reduction and error suppression. Our estimation of the system's intrinsic accuracy with the low-cost camera revealed RMS-errors of 0.62 mm and 0.71 mm for movements parallel to the camera. The depth axis contained a systematic error of 2.7%. If calibrated decently, the RMS error on the X-axis reduces to 0.34 mm. Our prototype has the potential for submillimeter-accuracy and is thus a promising setup for compensating head motions in medical applications. Low-cost cameras are problematic but can be used if calibrated correctly. Nevertheless, the determined error is a theoretical value as all measurements were averaged over 20 seconds. Besides, the elastic deformation of the skin remains a source of registration errors. To resolve the named issues, our institute is developing a highly accurate laser scanner capable of measuring subcutaneous tissue thickness [5].

References

1. Kooy HM, Dunbar SF, Tarbell NJ, et al. Adaptation and verification of the relocatable Gill-Thomas-Cosman frame in stereotactic radiotherapy. Int J Radiat Oncol. 1994;30(3):685–91.
2. Pan H, Cerviño LI, Pawlicki T, et al. Frameless, real-time, surface imaging-guided radiosurgery: clinical outcomes for brain metastases. Neurosurgery. 2012;71(4):844–52.
3. Wiersma RD, Tomarken SL, Grelewicz Z, et al. Spatial and temporal performance of 3D optical surface imaging for real-time head position tracking. Med Phys. 2013;40(11):111712.
4. Rusu RB, Blodow N, Beetz M. Fast point feature histograms (FPFH) for 3D registration. Proc IEEE Int Conf Robot. 2009; p. 3212–7.
5. Ernst F, Bruder R, Wissel T, et al. Real time contact-free and non-invasive tracking of the human skull: first light and initial validation. Proc SPIE. 2013 Aug;8856:88561G–1–8.

Multiple Subviral Particle in Fluorecsence Microscopy Sequences

Christian Kienzle[1], Gordian Schudt[2], Stephan Becker[2], Thomas Schanze[1]

[1]KMUB, Technische Hochschule Mittelhessen, Germany
[2]Institut für Virologie, Philipps-Universität Marburg, Germany
christian.kienzle@kmub.thm.de

Abstract. To analyze the intracellular movements of subviral particles (nucleocapsids, NCs) of the Marburg virus, the viral protein VP30 has been labeled fluorescently. This makes the NCs observable by fluorescence microscopy under biosafety level 4 conditions. An algorithm has been developed, aiming to allow the automated detection and tracking of the NCs . The specific feature of this approach is the inclusion of expertise about the NCs' appearance and movement characteristics, what gives more reliable results than a simple nearest neighbor linking of the detected NCs.

1 Introduction and state of the art

To understand the mechanisms and characteristics of the intracellular movements of Marburg virus NCs, virologists from the Institute for Virology in Marburg have visualized them by the means of fluorescence microscopy. In order to do that, the viral nucleocapsid-associated protein VP30 was fused with a fluorescent protein. By expression of this fusionprotein during infection, NCs can now be detected in fluorescence microscopy sequences [1]. Due to the multiplicity of the NCs that occur in just one recorded cell, the manual tracking is a very time consuming process. Aiming to allow automated detection and tracking of the NCs, an algorithm has been developed in this work. The specific feature of this approach, in contrast to current free accessible tracking tools, is the inclusion of expert knowledge about the NCs' movement characteristics.

Common algorithms that allow an automated tracking of objects in image sequences typically consist of two subsequent steps [2]. The first step is the detection the objects with their features. The second step is the linking of the objects between subsequent frames [3, 4]. For the detection of the objects many different methods can be used. Depending on the objects' characteristics, intensity thresholding, feature detection or morphological filtering are possible approaches, amongst other techniques [5]. The linking of the objects can be done in a deterministic or in a probabilistic way [6]. An overview, concerning the tracking of viral particles in fluorescence microscopy sequences, is given by Godinez et al. [7].

A straightforward, deterministic approach for the linking of the objects between subsequent frames is the nearest neighbor search. The algorithm that was developed in this work uses a restricted nearest neighbor tracking approach, which includes expertise about the NCs shape and movement characteristics. The NCs, which are to be tracked, show an ellipsoid form and move mainly in direction of one of their tipped ends (Fig. 1). Including this information in the developed algorithm, the linking of the NCs is done more robustly than with a simple nearest neighbor approach. In order to close gaps in the detected tracks, a probabilistic assignment, based on models of the expected dynamics of the objects, could be done in further steps.

2   Materials and methods

For a robust tracking of the NCs, the inclusion of expertise about their movement characteristics and image representation is essential [8]. Therefore, in the next sections, the relevant knowledge is summed up before the algorithmic methods are explained in detail.

2.1   Characteristics of the NCs

The analyzed image sequences (> 20) consist of 20 up to 600 images. These images contain mostly one, sometimes two cells (Fig. 1, top). The small elongated structures within the shown cell are the NCs, which are to be tracked (Fig. 1). The size of NCs is about 900 by 90 nm. The NCs move mainly in direction of

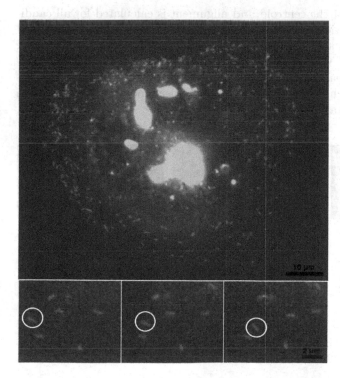

Fig. 1. Top: Sample frame from one of the analyzed image sequences. Small elongated objects are the NCs, which are to be tracked. Some other small, but spherical objects can be vesicles. Big bright objects, called inclusion bodies, represent viral induced replication compartments around the nucleus. Bottom: NCs in subsequent frames (dt = 3 s). The white circle marks one NC within these three frames, to show the NCs' movement mainly in direction of their tips.

their tips (Fig. 1, bottom). This information is used for a robust algorithmic linking of the detected objects in subsequent video frames [1].

Although the NCs move in special flat cells [1], there is still an expansion perpendicular to the focal plane. This issue often causes a defocussing of the NCs during their movement in particular in the thicker cell center. The defocussing of the NCs causes a considerable variation of their image representations along their tracks and has to be taken into account for the tracking (Fig. 2.1).

2.2   Multiple object tracking

The tracking algorithm consists of three main steps. The first step is the detection of possible NCs. The second step is the bf characterisation of all candidates. The extracted information is used in the final step, the linking, to track the NCs through the image sequences. These three steps will be explained in more detail in the following.

Detection Since the NCs are non spherical objects they have to be aligned to allow the extraction of further features. That is why the first algorithmic step is the extraction of a set of possible NCs that can then be aligned and analyzed. A size-selective grayscale tophat operation followed by a global thresholding yields appropriate small objects. These so called candidates are analyzed in the subsequent step.

Characterisation First the centroid and alignment is calculated for all candidates using a two-dimensional Principal Component Analysis (PCA). All aligned and centered candidates are then compared to an aligned template created from a manual selected set of NCs via multidimensional PCA. That way different parameters e.g. center of mass, similarity to the template, alignment and brightness can be computed for each detected object. These object specific parameters can then be used to achieve a robust linking of the NCs.

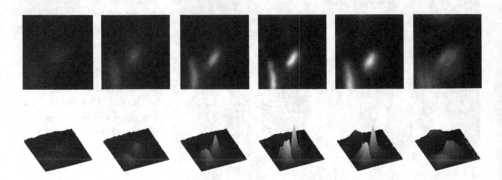

Fig. 2. Defocussing of the NCs. NCs recorded at different focal planes (dx = 600 nm). Top: image samples. Bottom: surface plots.

Linking To reduce the amount of misdetections, objects with a similarity to the template lower than a threshold, found by a bootstrap method, are ignored during subsequent linking. Based on the above mentioned expertise in the NCs' movement characteristics, the linkage uses a nearest neighbor linking with restricted freedom of lateral movement of the NCs (Fig. 3). Furthermore, the change of similarity and brightness is restricted by thresholds. These additional conditions allow a robust linking even with a high object density. The restricted change of similarity also leads to the disruption of the tracks if the tracked objects are intersecting and, for that reason, cannot be characterized individually.

2.3   Validation of the tracks

The first step of the validation of the detected tracks is the verification of 800 linkages randomly selected from four different image sequences. The question was not whether the linked objects are NCs, but only if the objects are linked properly to the corresponding objects in the subsequent frames. It has been shown that experts could not find any incorrect link within this sample. Therefore it can be assumed that the found tracks are congruent with real objects' tracks. Considering the samples binomially distributed, this leads to an error rate lower than 0.37 % with a probability of 95 %.

The next question was which tracks are to be chosen to extract only the NCs' tracks. The classifier that was used to separate the NCs from other candidates was the similarity to the template. In order to find an appropriate threshold, a receiver operating characteristic (ROC) analysis was performed [9]. To generate a set of known instances, all objects from multiple frames with known similarities have been classified by an expert as NCs or Not-NCs. The outcome of this analysis was that a threshold of 0.9 leads to a specificity bigger than 0.98 with a sensitivity of about 0.22, regarding single objects [9]. As the image representation of the NCs and therefore their similarity values vary along the tracks, tracks with at least one object with a similarity of 0.9 or bigger have been classified as NCs' tracks. Due to the good linking performance this leads to a much higher sensitivity, than showed in the ROC analysis for single frames (Fig. 4).

3   Results

The developed algorithm allows automated detection and tracking of NCs in fluorescent microscopy image sequences (Fig. 2.3). A big amount of tracks,

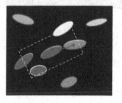

Fig. 3. The object in the center of the rectangle will be linked to an object in the subsequent frame. All objects within the rectangle are potential candidates in the subsequent frame. The yellow objects are dismissed due to differences to the current object (similarity to the template or energy). Out of the remaining green objects the closest one is linked.

Fig. 4. Detail of the ROC curve for the similarity to the template (TP, true positive rate; FP, false positive rate). Analyzed was a set of 1805 objects classified by an expert. The set contains 1109 NCs and 696 Not-NCs. Choosing a threshold of 0.9 gives a very good specificity (=1-FP) of 0.98 and a sensitivity of about 0.22.

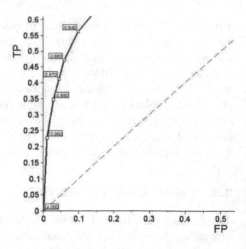

providing data for reliable statistics, can be extracted in a short period of time. Introducing a threshold for the similarity to the template, which had to be reached by one object in a detected track to classify the track as an NC-track, a sensitivity greater than 0.62 could be reached, keeping the specificity above 0.95.

An illustrative example for subviral particles velocities provides Fig. 2.3. Here, all tracks detected in a sequence of 600 frames are plotted over a maximum intensity projection of the same sequence. The maximum intensity projection provides an image with bright lines that correspond to bright objects moving through the sequence. For this particular sequence, containing mainly NCs,

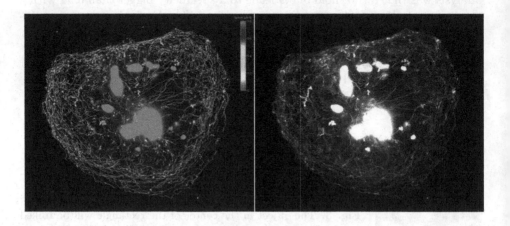

Fig. 5. Left: NCs' tracks. Speed of the objects color-coded. The underlying image is a maximum intensity projection over 600 frames. The bright lines in the maximum projection correspond mainly to the paths of the NCs. A good congruence between the bright lines and the tracks can be found. Right: Maximum intensity projection.

most of the bright lines represent NCs' tracks. Fig. 2.3 shows, that a good congruence between the bright lines and the detected tracks can be found.

4   Discussion and conclusion

A good performance of the subviral particle tracking algorithm was obtained for different recording parameters. It was not necessary to adapt the parameters for most of the analyzed sequences. The now accessible tracks open up many possibilities for biomedical driven analysis, e.g. mean velocities for different areas and periods, curvature or acceleration.

Some of the detected tracks are fractional and could be linked by statistical means in further steps, using the gotten information as an initialization for probabilistic tracking approaches. There are many algorithmic steps that can be optimized for possibly generating better results, but the goal of extracting reliable data that only contains a small amount of misdetections was reached. In future much work has to be done to illustrate and analyze the extracted data with regard to appropriate and relevant biological issues.

References

1. Schudt G, Kolesnikova L, Dolnik O, et al. Live-cell imaging of Marburg virus-infected cells uncovers actin-dependent transport of nucleocapsids over long distances. Proc Natl Acad Sci. 2013;110(35):14402–7.
2. Smal I, Draegestein K, Galjart N, et al. Particle filtering for multiple object tracking in dynamic fluorescence microscopy images: application to microtubule growth analysis. IEEE Trans Med Imaging. 2008;27(6):789–804.
3. Meijering E, Dzyubachyk O, Smal I. Methods for cell and particle tracking. Methods Enzymol. 2012;504:183–200.
4. Cheezum MK, Walker WF, Guilford WH. Quantitative comparison of algorithms for tracking single fluorescent particles. Biophys J. 2001;81(4):2378–88.
5. Meijering E. Cell segmentation: 50 years down the road [life sciences]. IEEE Signal Process Mag. 2012;29(5):140–5.
6. Arulampalam MS, Maskell S, Gordon N, et al. A tutorial on particle filters for online nonlinear/non-Gaussian Bayesian tracking. IEEE Trans Signal Process. 2002;50(2):174–88.
7. Godinez WJ, Lampe M, Wörz S, et al. Deterministic and probabilistic approaches for tracking virus particles in time-lapse fluorescence microscopy image sequences. Med Image Anal. 2009;13(2):325–42.
8. Kienzle C, Schudt G, Becker S, et al. Subviral particle tracking. Biomed Eng / Biomed Tech. 2013;58(s1-keynote):1–4.
9. Fawcett T. An introduction to ROC analysis. Pattern Recognit Lett. 2006;27(8):861–74.

Alae Tracker
Tracking of the Nasal Walls in MRI

Katharina Breininger[1], Andreas K. Maier[1], Christoph Forman[1],
Wilhelm Flatz[2], Catalina Meßmer[3], Maria Schuster[3]

[1]Pattern Recognition Lab, Friedrich-Alexander-Universität Erlangen-Nürnberg
[2]Institute of Clinical Radiology, Ludwig-Maximilians-University, Munich
[3]Dept. of Otorhinolaryngology, Head and Neck Surgery, University of Munich
`katharina.breininger@studium.fau.de`

Abstract. MR imaging opens the opportunity to image soft materials
in the human body non-invasively and to observe the behavior of organs
and muscles over a period of time. In this paper, a simple and easy-
to-use method to track and measure the movement of the nasal walls
during breathing is presented that uses a sum of three Gaussian functions as an estimator for the intensity distribution of the MR image. By
post-processing MR-data it is possible to quantify internal nasal movement in a non-invasive manner. The approach shows very good results in
comparison to manual segmentation and with respect to stability. Deviations of $\pm 10°$ of the ROI still lead to sub-pixel accuracy. The software
is available at http://www5.cs.fau.de/research/software/alae-tracker.

1   Introduction

For sufficient breathing human nostrils are kept stable by small cartilages in the
nasal alae forming the outer nasal lateral walls. When instability of the cartilages
occur, the nostrils can collapse during breathing leading to an obstruction of the
upper airway. Until now there is no reliable diagnostic method to evaluate the
stability of the outer nasal walls.

We propose to use MR Cine series [1] and a semi-automatic segmentation
technique. In contrast to other methods no device needs to be inserted into the
nose which has the risk of changing the nasal movement. It provides a non-
invasive approach to track and measure the movement of the nasal septum and
cartilages during breathing [2].

The method can be used to examine the movement of the inner nose in various
applications including fundamental research, assessment of nasal function and
monitoring of the rehabilitation process after nasal surgeries. The idea of this
approach is to model the intensity distribution along a line through the human
nose with a sum of three scaled Gaussian functions, such that the optima of the
function coincide the intensity peaks of the nasal walls.

The approach as well as the mathematical background is more extensively
described in Sec. 2. Here, the used data is described as well as the process to
extract the necessary information from the MR image sequence and the tracking

itself. In Sec. 3 the achieved tracking results are evaluated and the stability with respect to the position of the user-defined selection analyzed. Furthermore the results of the approach are compared with manual tracking of the nasal walls. Sec. 4 sums the results up.

2 Materials and methods

We collected data with the following structure with the following properties: The image sequence shows the temporal progress during forced breathing in a cross section through the human head, such that the movement of the nasal walls can be observed. An example of one image is depicted in Fig. 1. In-vivo experiments were performed in one healthy volunteer on a 3T clinical MR scanner (MAGNETOM Verio, Siemens AG, Healthcare Sector, Erlangen, Germany), with software release syngo MR B17. Imaging was performed with the following parameters: TR/TE 2.45/155.31 ms, radio frequency excitation angle 10°, FOV $192 \times 192\,\mathrm{mm}^2$, acquired matrix 96×93, reconstructed matrix 96×96, pixel-size $2\,\mathrm{mm}^2$, slice thickness 12 mm and a receiver bandwidth of 1021 Hz/Px.

The processing and evaluation of the image data consists of four steps: The line selection by the user, the reslicing of the image sequence, the estimation process and the extraction of the tracking result. For all steps the image processing framework ImageJ is used [3].

The first step of this semi-automatic segmentation process is user-driven: The user chooses a line in the above described image sequence centered through the nose. The line should be positioned in the center between the tip and the cheeks, approximately at right angle to the septum. Fig. 1 shows an example of the correct placement. The line selection denotes where the movement of the nasal alae will be observed.

The given image sequence is then resliced: For image $i, i = \{1, ..., n\}$ the intensities values along the line selections composed to the i-th image line of the

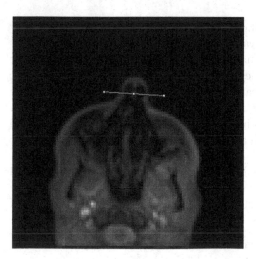

Fig. 1. Position of the cross section through the human head as well as an example for a line selection through the nose.

resliced image [4]. The necessary information for the estimation is compressed into this one resliced image. The result can be seen in Fig. 3. This image is used for the estimation process and later to compactly display the tracked movement of the nasal alae, since each image line now depicts the position of the nasal walls at one point in time.

Based on the resliced image data, the estimation process is carried out for each image line i: The intensities are fitted to a sum of three scaled Gaussian functions. The idea is to model the intensity peaks that are the nasal walls each with a Gaussian bell function. The model function has the following form

$$g_s(x) = \sum_{k=1}^{3} \alpha_k \mathcal{N}(x; \mu_k, \sigma_k) \tag{1}$$

where

$$\mathcal{N}(x; \mu, \sigma) = \frac{1}{\sigma\sqrt{2\pi}} e^{-\frac{1}{2}\left(\frac{x-\mu}{\sigma}\right)^2} \tag{2}$$

The measured intensities and the model function are then fitted using mean squared error. The function

$$\sum_{i=1}^{N} \left(f(x) - \sum_{k=1}^{3} \alpha_k \mathcal{N}(x; \mu_k, \sigma_k)\right)^2 \to min \tag{3}$$

is minimized with respect to the free parameters mean μ_k, standard deviation σ_k and scaling factor α_k for $k = \{1, 2, 3\}$. In (3) the term $f(x), x \in 1, ..., N$ denotes the image intensity of the x-th pixel of the current image line, where N is the length of an image line.

For the optimization process, a gradient-decent method provided in the JPOP (Java Parallel Optimization Package) library is used[1]. As mentioned above the optimization and estimation process is performed for every point in time resp. for every image line in the resliced image, resulting in a temporal tracking of the motion.

Since the peaks of the Gaussian function are supposed to model the intensity peaks of the nasal walls, the mean values $\mu_k, k = \{1, 2, 3\}$ are the estimates positions of the nasal walls. The estimated mean values for each image line are drawn into the resliced image and the distances between the mean values are calculated (in mm) and put into a measurement table. This measurement table can be exported out of the ImageJ framework and used for further evaluation. Furthermore if the estimation process has failed, optionally interpolation can be used on the original image data set to artificially increase the resolution and/or a manual refinement of the tracking can be applied to improve the results.

To evaluate the method, a manual tracking of the motion of septum and cartilages has been performed on the available data set. Furthermore different initial manual selections for the tracking process were set to test the stability of the semi-automatic tracking and measurements.

---

[1] http://www5.cs.fau.de/research/software/java-parallel-optimization-package/

Fig. 2. Estimation of the intensity distribution (red) with three scaled Gaussian functions (blue) for one point in time.

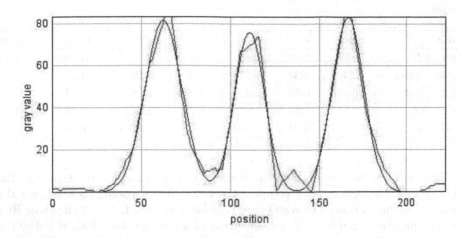

3   Results

The achieved results reveal a very good agreement of the semi-automatic tracking with the intensity distribution of the MR-image. An example of the intensity distribution across the nasal septum and cartilages and the corresponding estimation with Gaussian functions is depicted in Fig. 2.

In Fig. 3 the complete estimate for points in time and the movement of the cartilages during breathing is shown. Again, we visually observe a good agreement between the automatic method and the image data. Note that the left nasal wall shows much more motion that the right nasal wall. The left wall has a maximum distance to the septum of 12.2 mm and a minimal distance of 5.4 mm. The maximal distance of the right wall to the septum is 11.4 mm while the minimal distance was 9.0 mm.

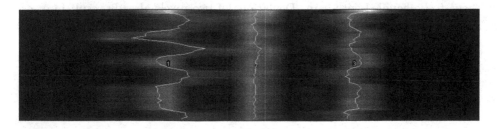

Fig. 3. The result of the reslicing (background) and the estimation process (yellow lines).

Table 1. RMSE with respect to manual segmentation. Using the same ROI as for the manual segmentation, we observe sub-pixel accuracy. Also small deviations still preserve the sub-pixel accuracy. Larger deviations lead to an accuracy of about one pixel.

ROI	Same	$-5°$	$+5°$	$-12°$	$+11°$	$+4\,$mm	$-4\,$mm
pos. left	0.54	0.68	0.85	0.89	1.10	1.48	1.41
pos. septum	0.42	0.33	0.51	0.38	0.90	1.07	1.10
pos. right	0.23	0.33	0.24	0.50	0.60	0.47	1.67
dist. left	0.85	0.81	1.21	0.95	1.46	2.26	1.48
dist. right	0.46	0.34	0.50	0.45	1.60	0.94	2.76

In addition, we investigated the stability of our method with respect to the manual ROI selection. We compared seven different configurations with the manual segmentation. The results are tabulated in Tab. 1. Using the same ROI as the manual segmentation, we get errors of about 0.5 mm which is below the pixel size of 2 mm. Also a slight change of orientation of $\pm5°$ is still handled robustly by the method. In these cases the error is most at 1.21 mm. Even deviations of more than $\pm10°$ still results in sub-pixel accuracy. With a shift of ±4 mm the accuracy is reduced more. The highest error is 2.76 mm.

4   Conclusion

We presented a method for semi-automatic tracking of the nasal wall in MR Cine sequences. This is the first approach to objectively detect a collapse of the nasal alae and measure the stability of the nose during breathing. The method was based on modeling the intensity profiles as Gaussian bell curves. We could show that the fitting procedure worked well compared to a manual segmentation. The error was below one pixel. Also slight modifications as they occur in the manual ROI selection process were handled by the method robustly. Small deviations resulted in only a small increase of the error. Deviations of up to 10° yielded sub-pixel accuracy. However, shifts perpendicular to the orientation of the ROI line have to be handled with care. Deviations of two pixels already result in errors of about one pixel. We regard this problem as rather minor as the position in this direction can be selected robustly from the anatomical information in the image. To further improve the results we suggest Kalman Filtering to reduce the influence of noise in the MR data.

References

1. Haacke EM, Brown RW, Thompson MR, et al. Magnetic Resonance Imaging: Physical Principles and Sequence Design. New York, Chichester, Weinheim, Brisbane, Singapore, Toronto: Wiley-Liss; 1999.

2. Gray H. Anatomy of the Human Body. Philadelphia, NJ, United States: Lea & Febiger; 1918.
3. Collins TJ. ImageJ for microscopy. Biotechniques. 2007;43(1 Suppl):25–30.
4. Gonzalez RC, Woods RE. Digital Image Processing. Upper Saddle River, NJ, United States: Prentice Hall International; 2007.

Erzeugung von Referenzdaten für Kopfbewegungskorrektur in Diffusion-MRI

Jan Hering[1,2], Peter F. Neher[1], Hans-Peter Meinzer[1], Klaus H. Maier-Hein[1,3]

[1]Abteilung für Medizinische und Biologische Informatik, DKFZ Heidelberg
[2]Medizinische Informatik, Hochschule Mannheim
[3]Quantitative bildgebungsbasierte Krankheitscharakterisierung, DKFZ Heidelberg
j.hering@dkfz.de

Kurzfassung. Die fehlenden Referenzdaten für in vivo diffusion-MR Aufnahmen verhindern eine quantitative Auswertung von Vorverarbeitungsschritten wie der Korrektur der Kopfbewegung. Eine Simulation der Bewegung durch das nachträgliche Hinzufügen von Headmotion-Effekten durch Transformation der einzelnen Bildvolumen ist nur mit Translation möglich, da das diffusion-gewichtete Signals von der Orientierung der Faser abhängt. Um komplexere Bewegungen zu simulieren, stellen wir eine Erzeugung von Daten mit Kopfbewegung vor, auf Basis von Fiberfox, einem Werkzeug für die Generierung von Software-Phantomdaten. Wir zeigen, dass die Rotationskomponente verglichen zur Translation einen signifikanten ($p < 0.01$) Einfluss auf den resultierenden target registration error (TRE) hat und bei der Evaluation von Korrekturansätzen nicht vernachlässigt werden darf. Für höhere Diffusionswichtungen ($b \geqslant 2000\,\text{s/mm}^2$) übersteigt der TRE auf den durch Rotation augmentierten Daten die Voxelgröße. Fehler von solcher Größe beeinflussen jede weitere Auswertung, insbesondere die immer stärker im Fokus stehende genaue Analyse von mikro-strukturellen Gewebecharakteristiken.

1 Einleitung

Die Kopfbewegungskorrektur gehört zu den wichtigsten Vorverarbeitungsschritten bei Diffusion MR Bilddaten, da Bewegungsartefakte die in vielen Studien verwendete Kenngrößen wie die fraktionelle Anisotropie (FA) stark beeinflussen [1]. Eine quantitative Auswertung der retrospektiven Korrektur der Kopfbewegung während einer diffusiongewichteten (DW) MR Aufnahme ist in den meisten Fällen nicht durchführbar, da keine Referenzdaten zur Verfügung stehen. Eine manuelle Identifikation von anatomischen Landmarken für eine quantitave Auswertung des target registration errors (TRE) ist aufgrund der hohen Anzahl von Bildern nicht praktikabel. Bisherige Arbeiten bewerten daher die Verfahren nur qualitativ anhand von illustrierenden Bildern [2, 3] oder es werden deskriptive Maße verglichen, wie die Varianz in den Intensitäten [3]. Eine quantitative Auswertung des TREs ist nur begrenzt möglich, z.B. indem man bereits bewegungsfreie Daten künstlich mit Bewegung augmentiert [4]. Bei der Augmentierung kommt es jedoch zu Interpolationsartefakten und Rotationen sind aufgrund der Richtungsabhängigkeit der Daten nur über Umwege und Modellannahmen zu simulieren.

Als Teil der open-source Bibliothek MITK wurde kürzlich das Werkzeug Fiberfox veröffentlicht [5], welches die Erzeugung von realistichen Phantomdaten ausgehend von einer beliebig komplexen Faserkonfiguration ermöglicht.

Wir präsentieren in unserem Beitrag eine Erweiterung von Fiberfox um die Simulation von Kopfbewegung während der Aufnahme, welche auch Rotationen einschließt und demonstrieren, dass gerade diese Rotation bei Evaluationen von Korrekturansätzen nicht vernachlässigt werden sollte.

2 Material und Methoden

2.1 Daten

Die Testdaten wurden aus der Human Connectome Project (HCP) Datenbank entnommen [6], da diese hoch aufgelöste DW Datensätze bereitstellt, die mit vielen Gradientenrichtungen bei unterschiedlichen $b-$Werten aufgenommen wurden. Ein Datensatz besteht aus 18 ungewichteten Aufnahmen ($b = 0\,\mathrm{s/mm^2}$) und aus jeweils 90 Richtungsaufnahmen für jeden $b-$Wert ($b = 1000, 2000$ und $3000\,\mathrm{s/mm^2}$) mit einer isotropen Auflösung von $1.25\,\mathrm{mm}$.

2.2 Bewegungssimulation

Auf Basis einer beliebigen Faserkonfiguration als Eingabe generiert Fiberfox, mittels State of the Art multi-compartment Modellierungstechniken und der

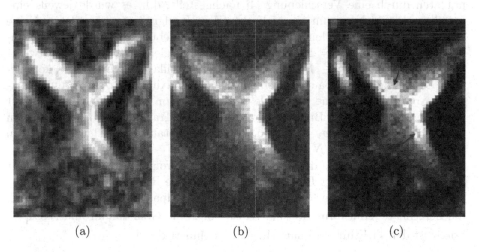

(a)   (b)   (c)

Abb. 1. Simulierte Daten. Der Hirnbalken als Beispielstruktur in einer axialen Schicht der Originaldaten (a), der mit Fiberfox generierten Daten ohne Bewegung (b) und mit Bewegung (c). Eine durch die Rotation bedingte Änderung des DW Signals (markiert durch rote Pfeile) ist sichtbar im Bild (c). Diffusionwichtung $b = 3000\,\mathrm{s/mm^2}$. Fensterung: (a) 122-1324, (b) und (c) 2-348.

realistischen Simulation der k-Raum Akquisition, ein diffusionsgewichtetes MR Signal [5]. Die Signalgenerierung auf Basis eines Modells der zugrundeliegenden Faserkonfiguration erlaubt das Erzeugen von Bewegungseffekten auf eine realistische und natürliche Art und Weise, indem das Fasermodell während der Signalsimulation rigide transformiert wird. Fiberfox ermöglicht die Fasertransformation mittels zufälliger Translations- und Rotationsbewegungen sowie durch gleichförmige Bewegungen, welche sich über die gesamte Akquisitionszeit erstrecken und durch eine maximale Translation und Rotation vollständig definiert sind. Die Transformation des Fasermodells wird zu diskreten Zeitpunkten, jeweils nach der Simulation eines vollständigen Gradientenvolumens, durchgeführt. Die Abb. 1 zeigt ein Beispiel der simulierten Daten.

2.3   Bewegungskorrektur

Die Bewegung wurde mittels parametrischer Registrierung korrigiert. Hierfür wurde ein Pyramidenansatz mit Gradientenverfahren aus der ITK Bibliothek [7] verwendet (Mindestgröße 12 Voxel). Wie in den meisten Studien üblich, wurden alle Bilder der Aufnahme auf das erste ungewichtete Bild unter der Optimierung der Mutual Information (MI) Fehlermetrik registriert [8].

2.4   Evaluation

Ausgehend von einer, anhand der Originaldaten berechneten Faserkonfiguration wurden zwei unterschiedliche Bewegungsarten simuliert. In der ersten Simulation wurde die nachträgliche Augmentierung der bewegungsfreien Originaldaten durch eine Verschiebung [4] nachgestellt, d.h. es wurde jeweils eine zufällige Verschiebung um ein vielfaches der Voxelgröße angewendet um eine Interpolation zu vermeiden. Jeder der drei Verschiebungsparameter wurde daher als $p_i = 1.25 \cdot n_i, i = 1, 2, 3$ berechnet, mit n_i gleichmäßig zufällig gewählt aus $\{-5 \leq n \leq 5, n \in \mathbb{N}\}$. In der zweiten Simulation wurde eine komplexere Bewegung nachgebaut. Dafür wurde eine maximale Rotation um die z-Achse von $15°$ sowie eine maximale Translation von $10\,\mathrm{mm}$ gewählt, d.h. für das k-te der $N = 287$ Bildvolumen wurde eine Translation mit Parametern $p_1 = k \cdot 10/N$, $p_2 = p_3 = 0\,(\mathrm{mm})$ und eine Rotation mit den Parametern $p_4 = p_5 = 0$, $p_6 = k \cdot 15/N$ (Grad) angewendet.

Als Fehlermaß wurde der target registration error (TRE) ausgewertet über die Eckpunkte $p \in P$ der Bounding-Box des für die Registrierung verwendeten Referenzdatensatzes. Die Registrierung für ein Bildpaar ist repräsentiert durch die berechnete Transformationsmatrix A_i sowie die Goldstandardmatrix $A_i^{(gt)}$. Somit ist der TRE für ein Paar $(A_i, A_i^{(gt)})$ definiert durch

$$1/|P| \cdot \sum_{\mathbf{x} \in P} \|A_i\,\mathbf{x} - A_i^{(gt)}\,\mathbf{x}\|_2 \tag{1}$$

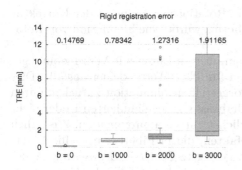

Abb. 2. Registrierungsfehler (TRE). Abgebildet ist der Registrierungsfehler für die Korrektur der durch zufällige Translationen augmentierte Originaldaten für die unterschiedlichen b-Werte (0, 1000, 2000 und 3000 s/mm^2).

3 Ergebnisse

Die Abb. 2 zeigt den TRE einer Translationskorrektur auf den nachträglich modifizierten Originaldaten. Der Fehler steigt mit höherer Diffusionswichtung und übersteigt für b-Werte ab 2000 s/mm^2 die Voxelgröße.

Die Abb. 3 (a) zeigt den TRE bei einer Translationskorrektur auf simulierten Daten. Ähnlich wie auf den modifizierten Originaldaten lässt sich ein steigender Fehler für steigende b-Werte feststellen. Allerding übersteigt der TRE für keinen der b-Werte die Voxelgröße.

Die Abb. 3 (b) zeigt den TRE bei der Korrektur einer Rotationsbewegung, der signifikant ($p < 0.01$) schlechter ausfällt als bei der Translationsbewegung.

4 Diskussion

Wir haben die Erzeugung von Referenzdaten für die Evaluation von Bewegungskorrektur in Diffusion MR Bildern mit Hilfe des DWI Simulationsframeworks

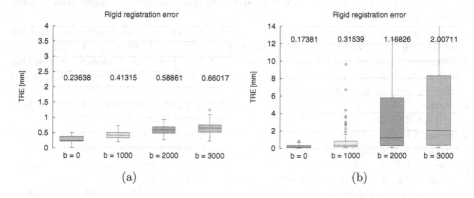

(a)   (b)

Abb. 3. Registrierungsfehler (TRE). Abgebildet ist der Registrierungsfehler für die unterschiedlichen b-Werte (0, 1000, 2000 und 3000 s/mm^2) entstanden bei der Korrektur der von Fiberfox simulierten Translationsdaten (a) und Rotationsdaten (b). Für $b > 0$ ist der TRE auf den Rotationsdaten signifikant ($p < 0.01$) höher.

Fiberfox vorgestellt und gezeigt, dass die Rotationsbewegung in der Korrektur nicht vernachlässigt werden darf. Mit Fiberfox wurde eine Simulation von Rotationen erst möglich gemacht.

Es fällt auf, dass der Fehler auf den simulierten Daten mit Verschiebung gegenüber den augmentierten Originaldaten für alle b-Werte kleiner ausfällt. Dies könnte auf den Einschränkungen der vorgestellten Simulation zurückzuführen sein. Zum einen wurden die Kontrastverhältnisse in den simulierten Bilder nicht darauf optimiert die Originaldaten möglichst gut zu approximieren. Zusätzlich simulieren wir von allen Aufnahmeartefakten, die in Fiberfox modelliert werden, nur das thermische Rauschen. Der geringere Fehler in der Korrektur der Translation stammt daher vermutlich von einem zu hohen SNR der Gradientenbildern. Umso deutlicher wird die Bedeutung der Simulation von Rotation für die Evaluation von Verfahren zur Bewegungskorrektur. Des weiteren wird die simulierte Bewegung nur zwischen den einzelnen Volumenaufnahmen ausgeführt. Eine geplante Erweiterung ist die Simulation einer realistischen, kontinuierlichen Bewegung auch während der Bildformation.

Das vorgestellte Verfahren ermöglicht die Simulation von Kopfbewegung inklusive Rotation und liefert somit wertvolle Referenzdaten für die vergleichende Evaluation verschiedener Korrekturmethoden wie des gruppenbasierten [3] oder der modelbasierten [4] Ansatzes. Die bisherigen Simulationen sind sehr limitiert [4, 3] oder benötigen aufwändige Bauten mit Headtracking während der Aufnahme [9] und damit verbundenem Aufwand.

Danksagung. Dr. Maier-Hein (né Fritzsche) und Jan Hering wurden durch die DFG gefördert, und zwar über die Projekte ME 833/15-1 bzw. WO 1218/3-1.

Literaturverzeichnis

1. Kim DJ, Park HJ, Kang KW, et al. How does distortion correction correlate with anisotropic indices? a diffusion tensor imaging study. Magn Reson Med. 2006;24(10):1369–76.
2. Ben-Amitay S, Jones DK, Assaf Y. Motion correction and registration of high b-value diffusion weighted images. Magn Reson Med. 2012;67(6):1694–702.
3. Huizinga W, Metz CT, Poot DHJ, et al. Groupwise registration for correcting subject motion and eddy current distortions in diffusion MRI using a PCA based dissimilarity metric. Proc CDMRI. 2014; p. 163–74.
4. Hering J, Wolf I, Meinzer HP, et al. Model-based motion correction of reduced field of view diffusion MRI data. Proc SPIE. 2014.
5. Neher PF, Laun FB, Stieltjes B, et al. Fiberfox: an extensible system for generating realistic white matter software phantoms. Proc CDMRI. 2014; p. 105–12.
6. Essen DCV, Ugurbil K, Auerbach E, et al. The human connectome project: a data acquisition perspective. Neuroimage. 2012;62(4):2222–31.
7. Ibanez L, Schroeder W, Ng L, et al.. The ITK Software Guide. http://www.itk.org/ItkSoftwareGuide.pdf: Kitware, Inc.; 2005.
8. Rohde GK, Barnett AS, Basser PJ, et al. Comprehensive approach for correction of motion and distortion in diffusion-weighted MRI. Magn Reson Med. 2004;51(1):103–14.

9. Aksoy M, Forman C, Straka M, et al.   Real-time optical motion correction for diffusion tensor imaging. Magn Reson Med. 2011;66(2):366–78.

Ein System zur situationsbezogenen Unterstützung in der Dentalimplantologie

Darko Katić[1], Patrick Spengler[1], Sebastian Bodenstedt[1],
Gregor Castrillon-Oberndorfer[2], Robin Seeberger[2], Jürgen Hoffmann[2],
Rüdiger Dillmann[1], Stefanie Speidel[1]

[1]Institut für Anthropomatik, KIT Karlsruhe
[2]Mund-Zahn-Kiefer-Klinik, Universitätsklinikum Heidelberg
katic@kit.edu

Kurzfassung. Erweiterte Realität(ER) hat großes Potential die Patientenversorgung in der Dentalimplantologie zu verbessern. Ein offenes Problem ist die Anpassung der Visualisierungen an die aktuelle Situation. Unser Ziel ist die Entwicklung eines Systems zur intraoperativen, situationsbezogenen Unterstützung dieses Eingriffs. Die Assistenz erfolgt dabei durch Einblendung von Informationen über eine Durchsichtbrille mit ER. Die Auswahl der Visualisierungen wird automatisch durch eine Interpretation der Situation im OP ermittelt, um so nur aktuell relevante Informationen anzubieten. Der Anspruch besteht darin, die Belastung des Chirurgen durch eine Minimierung des Bedienungsaufwandes zu verringern. Das System wurde in einem Kadaverversuch an einem Schweinekiefer mit postoperativen Messungen und einem Fragebogen evaluiert.

1 Einleitung

Gerade in der Mund-Kiefer-Gesichtschirurgie haben computergestützte Assistenzsysteme ihr Potential zur Verbesserung der Patientenversorgung bewiesen [1, 2]. Ein Problem dabei ist es, die Planungs- und Navigationsinformationen in den OP zu bringen. Dabei sind zwei Hürden zu bewältigen. Zum einen ist eine Methode notwendig, um dem Chirurgen intuitiv Informationen anzuzeigen. Zum anderen muss der Bedienungsaufwand möglichst gering sein, so dass sich der Chirurg, gerade in schwierigen Situationen, voll auf die Operation konzentrieren kann. Die Erweiterte Realität(ER) ist dabei ein vielversprechendes Paradigma zur Visualisierung [3]. Durch die ER ist es möglich reale Strukturen überdeckt mit virtuellen Bildern direkt im Blickfeld des Chirurgen darzustellen. Dadurch ist eine intuitive Darstellung möglich, die kein Abwenden des Blickes vom Patienten erfordert. Durch die zusätzlichen Einblendungen besteht allerdings auch die Gefahr sensorischer Überlastung [4]. In dem Fall ist Information zwar verfügbar, aber nicht effektiv nutzbar, weil es zu schwierig ist die notwendige Information in der Flut an Daten zu erkennen [5]. Positionen von Vitalstrukturen, wie bspw. des Mandibularnervs, sollten nur eingeblendet werden, wenn sie gefährdet sind. In anderen Fällen ist die Visualisierung aber eher störend. Manuelle Anpassungen sind aufwändig und gerade bei unerwarteten Risikosituationen zu langsam.

Die Idee hinter Sitautionsbezogener ER (SER) ist es deshalb den Operationsverlauf mit Sensoren zu beobachten und automatisch die Operationsphase zu erkennen. So wird das Informationsbedürfnis des Chirurgen bestimmt und die Visualisierung angepasst. Gerade in der Chirurgie, in der verschiedene Informationen selektiv zur Entscheidungsfindung berücksichtigt werden müssen, kann so die kognitive Belastung des Chirurgen vermindert werden [6]. Dazu wurden diverse Verfahren zur Wissensakquisation und Situationsinterpretation entwickelt und erste Systeme evaluiert [7, 8, 9]. Die besondere Schwierigkeit liegt dabei in den Echtzeitbedingungen und der Einbettung in den OP-Prozess.

Wir haben ein SER-System für das Setzen von Dentalimplantaten entwickelt und evaluiert. Die Unterstützung erfolgt durch Einblendungen über eine Durchsichtbrille. Die Auswahl der Visualisierungen wird automatisch durch Interpretation der aktuellen Situation ermittelt, so dass nur die aktuell relevante Untermenge der verfügbaren Informationen angeboten wird. So wird eine Reizüberflutung vermieden, ohne dass kritische Informationen verlorengehen. Konkret werden dazu Posen der Instrumente und des Kiefers mit dem NDI Polaris System räumlich verfolgt. Darauf aufbauend findet die Situationsinterpretation statt. Das System wurde in einer Kadaverstudie evaluiert.

2 Materialen und Methoden

Zur Bereitstellung der Assistenz müssen relevante Situationen identifiziert und geeignete Visualisierungen gefunden werden. Des Weiteren muss die aktuelle Situation im Rechner modelliert und interpretiert werden. Konkret soll in folgenden Situationen assistiert werden. Bei der Realisierung der Implantatspositionen wird mit dem Handstück an einer präoperativ bestimmten Stelle im Kiefer ein Loch ausgebohrt, in dem später das Implantat befestigt wird. Dabei sind Bohrtiefe, Position und Ausrichtung determinierende Faktoren. Entsprechend sollen diese Größen visualisiert und der Chirurg bei zu großer Abweichung gewarnt werden. Zur Vermeidung von Komplikationen soll des Weiteren auf die Gefährdung des Mandibularnervs durch zu tiefes Eindringen des Handstücks hingewiesen werden. Zuletzt soll Hilfestellung bei der Auswahl des Bohraufsatzes gegeben werden, wenn ein Wechsel notwendig ist.

Die zugehörigen Visualisierungen müssen intuitiv und unaufdringlich sein und nicht störend wirken. Das Problem bei der an sich intuitiven ER ist, dass die Sicht auf den Patienten eingeschränkt wird. Deshalb soll das System für jede Assistenzfunktion unterschiedliche Visualisierungen anbieten. Konkret sollen statische Visualisierungen fest an eine Stelle am Rande des Blickfeldes des Chirurgen platziert werden, um freie Sicht auf den Patienten sicherzustellen. Gleichzeitig soll eine alternative, kontaktanalog Darstellung angeboten werden. In diesem Fall werden die Einblendungen auf reale Strukturen überlagert.

2.1 Situationserkennung

Die Situationserkennung erfolgt über einen wissensbasierten Ansatz mit Beschreibungslogiken im OWL Standard [10]. Die Idee ist es, medizinisches Hintergrundwissen ontologisch zu formalisieren und für den Rechner nutzbar zu machen. Eine Situation wird dabei durch eine Menge von Situationsmerkmalen modelliert, wobei eine Merkmal, analog zu [7], ein Tupel der Form <Instrument, Relation, Anatomische Struktur> ist. So wird bspw. das Realisieren der Implantatsposition durch <Handstück, nah, Implantsposition1> dargestellt. Eine Phase ist eine Sequenz von Merkmalen, die medizinisch zusammengehören. Für die Erkennung werden jeweils über Regeln typische Situationsmerkmale gesucht und so die Phase inferiert. So wird die Gefährdung des Mandibularnervs erkannt, wenn das Handstück dieser Vitalstruktur zu nahe kommt, also das Merkmal <Handstück, nahe, Mandibularnerv> vorliegt. Die Realisierung einer Position wird angenommen, wenn das Handstück sich im relevanten Bereich befindet, also <Handstück, nahe, Implantatsposition1> detektiert wird. Ein Problem dabei ist, dass die Messwerte zunächst in numerischer Form vorliegen und erst in eine logische Darstellung überführt werden müssen. Dazu wenden wir eine Werteaufteilung (value partition) mit unscharfen Mengen an [11]. Die Grundidee dabei ist es über ein Lernverfahren unscharfe Mengen zu generieren, welche die Zugehörigkeit von Abstandswerten zu „nah" und „fern" erfassen. Ein Messwert wird dann der unscharfen Menge mit dem höchsten Zugehörigkeitswert zugeordnet. Der Ansatz, und die zugehörigen Situationsmerkmale, wird in [12] erläutert.

2.2 Visualisierung

Für jede Information steht eine kontaktanaloge und statische Visualisierung zur Verfügung. In Abb. 1.a ist die aktuelle Ausrichtung und erreichte Bohrtiefe, jeweils in Relation zu der Vorgabe, dargestellt. Der Grad der Abweichung ist farblich kodiert. Rot signalisiert eine schlechte Ausrichtung, grün eine gute (Abb. 1.b). Abb. 1.c zeigt die Bedrohung des Mandibularnervs. In der statischen Variante sind Nerv und Spitze des Handstücks sowie deren Abstand auf der linken Seite des Sichtfeldes zu sehen. In der kontaktanalogen werden diese Informationen direkt über den realen Objekten dargestellt.

3   Ergebnisse

Um die medizinische Eignung zu bewerten, wurde ein Versuch am Tierkadaver durchgeführt, bei dem Implantatspositionen in einem Schweinekiefer umgesetzt

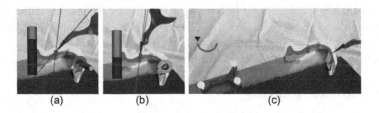

(a)   (b)   (c)

Abb. 1. Visualisierung mittels statischer und kontaktanaloger Erweiter Realität.

wurden. Im Gegensatz zum in [12] vorgestelltem Ansatz wird auf den Fallbasierten Ansatz verzichtet und die Situation nur mit Regeln erkannt. Zur Versuchsdurchführung wurden Cone-Beam-CT-Aufnahmen erstellt und segmentiert. Die Segmentierung ist dabei einfach und halbautomatisch durchführbar, da nur knöcherne Strukturen berücksichtigt werden müssen, die einen guten Kontrast zum umliegenden Gewebe haben. Darauf aufbauend wurden die Implantatspositionen geplant. Zur intraoperativen Unterstützung kamen die oben genannten Visualisierungen zum Einsatz. Der Versuchsaufbau ist in Abb. 2.a dargestellt. Der Chirurg trägt eine optische Durchsichtbrille mit künstlichen Landmarken, welche über das NDI Polaris räumlich verfolgt werden. Ebenso werden Posen von Handstück, Bohreraufsätzen und Patient bestimmt. Die Aufgabe ist es, die zwei geplanten Implantatspositionen zu realisieren. In Abb. 2 ist der Ablauf des Versuchs und die Visualisierung, wie sie der Chirurg sah, abgebildet.

3.1 Genauigkeit der Umsetzung

Die Bestimmung der Genauigkeit erfolgte über ein post-operatives Cone-Beam-CT. Bei der ersten Implantatsposition wurde eine Abweichung von 1,1 mm von der intendierten Position erreicht, mit einem Winkelfehler von 2°. Damit konnte die Planung an dieser Stelle zufriedenstellend realisiert werden. Bei der zweiten Implantatsposition kam es zu größeren Problemen, da sich unter der Position ein Milchzahn befand. Dieser Umstand wurde in den Cone-Beam-CT-Aufnahmen nicht erkannt. Dadurch konnte die Position nicht korrekt realisiert werden. Insgesamt kam es zu einer Abweichung von 2,48 mm in der Positionierung. Der Feh-

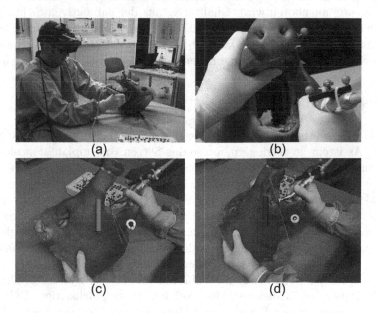

(a)   (b)

(c)   (d)

Abb. 2. Visualisierungen während der Kadaverexperimente.

ler im Winkel ließ sich nicht bestimmen, da kein vollständiges Loch entstand, sondern nur ein dünner Eingang in den Hohlraum über dem Milchzahn.

3.2 Benutzbarkeit des Systems

Die Evaluierung des medizinischen Nutzens wurde mit eine Fragebogen durchgeführt. Dabei stellte sich die automatische Anpassung der Visualisierung sowie die Visualisierungen an sich als sehr hilfreich heraus. Besonders die Anzeige der Bohrachse wurde positiv erwähnt. Die farbliche Kodierung, die zur Bewertung der Ausrichtung verwendet wird, wurde als sehr hilfreich eingestuft. Als besonderer Vorteil der statischen Variante wurde hervorgehoben, dass durch die Draufsicht der Kopf nicht gekippt werden muss, um die Achse korrekt auszurichten. Die ergänzende, kontaktanaloge Anzeige zwecks optischer Kontrolle wird allerdings begrüßt. Bemängelt wurde, dass weder die Drehzahl des Motors noch das Drehmoment angezeigt werden. Ansonsten waren alle notwendingen Informationen klar und verständlich verfügbar. Die Visualisierung des Mandibularnervs wurden ebenfalls begrüßt und tatsächlich wurde der Nerv nicht verletzt. Der Chirurg gab an, aus Sicherheitsgründen immer einen zusätzlichen Sicherheitsabstand einhalten zu wollen, um die Grenzen, wie sie durch die Visualisierung dargestellt werden, nicht auszureizen. Bei der Wahl zwischen statisch und kontaktanalog fiel die Entscheidung zu Gunsten der statischen Darstellung aus. Bei der kontaktanalogen Variante wurde die Beeinträchtigung der Sicht auf den Operationsbereich bemängelt, die Übersichtlichkeit der statischen Variante hingegen gelobt. Wichtig für die Akzeptanz des System ist auch eine geringe Anzahl Fehlerkennung, so dass sichergestellt werden kann, dass möglichst immer die korrekte Visualisierung angeboten wird. Qualitativ, aus der subjektiven Sicht des Chirurgen, wurden die Fehlerkennungen während des Versuchs als unproblematisch angesehen, weil sie sehr selten auftraten. Dies deckt sich mit der quantitiven Untersuchung in [12], bei der eine Erkennungsrate von 85% erreicht wurde.

4 Diskussion

Unser Ziel besteht darin, die Belastung des Chirurgen durch eine situationsangepasste Assistenz zu verringern, um so das Setzen von Implantatspositionen im Kiefer zu unterstützen. Im Experiment am Tierkadaver stellte sich die Visualisierung mittels SER als vielversprechendes Paradigma zur bildbasierten Navigation und Vermeidung von Komplikationen heraus. Gerade der situationsbezogene Aspekt trug stark zur Akzeptanz bei, da der intraoperative Bedienaufwand praktisch komplett entfällt. Im Sinne einer Personalisierung sind Möglichkeiten zur Anpassung der Visualisierung, wahlweise statisch oder kontaktanalog, ein wichtiger Schritt hin zur klinischen Anwendung.

Im Vergleich zu rigiden Bohrschablonen bietet das System größtmögliche Flexibilität bei der Realisierung der Positionen bei gleichzeitiger Führung des Chirurgen gemäß seiner Planung und Unterstützung bei der Vermeidung von Verletzungen des Mandibularnervs. Durch die kontextbezogene Assistenz wird gleichzeitig die kognitive Belastung vermindert. Ein offenes Problem bleibt die Genauigkeit. Zwar kann das NDI Polaris Positionen submillimeter genau messen, allerdings sind durch die vielen Kalibierungsvorgänge und Verknüpfungen mehrerer Messungen Fehlerquellen enthalten, die zu einer höheren Ungenauigkeit führen. Im Fokus der weiteren Arbeiten sollen Methoden zur genaueren Verfolgung von Objektposen untersucht werden, um das bisherige Polaris System zu ergänzen. Dies kann etwa durch Beschleunigungssensoren geschehen.

Danksagung. Diese Arbeit entstand im im DFG-geförderten „SFB/Transregio 125 Cognition-Guided Surgery - Wissens- und modellbasierte Chirurgie" und im Projekt „Situationsbezogene Erweiterte Realität im Operationssaal (DI 330/23-2)" .

Literaturverzeichnis

1. Ewers R, Schicho K, Truppe M, et al. Computer-aided navigation in dental implantology: 7 years of clinical experience. J Oral Maxillofac Surg. 2004;62(3):329–34.
2. Hassfeld S, Mühling J. Computer assisted oral and maxillofacial surgery A review and an assessment of technology. J Oral Maxillofac Surg. 2001;30(1):2–13.
3. Kersten-Oertel M, Jannin P, Collins DL. The state of the art of visualization in mixed reality image guided surgery. Comput Med Imaging Graph. 2013;37(2):98–112.
4. Woods D, Patterson E, Roth E. Can we ever escape from data overload? A cognitive systems diagnosis. Cognition Technology & Work. 2002;4(1):22–36.
5. Joyce J, Lapinski G. A history and overview of the safety parameter display system concept. IEEE Nucl Sci. 1983;30(1).
6. Cleary K, Chungand H, Mun S. OR 2020: the operating room of the future. J Laparoendosc Adv Surg Tech. 2005;1281(1):832–8.
7. Neumuth T, Strauß G, Meixensberger J, et al. Acquisition of process descriptions from surgical interventions. Proc DEXA. 2006;LNCS(4080):602–11.
8. Blum T, Padoy N, Feußner H, et al. Workflow mining for visualization and analysis of surgeries. Int J Computer Assist Radiol Surg. 2008;3(5):379–86.
9. Nicolau S, Diana M, Agnus V, et al. Semi-automated augmented reality for laparoscopic surgery: first in-vivo evaluation. Int J Computer Assist Radiol Surg. 2013;8(1):109–13.
10. Baader F, Calvanese D, McGuinness DL, et al. The Description Logic Handbook: Theory, Implementation, Applications. Cambridge: Cambridge University Press; 2003.
11. Katic D, Wekerle AL, Gärtner F, et al. Ontology-based prediction of surgical events in laparoscopic surgery. Proc SPIE. 2012;8671(1A):531–40.
12. Katic D, Sudra G, Speidel S, et al. Knowledge-based situation interpretation for context-aware augmented reality in dental implant surgery. Lect Notes Comput Sci. 2010;6326:531–40.

Segmentierung von Knochenfragmenten in typischen Kontaktsituationen

Berechnung optimaler Schnitte verbundener Objekte durch Graph-Cut Verfahren

Ralf Westphal, Martin Mikolas, Friedrich M. Wahl

Institut für Robotik und Prozessinformatik, Technische Universität Braunschweig
ralf.westphal@tu-bs.de

Kurzfassung. Für die Visualisierung, Korrekturplanung und Navigation von Frakturen sind präzise Computermodelle der Knochenfragmente erforderlich. Zwar stellt die Segmentierung knöcherner Strukturen aus CT-Daten im Allgemeinen kein Problem dar; gerade bei Frakturen stehen aber häufig die einzelnen Fragmente in direkten Kontakt miteinander, wodurch eine automatische Separierung der Fragmente während des Segmentierungsprozesses erschwert wird. Es wird ein auf Graph-Cuts basierender Segmentierungsalgorithmus vorgestellt, mit dem es möglich ist, Knochenfragmente mit direktem Kontakt mit geringer Nutzerinteraktion semiautomatisch, effizient und optimal zu separieren.

1 Einleitung

Im Allgemeinen ist aufgrund des hohen Kontrastes die Segmentierung knöcherner Strukturen von umgebenem Weichteilgewebe im CT mit einfachen, wie z.B. schwellwertbasierten Verfahren relativ einfach und zuverlässig möglich. Sollen jedoch mehrere Knochen oder Knochenfragmente, die in direktem Kontakt zueinander stehen separat segmentiert werden, sind in der Regel komplexere Verfahren erforderlich. Schwellwertbasierte Verfahren scheitern hier, da bei der Wahl eines Schwellwertes, der hoch genug ist, die Fragmente voneinander zu trennen, in der Regel auch ein signifikanter Anteil an Oberflächeninformationen verloren geht (Abb. 1).

Computerassistierte Planungsverfahren z.B. für die automatische Planung von Frakturkorrekturen [1] oder etwa einer roboterassistierten Frakturreponierung [2] erfordern zum einen eine möglichst automatische Trennung der Knochenfragmente und zum anderen eine präzise Darstellung bzw. Segmentierung der Frakturflächen. Beides wird im klinischen Alltag durch den Weichteilmantel erschwert, der die Knochenfragmente in Kontakt drückt und dadurch eine vollautomatische Segmentierung beeinträchtigt. Wünschenswert ist ein Segmentierungsansatz, in den unterschiedliche Informationsquellen integriert werden können. Ein Framework für die integrative Berücksichtigung von z.B. Grauwerten, Kanten/Gradienten, Abständen zu umgebenen Strukturen (Distanzkarten) und auch manuelle Benutzervorgaben ist daher ein Ziel unserer Arbeiten. Im Rahmen dieses Beitrags soll untersucht werden, inwieweit sich Graph-Cut-Ansätze eignen, diese Vorgaben zu erfüllen. Durch die Graphenstruktur ist es möglich, Segmentierungsvorgaben als Kantengewichte bereitzustellen. Diese Vorgaben und Parameter können aus verschiedenen Quellen stammen und werden durch die Graphenstruktur im Sinne eines einheitlichen Frameworks integriert.

Das Graph-Cut-Verfahren ist im Allgemeinen eine Methode zur Bestimmung des Minimums einer gegebenen Energiefunktion. Diese Funktion wird in Form eines gerichteten Graphen repräsentiert. Nach dem Max-Flow/Min-Cut-Prinzip kann aus dem maximalen Fluss durch einen Graphen von einer Quelle zur Senke der minimale Schnitt, der den Graphen in zwei Teilgraphen separiert, berechnet werden. Der maximale Fluss wiederum hängt von den Kantengewichten ab. Algorithmen für die effiziente Lösung des Max-Flow/Min-Cut-Problems wurden bereits Mitte der 1950er Jahre entwickelt [3]. Die erste Verwendung des Graph-Cut im Computervision-Bereich erfolgte 1989 [4]. Heute werden solche Graph-Cuts-Verfahren unter anderem für Segmentierungsaufgaben verwendet [5], wobei es sich dabei aber typischerweise um unterscheidbare Bildregionen handelt.

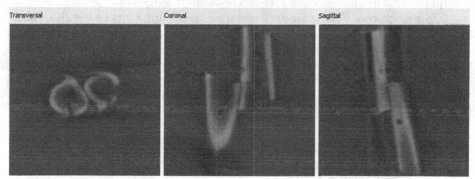

(a) CT Schnitte eines gebrochenen Femurs mit seitlichem Kontakt.

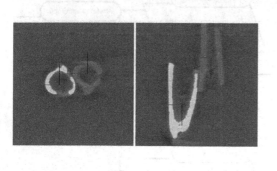
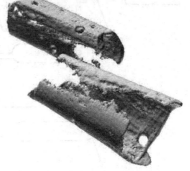

(b) Ergebnis einer schwellwertbasierten Segmentierung: Es sind deutliche Lücken in der segmentierten Knochenoberfläche zu sehen.

Abb. 1. Problematik der Segmentierung mehrerer Knochenfragmente bei typischen Kontaktsituationen zwischen den Fragmenten.

2   Material und Methoden

Der Ablauf des vorgestellten Segmentierungsprozesses ist in Abb. 2 dargestellt. Ausgangsbasis ist ein DICOM-Datensatz der zu segmentierenden Struktur. Dabei kann es sich um einen CT-Datensatz oder z.B. auch um einen mittels intraoperativen 3D-Röntgenscan erstellten Datensatz handeln. In einem ersten Verfahrensschritt „Klassifizierung" werden Hintergrundvoxel von den Voxeln der Knochenfragmente segmentiert. Dies erfolgt mittels Schwellwertverfahren, wobei der Schwellwert entweder manuell vorgegeben werden muss oder z.B. mittels des Verfahrens von Otsu automatisch bestimmt werden kann. Dem nachgeschaltet wird eine „Etikettierung" durchgeführt, um zusammenhängende Regionen zu identifizieren. Im dritten Verfahrensschritt „Artefakte entfernen" werden Regionen entfernt, die nicht zu den Knochenfragmenten gehören. Hierzu müssen zunächst die für den Graph-Cut erforderlichen Seedpunkte bzw. Seedbereiche in den einzelnen Fragmente manuell vorgegeben werden. Anschließend werden automatisch alle Regionen entfernt, die nicht mit einem Seedbereich verbunden sind. Aus den verbleibenden Regionen wird im Schritt „Graph generieren" die Graphenstruktur anhand einer 6-er-Nachbarschaft aufgebaut.

Ein wesentlicher Faktor für die Ergebnisse des Graph-Cuts ist die „Kantengewichtung", nach der sich der Fluss durch den Graphen berechnet. Wir verwenden dafür im Wesentlichen den Hounsfieldwert, da sich gezeigt hat, dass dieser auch bei Kontaktsituationen zwischen den Fragmenten leicht abfällt und daher ein guter Indikator für den möglichen Separierungsbereich darstellt. Zusätzlich wird dieser Hounsfieldwert mit einem Gewichtungsfaktor multipliziert, durch den Be-

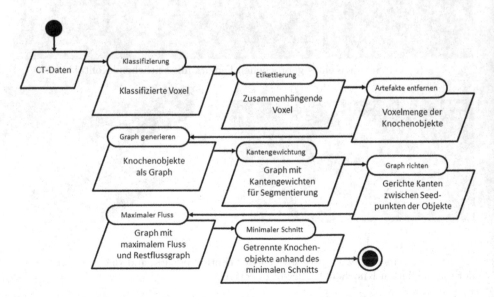

Abb. 2. Der komplette Segmentierungsprozess ausgehend von CT-Daten mit dem Resultat separierter Knochenobjekte.

nutzervorgaben für die vorgesehenen Schnittregionen berücksichtigt werden können.

Nachdem die Initialisierung des Graphen abgeschlossen ist, muss dieser vom Seedbereich eines Fragments zum Seedbereich eines zweiten Fragments im Prozessschritt „Graph richten" gerichtet werden, um die Pfadsuche im darauf folgende Graph-Cut-Verfahren zu ermöglichen. Nach dem Max-Flow/Min-Cut-Prinzip unter Verwendung einer eigenen Implementierung des Algorithmus von Ford and Fulkerson [3] wird zunächst ein Maximaler Fluss im Graphen berechnet anhand dessen schließlich ein Minimaler Schnitt durchgeführt werden kann. Dieser minimale Schnitt trennt die Region des einen Seedbereichs in optimaler Weise von der Region des zweiten Seedbereiches. Die Trennung erfolgt subpixelgenau anhand der Hounsfieldwerte.

Zu Testzwecken standen vier DICOM-Datensätze von gebrochenen menschlichen Femora ohne umgebenes Weichteilgewebe, aufgenommen mit dem Siemens Siremobil IsoC 3D, zur Verfügung. mit diesen Datensätzen wurden vier typische Kontaktsituationen nachgestellt, die bei Frakturen langer Röhrenknochen auftreten (Abb. 3): Kontakt zweier Fragmente direkt im Frakturbereich, seitlich flächiger Kontakt zweier Fragmente, Punktkontakt zweier Fragmente und der Kontakt mehrerer kleinerer Fragmente im Frakturbereich.

3 Ergebnisse

Die Segmentierungsergebnisse für die vier Testdatensätze sind in Abb. 4 dargestellt. Es war für alle Kontaktsituationen möglich, die einzelnen Knochenfragmente an den korrekten Grenzflächen zu separieren. Eine Übersicht über die Ergebnisse und die Berechnungszeiten können Tab. 1 entnommen werden. Die in der Tab. 1 aufgelisteten Ausführungszeiten wurden mit einem handelsüblichen PC mit 4 GB Arbeitsspeicher und einem Intel Core i5-2430M Prozessor mit 2,40 GHz erreicht. Die DICOM-Datensätze hatten eine Auflösung von

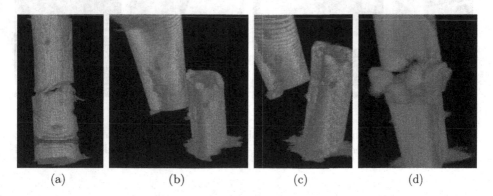

(a)   (b)   (c)   (d)

Abb. 3. DICOM-Datensätze typischer Kontaktsituationen: Kontakt im Frakturbereich (a), Seitlicher, flächiger Kontakt (b), Punktkontakt (c) und Mehrfragmentkontakt (d).

358   Westphal, Mikolas & Wahl

Tabelle 1. Ergebnisse im Detail für die einzelnen Testdatensätze: Kontakt im Frakturbereich (a), Seitlicher, flächiger Kontakt (b), Punktkontakt (c) und Mehrfragmentkontakt (d).

	(a)	(b)	(c)	(d)
Schwellwertberechnung (Otsu)	1684 ms	1685 ms	1700 ms	1732 ms
Klassifizierung (Schwellwert)	1326 ms	1357 ms	1523 ms	1232 ms
Etikettierung	421 ms	453 ms	765 ms	296 ms
Graphenerstellung	343 ms	358 ms	474 ms	312 ms
Graphengewichtung	343 ms	458 ms	546 ms	281 ms
Graph-Cut	25210 ms	23447 ms	4660 ms	36785 ms
Gesamtlaufzeit	**30342 ms**	**28891 ms**	**11454 ms**	**41777 ms**
Anzahl Seedpunkte	2	2	2	6
Anzahl Voxel nach Etikettierung	520368	603816	763678	419913
Anzahl Kanten im Graphen	1469113	1699831	2165825	1196066
Anzahl Schnittkanten	845	620	76	846
Speicherbedarf	∼66,6 MB	∼77,2 MB	∼97,7 MB	∼53,7 MB

255x255x255 Voxeln. Wie der Tab. 1 zu entnehmen ist, konnten drei der vier Datensätze im Schnitt in etwa 30 s segmentiert werden. Lediglich der Punktkontakt konnte deutlich schneller in etwa fünf Sekunden segmentiert werden. Die zur Speicherung und Bearbeitung des Graphen erforderlichen Arbeitsspeichergröße lag bei unter 100 MB.

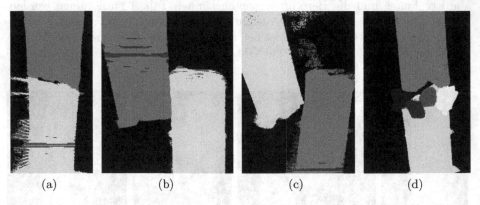

(a)   (b)   (c)   (d)

Abb. 4. Segmentierungsergebnisse für typische Kontaktsituationen mittels Graph-Cut: Kontakt im Frakturbereich (a), Seitlicher, flächiger Kontakt (b), Punktkontakt (c) und Mehrfragmentkontakt (d).

4 Diskussion

Insgesamt sind mit dem vorgestellten Segmentierung-/Separierungsverfahren basierend auf Graph-Cuts gute Ergebnisse zu erzielen. Die Ausführungszeiten von deutlich unter einer Minute für die verwendeten Datensätze sind für einen routinemäßigen Einsatz akzeptabel. Hinzu gerechnet werden muss für einen realen Einsatz noch die manuelle Vorgabe der Seedpunkte sowie unter Umständen eine grobe Platzierung der Schnittregion. Diese manuellen Arbeiten können in der Regel innerhalb von ein bis zwei Minuten erfolgen, sodass inklusive einer Zeit für die Begutachtung des Datensatzes mit einer Bearbeitungszeit von etwa fünf Minuten zu rechnen ist. Dies scheint akzeptabel für eine klinische Anwendung des Verfahrens.

Über die vorgestellte Anwendung auf Femurfrakturen hinaus, sind die Ansätze auch auf andere Frakturformen wie etwa intraartikulärer Frakturen oder Frakturen im MKG Bereich übertragbar. Auch die Segmentierung/Separierung anatomisch unveränderter Strukturen, wie z.B. aneinander anliegende Knochen, kann mit solchen Ansätzen unterstützt werden. Die gute Integrierbarkeit unterschiedlicher Datenquellen, insbesondere auch von manuellen Segmentierungsvorgaben, in ein einheitliches Framework ist ein wesentlicher Vorteil der gewählten Methode. So ist es ohne weiteres möglich, weitere Gewichtungsmaße, wie z.B. Distanzkarten zu umgebenen Strukturen, Oberflächenmerkmale oder Modellinformationen, zu integrieren.

Obwohl es sich hierbei um eine erste Studie mit einer begrenzten Testdatenmenge handelt, sind die ersten Ergebnisse bereits vielversprechend, sodass sich eine weitere Betrachtung der Ansätze lohnt. In zukünftigen Arbeiten müssen weitere Testfälle auch mit realen Patientendaten erprobt und analysiert werden, die Artefaktreduktion muss weiter verbessert werden (Abb. 4) und der vorgestellte Ansatz muss mit alternativen Verfahren verglichen werden.

Die vorgestellte Arbeit entstand im Rahmen des DFG Projekts „Roboterassistierte Reponierung von Frakturen der Röhrenknochen".

Literaturverzeichnis

1. Winkelbach S, Westphal R, Gösling T. Pose Estimation of Cylindrical Fragments for Semi-automatic Bone Fracture Reduction. Lect Notes Comput Sci. 2003;2781:566–73.
2. Westphal R, Winkelbach S, Wahl F, et al. Robot-assisted long bone fracture reduction. Int J Rob Res. 2009;28(10):1259–78.
3. Ford LR, Fulkerson DR. Maximal flow through a network. Canad J Math. 1956;8:399–404.
4. Greig DM, Porteous BT, Seheult AH. Exact maximum a posteriori estimation for binary images. J R Stat Soc Series B Stat Methodol. 1989;51:271–9.
5. Boykov YY, Jolly MP. Interactive graph cuts for optimal boundary amp; region segmentation of objects in N-D images. Proc IEEE ICCV. 2001;1:105–12.

Kabelloses elektromagnetisches Tracking in der Medizin
Standardisierte Genauigkeitsuntersuchung des Calypso-Systems

A. M. Franz[1], D. Schmitt[2], A. Seitel[1], M. Chatrasingh[3], G. Echner[2],
H.-P. Meinzer[1], S. Nill[4], W. Birkfellner[3], L. Maier-Hein[1]

[1]Juniorgruppe Computer-assistierte Interventionen, DKFZ Heidelberg
[2]Abteilung Medizinische Physik in der Strahlentherapie, DKFZ Heidelberg
[3]Zentrum für medizinische Physik und biomedizinische Technik,
Medizinische Universität Wien
[4]Joint Department of Physics, The Institute of Cancer Research and The Royal
Marsden NHS Foundation Trust, Downs Road, Sutton, Surrey, SM2 5PT, UK
a.franz@dkfz.de

Kurzfassung. Elektromagnetisches (EM) Tracking ist der Oberbegriff
für verschiedene Trackingtechnologien, die EM Felder nutzen um Objekte im Raum zu lokalisieren. Verbreitet sind die Techniken Magnetische
Ortung (MO) und Transponderlokalisierung (TL). Während MO schon
in vielen Studien untersucht wurde gibt es für TL noch wenige Veröffentlichungen, obwohl TL ohne Kabelverbindung zum getrackten Objekt
auskommt. In dieser Studie untersuchen wir erstmalig die Genauigkeit
und Präzision des TL Systems Calypso nach einem standardisierten Protokoll und vergleichen es mit dem etablierten MO System NDI Aurora®.
Die Ergebnisse zeigen eine hohe Genauigkeit und Präzision von unter
1 mm für beide Systeme. TL sollte für künftige Entwicklungen im Bereich Computer-assistierter Interventionen als Alternative in Betracht
gezogen werden.

1 Einleitung

Computer-assistierte Interventionen (CAI) gewinnen zunehmend an Bedeutung
für die Medizin [1]. Dabei werden üblicherweise medizinische Bilddaten und Po-
sitionsdaten von Instrumenten und Patient in Relation gesetzt um dem Arzt
während der Intervention eine bestmögliche Hilfestellung zu geben. Die Positi-
onsdaten werden meist durch so genannte Trackingsysteme gewonnen. Tracking
ist daher eine Schlüsseltechnologie für CAI [1].

Optisches Tracking ist die verbreitetste Technik, benötigt jedoch eine freie
Sichtlinie. Ist die Sicht zum Instrument versperrt, wie z.B. bei minimal-invasiven
Eingriffen, kommen Technologien die unter dem Oberbegriff Elektromagnetisches (EM) Tracking zusammengefasst werden zum Einsatz [1]. Bisherige Arbeiten zu EM Tracking hatten zumeist das Prinzip der Magnetischen Ortung (MO)

im Fokus, wobei eine Kabelverbindung zum getrackten Sensor benötigt wird. Daneben existiert jedoch die Technik der Transponderlokalisierung (TL), die bisher nur selten und nie standardisiert untersucht wurde. In dieser Studie wenden wir daher erstmalig ein standardisiertes Protokoll an um die Genauigkeit und Präzision des TL Systems Calypso GPS for the Body® zu untersuchen und vergleichen es mit dem etablierten MO System NDI Aurora®.

Im ersten Teil dieser Arbeit gehen wir zunächst auf die grundlegende Funktionsweisen der EM Trackingtechnologien ein, da diese in bisherigen Veröffentlichungen [2, 3, 4] nie übergreifend betrachtet wurde. Im zweiten Teil folgen die Beschreibung der standardisierten Genauigkeitsuntersuchung des Calypso-Systems sowie die Präsentation der Ergebnisse und eine abschließenden Diskussion.

2   Funktionsweise von EM Tracking

EM Tracking, teilweise auch als magnetisches Tracking bezeichnet, nutzt die Eigenschaften von Magnetfeldern um spezielle Objekte, z.B. Magnetfeldsensoren, im Raum zu lokalisieren. Verbreitet sind die Technologien MO (Abschnitt 2.1) und TL (Abschnitt 2.2) [1]. Weitere Techniken, wie zum Beispiel die Lokalisierung von Permanentmagneten durch spezielle Sensoren [2], spielen für die Praxis eine untergeordnete Rolle, da keine kommerziellen Systeme verfügbar sind.

2.1   Magnetische Ortung (MO)

Bei dieser Trackingtechnologie werden EM Felder mit bekannter Geometrie aufgebaut und genutzt um die Position von Magnetfeldsensoren im Raum zu bestimmen, wie in Abb. 1a schematisch dargestellt. Um die Magnetfelder zu erzeugen kommen Spulen zum Einsatz. Da die Trackingalgorithmen üblicherweise mehrere unterschiedliche Felder benötigen, werden zumeist mehrere Spulen in einer festen geometrischen Anordnung kombiniert [3]. Zusammen genommen wird diese Komponente als Feldgenerator (FG) bezeichnet.

Mit der verfügbaren Sensortechnologie kann das EM Feld nicht direkt gemessen werden. Magnetfeldsensoren messen vielmehr den Magnetischen Fluss Φ, also den Teil eines Magnetfeldes der durch einen spezifischen Punkt fließt. Fluxmeter verwenden eine Messspule um Φ als Funktion der Zeit zu bestimmen, wozu magnetische Wechselfelder benötigt werden. Fluxgate-Sensoren nutzen hingegen zwei gegensinnig angeordnete Spulen zur vektoriellen Bestimmung des Magnetfeldes und benötigen statische oder mit einer sehr geringen Frequenz alternierende Magnetfelder. Andere Sensortypen, wie zum Beispiel supraleitende Quanteninterferenzeinheiten (SQUIDs) oder Hall-Sensoren kommen in derzeitigen MO Trackingsystemen nicht vor. Je nach Sensortyp kommen quasi-statische (DC) oder wechselnde (AC) EM Felder zum Einsatz [1]. Auch wenn theoretisch einige Unterschiede zwischen diesen beiden Techniken der MO bestehen, haben Studien gezeigt, dass das Verhalten bzgl. Robustheit und Genauigkeit in der Praxis sehr ähnlich ist [5, 6]. Um eine Lokalisierung durchzuführen, muss der Sensor üblicherweise durch ein Kabel mit dem Trackingsystem verbunden werden, wobei miniaturisierte Sensoren mit Durchmessern von weniger als 1 mm verfügbar sind. Dann kann durch die Messung von Signalabschwächung oder -laufzeit[4] der Abstand zwischen Feldquelle und Sensor bestimmt werden. Sequentielle Messungen mit mehreren Quellen in bekannter geometrischer Anordnung ermöglichen die Berechnung der Position des Sensors durch Triangulation [7].

MO Trackingsysteme sind von verschiedenen Herstellern erhältlich. Die verfügbaren Modelle unterscheiden sich durch die Größe des Bereichs, in dem Sensoren getrackt werden können (Trackingvolumen), die Aktualisierungsraten und die Anzahl der trackbaren Sensoren. Typisch sind dabei Trackingvolumina bis zu ca. $1\,m^3$ Größe, Aktualisierungsraten von ca. 50 bis 250 Hz, und weniger als 10 trackbare Sensoren. In dieser Studie wurde das AC System NDI Aurora® (Northern Digital Inc., Waterloo, Canada) als Vergleichssystem genutzt.

2.2   Transponderlokalisierung (TL)

Bei dieser Art von EM Tracking werden Transponder durch ein EM Feld mit Energie versorgt und senden ein Lokalisierungssignal aus, wie in Abb. 1b dargestellt. Das Lokalisierungssignal wird von einem Sensorarray gemessen. Durch Signalintensität, -verzögerung, oder -phasenverschiebung kann die Entfernung des Transponders zu den Sensoren bestimmt werden. Aufgrund der bekannten Geometrie des Sensorarrays kann dann die Position im Raum berechnet werden [8]. Als Transponder, die mit Durchmessern von unter 1 mm verfügbar sind, kommen beispielsweise kleine Schwingkreise zum Einsatz, die ein Signal emittieren, wenn sie auf ihrer Resonanzfrequenz durch ein EM Feld angeregt werden. Der Vorteil von TL liegt darin, dass keine Kabelverbindung zum Transponder benötigt wird.

Das System Calypso GPS for the Body® (Varian Medical Systems Inc., Palo Alto, CA, USA) ist das einzige am Markt erhältliche System dieser Art, wobei das EM Trackingsystem in ein medizinisches Gesamtprodukt zur Strahlentherapie integriert ist, das nicht ohne Weiteres als stand-alone System verwendet werden

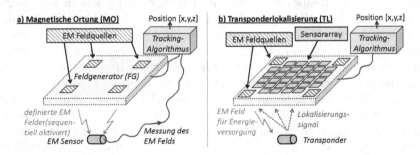

Abb. 1. Veranschaulichung des Funktionsprinzips der beiden verbreiteten EM Trackingtechnologien a) Magnetische Ortung und b) Transponderlokalisierung.

kann. Es ermöglicht die sequentielle Lokalisierung von drei analogen Transpondern, auch bezeichnet als Beacons, mit Resonanzfrequenzen von 300, 400 und 500 kHz und einer Updaterate von 10 Hz—d.h. ca. 3.3 Hz pro Beacon—in einem Trackingvolumen von 14 cm × 14 cm × 27 cm [8].

3 Standardisierte Untersuchung des TL Systems Calypso

3.1 Methoden

Um das TL System Calypso GPS for the Body® hinsichtlich seiner Präzision und Genauigkeit zu untersuchen wurde auf ein standardisiertes Protokoll von Hummel et al.[6] zurückgegriffen. Der Messaufbau und das Hummel-Phantom sind in Abb. 2 dargestellt. Für kleinere Trackingvolumina—wie in dieser Studie—kann das Protokoll, gemäß einem Vorschlag aus einer früheren Studie [9], auf einen kleineren Bereich angewandt werden. Dies führt im Fall des Calypso-Systems zu 3×3 Positionen, die auf 3 Ebenen (+5cm/0cm/-5cm) vermessen werden. Pro Position werden 150 Messwerte aufgezeichnet. Pro Ebene wird für die Genauigkeit der Fehler von $3(Spalten) \times 2 + 2(Reihen) \times 3 = 12$ Abständen à 5 cm und für die Präzision der mittlere quadratischer Fehler (engl. RMSE) an 9 Positionen ausgewertet [9]. Zum Vergleich wurde auf Daten des MO Systems NDI Aurora® mit einem 5 DoF Sensor (Aurora® 5D FlexCord 2.1×1200) und dem Compact FG (Typ 7-10) aus einer früheren Studie[9] zurückgegriffen, die für diese Arbeit auf den gleichen 9 Positionen ausgewertet wurden.

Das Sensorarray des Calypso-Systems wurde in einer festen Position belassen und die Beacons nur relativ zu diesem bewegt. Damit wurde sichergestellt, dass nur das EM Tracking—das Calypso-System enthält daneben noch ein optische Trackingkomponente[8]—untersucht wird. Um die Beacons mit dem Hummel-Phantom zu verwenden, wurde eine spezielle Beacon-Halterung angefertigt. Da für das Calypso-System ein festes Setup für die Bestrahlung vorgegeben ist, müssen immer alle drei Beacons getrackt werden, damit das System fehlerfrei läuft. Daher enthielt die Beacon-Halterung drei Beacons, zur Auswertung wurde aber nur auf die Trackingdaten eines Beacons zurückgegriffen um vergleichbare Werte für jeweils einen Beacon/Sensor zu erhalten. Bei allen Messungen wurde durch ein zusätzliches optisches Trackingsystem sichergestellt, dass sich weder Phantom noch Trackingsystem bewegen. Des Weiteren wurde bei den Messungen auf eine störquellenfreie Umgebung geachtet.

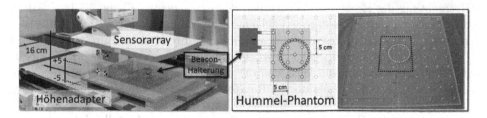

Abb. 2. Messaufbau (links) und Hummel-Phantom (rechts)[6].

Tabelle 1. Ergebnisse der Messungen mit dem standardisierten Hummel-Protokoll[6]. Für die Genauigkeit wurde pro Ebene über 12 Fehler von Abstandsmessungen à 5 cm gemittelt, für die Präzision über den RMSE an 9 Positionen.

Jeweils $\mu \pm \sigma$ [mm]	Ebene	NDI Aurora®	Calypso GPS for the Body®
Genauigkeit	oben	0.60 ± 0.59	0.07 ± 0.07
	Mitte	0.16 ± 0.12	0.07 ± 0.04
	unten	0.48 ± 0.48	0.08 ± 0.06
	gesamt	0.41 ± 0.47	0.07 ± 0.06
Präszision	oben	0.02 ± 0.01	0.22 ± 0.02
	Mitte	0.05 ± 0.03	0.14 ± 0.02
	unten	0.07 ± 0.02	0.57 ± 0.05
	gesamt	0.05 ± 0.03	0.31 ± 0.19

3.2 Ergebnisse

Die Ergebnisse der Messungen mit dem Hummel-Protokoll[9] sind in Tab. 1 dargestellt. Im Mittel zeigt das Aurora®-System mit 0.41 mm einen ca. 6-mal höheren Fehler als das Calypso-System mit 0.07 mm. Bezüglich der Präzision ist der mittlere Fehler des Aurora®-Systems mit 0.05 mm hingegen ca. 6-mal niedriger als der des Calypso-Systems mit 0.31 mm. Beide Systeme zeigen eine Abnahme der Genauigkeit und Präzision bei hohem Abstand (unten) zum FG/Sensor-Array.

4 Diskussion

EM Tracking wird schon seit einiger Zeit als Möglichkeit zur Lokalisation von Instrumenten und Patient bei CAI diskutiert, wenn keine freie Sichtlinie zur Verfügung steht. Der Begriff EM Tracking kann hierbei als Überbegriff verschiedene Trackingtechnologien gesehen werden [2]. In dieser Arbeit wurde das TL System Calypso, das ein kabelloses EM Tracking ermöglicht, erstmals nach einem standardisierten Protokoll untersucht und mit dem etablierten MO System NDI Aurora® verglichen. Die Ergebnisse zeigen für beide Systeme eine Genauigkeit und Präzision von unter 1 mm, wobei das Calypso-System die bessere Genauigkeit und das Aurora®-System die bessere Präzision aufweist. Bei genauerer Betrachtung der Ergebnisse hinsichtlich der untersuchten Ebenen fällt auf, dass die Werte nah am Sensorarray/Feldgenerator (oben) teilweise etwas schlechter sind als in der Mitte des Trackingvolumens, während sie bei großem Abstand (unten) wie zu erwarten wieder deutlich schlechter werden (Tab. 1). Eine mögliche Erklärung könnte sein, dass sich der Beacon/Sensor in unmittelbarer Nähe zum Sensorarray/Feldgenerator im Randbereich des Trackingvolumens befindet und einzelne Messwerte daher ungültig oder ungenau sind.

Bezüglich der Robustheit gegenüber Störquellen wie Metall zeigten die besser untersuchten MO Systeme bisher deutliche Schwächen [9, 5, 6]. Auch für das

Calypso-System wurde in einer nicht-standardisierten Studie bereits von derartigen Problemen berichtet. Künftig sollte untersucht werden, wie beide Technologien im Vergleich auf Metalle reagieren und ob ein Einsatz von TL zum Tracking von metallischen medizinischen Instrumenten überhaupt möglich ist.

Hinsichtlich der Größe des Trackingvolumens wurde für diese Studie eine Konfiguration des Aurora®-Systems gewählt, die dem Calypso-System nahe kommt. Allerdings ist der verwendete Compact FG deutlich kleiner und mobiler als das Sensorarray des Calypso-Systems, was als Vorteil des Aurora®-Systems gewertet werden kann. In diesem Zusammenhang ist ebenfalls zu erwähnen, dass das Calypso-System pro Beacon ausschließlich die 3D-Position, das Aurora®-System pro Sensor aber sowohl die 3D-Position als auch – je nach Sensortyp – zwei oder drei Freiheitsgrade der Orientierung misst.

Bei dem Calypso-System handelt es sich um ein Gesamtsystem für die Radiotherapie, TL ist davon nur eine Teilkomponente. Da es sich dabei um das einzige am Markt erhältliche TL System handelt, war diese Technologie daher bisher für viele CAI Anwendungen nicht verfügbar. Die guten Ergebnisse im Vergleich zu einem etablierten MO System sowie der Vorteil eines kabellosen Trackings legen jedoch eine Verwendung auch für andere Bereiche von CAI nahe.

Danksagung. Dieses Projekt wurde im Rahmen des DFG-geförderten Graduiertenkollegs 1126: Intelligente Chirurgie durchgeführt und durch das Intramurale Förderprogramm des DKFZ Radio-frequency identification (RFID) for wireless tracking of medical devices unterstützt.

Literaturverzeichnis

1. Peters T, Cleary K, editors. Image-Guided Interventions: Technology and Applications. Springer, Berlin; 2008.
2. Placidi G, Franchi D, Maurizi A, et al. Review on patents about magnetic localisation systems for in-vivo catheterizations. Recent Pat Biomed Eng. 2009;2:58–64.
3. Raab FH, Blood EB, Steiner TO, et al. Magnetic position and orientation tracking system. IEEE Trans Aerosp Electron Syst. 1979;AES-15(5):709–18.
4. Kuipers JB. SPASYN: an electromagnetic relative position and orientation tracking system. IEEE Trans Instrum Meas. 1980;29(4):462–6.
5. Yaniv Z, Wilson E, Lindisch D, et al. Electromagnetic tracking in the clinical environment. Med Phys. 2009;36:876–92.
6. Hummel JB, Bax MR, Figl ML, et al. Design and application of an assessment protocol for electromagnetic tracking systems. Med Phys. 2005;32(7):2371–9.
7. Plotkin A, Paperno E. 3D magnetic tracking of a single subminiature coil with a large 2D array of uniaxial transmitters. IEEE Trans Magn. 2003;39(5):3295–7.
8. Mate TP, Krag D, Wright JN, et al. A new system to perform continuous target tracking for radiation and surgery using non-ionizing alternating current electromagnetics. Proc CARS. 2004;1268(0):425–30.
9. Maier-Hein L, Franz AM, Birkfellner W, et al. Standardized assessment of new electromagnetic field generators in an interventional radiology setting. Med Phys. 2012;39(6):3424–34.

Semi-automatische Echtzeit-Konturierung

Ein vorlagenbasierter skalierungsinvarianter Ansatz

Jan Egger

Fachbereich Medizin, Universitätsklinikum Gießen und Marburg (UKGM)
egger@med.uni-marburg.de

Kurzfassung. In diesem Beitrag wird ein semi-automatischer und skalierungsinvarianter Segmentierungsalgorithmus zur Echtzeit-Konturierung vorgestellt. Dabei „verpackt" der Ansatz Parameter des Algorithmus in seiner Interaktivität für den Anwender. Dadurch wird vermieden, dass ein Anwender, um ein akzeptables Segmentierungsergebnis zu erzielen, ihm unbekannte Parametereinstellungen finden muss, die er im Gegensatz zum Entwickler des Algorithmus nicht ohne weiteres verstehen kann. Für die interaktive Segmentierung wurde ein spezieller graphbasierter Ansatz entwickelt, der sich insbesondere für eine interaktive Echtzeit-Konturierung eignet, da nur ein benutzerdefinierter Saatpunkt innerhalb der Zielstruktur benötigt wird und sich das Segmentierungsergebnis durch die besondere geometrische Konstruktion des Graphen sehr schnell berechnen lässt. Außerdem lassen sich die Grauwertinformationen, die für den Ansatz benötigt werden, automatisch aus dem Bereich um den benutzerdefinierten Saatpunkt herum extrahieren. Der Ansatz wurde über feste Saatpunkte in medizinischen 2D- und 3D-Daten evaluiert. Ein direkter Vergleich mit wesentlich zeitintensiveren manuellen Segmentierungen soll die praktische Anwendbarkeit des Ansatzes verdeutlichen.

1 Einleitung

Segmentierungsalgorithmen in der medizinischen Bildverarbeitung werden im Allgemeinen für eine ganz bestimmte Pathologie in einer ganz bestimmten Aufnahmemodalität entwickelt. Dennoch versagen (voll)automatische Segmentierungsalgorithmen bei neuen Daten immer wieder. Ganz wesentlich sind präzise Parametereinstellungen, um gute Ergebnisse zu liefern. Deshalb werden Konturierungen in der klinischen Routine immer noch rein manuell und Schicht für Schicht vorgenommen. Interaktive Segmentierungsansätze [1, 2], bei denen der Benutzer den Algorithmus mit intuitiven Informationen beim Segmentierungsprozess unterstützt, werden immer interessanter für die klinische Routine, insbesondere bei schwierigen Segmentierungsproblemen. In diesem Beitrag wird ein interaktiver graphbasierter Segmentierungsalgorithmus zur Konturierung von medizinischen Strukturen vorgestellt. Aufgrund der speziellen Graphkonstruktion benötigt der Ansatz nur einen Saatpunkt und eine Segmentierung kann sehr schnell berechnet werden. Dadurch eignet sich der Ansatz auch für eine interaktive Konturierung in Echtzeit.

2   Material und Methoden

Der Segmentierungsansatz funktioniert mit 2D- und 3D-Daten und beginnt mit der Graphkonstruktion, ausgehend von einem benutzerdefinierten Saatpunkt innerhalb der zu segmentierenden Struktur. Die Knoten $n \in V$ des Graphen $G(V, E)$ werden entlang von Strahlen abgetastet, die radial vom Saatpunkt ausgesandt werden. Zusätzlich ist $e \in E$ eine Menge von Kanten, die aus Kanten zwischen den Knoten bestehen und aus Kanten, die die Knoten mit einer Quelle s und einer Senke t verbinden, um die Berechnung eines minimalen s-t-Schnitts [3] zu ermöglichen. In Anlehnung an die Notation von Li et al. [4] verbindet eine Kante $< v_i, v_j > \in E$ zwei Knoten v_i, v_j. In der Kantenmenge gibt es zwei Arten von ∞-gewichteten Kanten: p-Kanten A_p und r-Kanten A_r. P ist die Anzahl der Knoten, die entlang eines Strahles $p = (0, \dots, P - 1)$ abgetastet wurden, und R ist die Anzahl der Strahlen, die radial ausgesandt wurden, mit $r = (0, \dots, R - 1)$. $V(x_n, y_n)$ ist als der Nachbar von $V(x, y)$ definiert (für weitergehende Details zur Graphkonstruktion wird an dieser Stelle auf [5, 6] verwiesen)

$$A_p = \{\langle V(x,y), V(x, y - 1)\rangle \mid y > 0\}$$
$$A_r = \{\langle V(x,y), V(x_n, \max(0, y - \Delta_r))\rangle\} \tag{1}$$

Die ∞-gewichteten Kanten für eine Oberfläche in 3D werden äquivalent zu den ∞-gewichteten Kanten für eine Kontur in 2D definiert

$$A_p = \{\langle V(x,y,z), V(x, y, z - 1)\rangle \mid z > 0\}$$
$$A_r = \{\langle V(x,y,z), V(x_n, y_n, \max(0, z - \Delta_r))\rangle\} \tag{2}$$

Ist der Graph konstruiert, wird der minimale s-t-Schnitt für den Graphen berechnet [3], der wiederum dem Segmentierungsergebnis entspricht. In Abb. 1 findet man verschiedene Beispiele für Vorlagen, mit denen unterschiedliche Pathologien in 2D und 3D segmentiert wurden. Bei allen Beispielen wurde der Graph von einem benutzerdefinierten Saatpunkt aus konstruiert, der innerhalb der Pathologie lag. Für die Segmentierung benötigt der Ansatz auch einen mittleren Grauwert der zu segmentierenden Struktur. Dieser mittlere Grauwert wird im Bereich des Saatpunktes automatisch bestimmt und jedes Mal neu berechnet, wenn der Benutzer ihn interaktiv auf dem Bild verschiebt. Das macht den Ansatz robuster gegen Segmentierungsfehler, wenn der Saatpunkt kurzfristig über Bereiche verschoben wird, die zwar innerhalb der zu segmentierenden Struktur liegen, aber nicht dem mittleren Grauwert der zu segmentierenden Struktur entsprechen, wie z.B. bei sehr hellen Kalzifikationen.

3   Ergebnisse

Der vorgestellte Ansatz wurde innerhalb der Plattform MeVisLab realisiert. Der spezielle Aufbau der Graphen ermöglichte eine Echtzeit-Konturierung auf einem Rechner mit Intel Core i5-750 CPU, 4x2.66 GHz, 8 GB RAM. Die Evaluierung erfolgte über feste Saatpunkte in medizinischen 2D- und 3D-Daten (Tab. 1). Abb. 2

gibt mehrere Screenshots aus einem Video wider, die die interaktive Echtzeit-Konturierung von Wirbelkörpern und Bandscheiben in einer sagittalen Schicht einer MRT-Aufnahme zeigen. Der Mittelpunkt des Graphen ist in Weiß dargestellt und kann vom Benutzer interaktiv auf dem Bild verschoben werden, die roten Punkte stellen das Ergebnis der Segmentierung dar. In Abb. 3 sieht man eine interaktive Prostata-Segmentierung mit einer Kreisvorlage in einer MRT-Aufnahme. Die oberen vier Bilder zeigen die resultierende Kontur (rot), wenn der benutzerdefinierte Saatpunkt näher an den Rand der Prostata verschoben wurde. Im oberen linken Bild zum Beispiel befindet sich der Saatpunkt näher am linken Rand der Prostata, daher tendiert das Segmentierungsergebnis auch zu einer Übersegmentierung im linken Bereich der Prostata. Allerdings ermög-

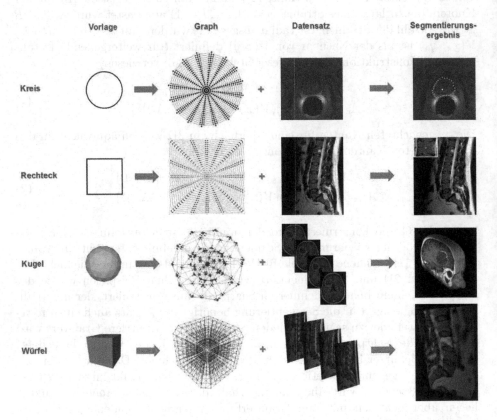

Abb. 1. Verschiedene Beispiele für Vorlagen, mit denen unterschiedliche Pathologien in 2D und 3D segmentiert wurden: Eine Kreisvorlage wurde dazu genutzt, einen Graphen aufzubauen und die Prostata zu segmentieren (erste Zeile), eine Rechteckvorlage wurde verwendet, um Wirbelkonturen in einzelnen 2D-Schichten zu bestimmen (zweite Zeile), eine Kugelvorlage diente dazu, Glioblastoma Multiforme (GBM) zu segmentieren (dritte Zeile), und für die Bestimmung ganzer Wirbelkörper in 3D kam eine Würfelvorlage zum Einsatz (untere Zeile). Bei allen Beispielen wurde der Graph vom benutzerdefinierten Saatpunkt innerhalb der Pathologie aus konstruiert.

Abb. 2. Mehrere Screenshots aus einem Video, die die interaktive Echtzeit-Konturierung von Wirbelkörpern und Bandscheiben in einer sagittalen Schicht einer Magnetresonanztomographie (MRT)-Aufnahme zeigen (von links nach rechts). Der Mittelpunkt des Graphen ist in Weiß dargestellt und kann vom Benutzer interaktiv auf dem Bild verschoben werden, die kleinen schwarzen Boxen zeigen die Ecken der Rechteckvorlage an, und die roten Punkte stellen das Ergebnis der Segmentierung da.

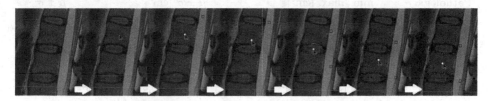

lichen das interaktive Verhalten und die Echtzeit-Rückmeldung des Ansatzes es dem Benutzer, schnell ein zufriedenstellendes Segmentierungsergebnis zu finden (linkes unteres Bild). Zum visuellen Vergleich des Segmentierungsergebnisses aus dem linken unteren Bild ist im rechten unteren Bild die Maske (blau) einer rein manuellen Segmentierung auf derselben 2D-Schicht dargestellt.

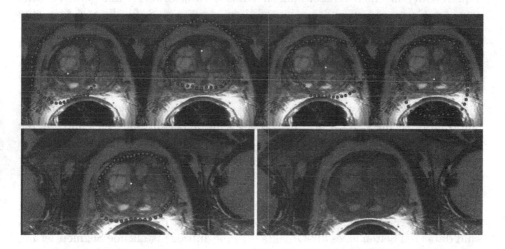

Abb. 3. Interaktive Prostata-Segmentierung mit einer Kreisvorlage in einer MRT-Aufnahme: Die oberen vier Bilder zeigen die resultierende Kontur (rot), wenn der benutzerdefinierte Saatpunkt näher an den Rand der Prostata verschoben wurde. Im oberen linken Bild z.B. befindet sich der Saatpunkt näher am linken Rand der Prostata, daher tendiert das Segmentierungsergebnis auch zu einer Übersegmentierung im linken Bereich der Prostata. Allerdings ermöglicht es die interaktive Echtzeit-Rückmeldung des Ansatzes dem Benutzer, schnell ein zufriedenstellendes Segmentierungsergebnis zu finden (linkes unteres Bild). Zum visuellen Vergleich des Segmentierungsergebnisses aus dem linken unteren Bild ist im rechten unteren Bild die Maske (blau) einer rein manuellen Segmentierung auf derselben 2D-Schicht dargestellt.

Tabelle 1. Ergebnisse: Mittelwert μ und Standardabweichung σ sind für manuell und automatisch segmentierte Volumina (cm^3) der Pathologien und für die Dice Similarity Koeffizienten (DSC) [7] zwischen den manuellen und automatischen Segmentierungen angegeben. Abkürzungen: Glioblastoma Multiforme (GBM), Hypophysenadenome (HA), Zerebrale Aneurysmen (ZA), Prostatadrüsen (PD) und Wirbelkörper (WK).

Pathologie	min./max. [cm^3]		$\mu \pm \sigma$ [cm^3]		$\mu \pm \sigma$
(Anzahl)	manuell	automatisch	manuell	automatisch	DSCs [%]
GBM (50)	0,47/119,28	0,46/102,98	23,66 ± 24,89	21,02 ± 22,90	80,37 ± 8,93
HA (10)	0,84/15,57	1,18/14,94	6,30 ± 4,07	6,22 ± 4,08	77,49 ± 4,52
ZA (3)	0,45/4,02	0,35/4,22	1,90 ± 1,88	2,02 ± 1,99	72,66 ± 10,71
PD (10)	13,67/66,16	13,29/67,56	31,32 ± 17,45	33,58 ± 18,88	78,94 ± 10,85
WK 2D (9)	0,25/0,51	0,24/0,49	0,42 ± 0,072	0,40 ± 0,073	90,97 ± 2,20
WK 3D (10)	15,42/33,83	16,64/28,78	24,97 ± 6,15	23,48 ± 5,12	81,33 ± 5,07

4 Diskussion

Der Fortschritt in diesem Beitrag besteht darin, dass Algorithmen (wie der Square-Cut) in einen echtzeitfähigen Ansatz transformiert und getestet wurden. Im Gegensatz zu anderen interaktiven Ansätzen [8, 9], die meistens eine aufwändige Initialisierung benötigen, wird durch diesen Ansatz eine interaktive Echtzeit-Segmentierung ermöglicht, da nur ein benutzerdefinierter Saatpunkt innerhalb des zu segmentierenden Objektes benötigt wird. Außerdem kann durch die spezielle geometrische Konstruktion des Graphen die Echtzeitfähigkeit (insbesondere in 3D) je nach Rechnerausstattung sichergestellt werden, z.B. durch eine geringere Strahlen- und Knotendichte. Darüber hinaus können Grauwertinformationen im Bereich des Saatpunktes automatisch analysiert und für die Segmentierung genutzt werden. Damit „verpackt" der Ansatz in seinem interaktiven Verhalten Parameter und verhindert dadurch, dass der Benutzer diese definieren muss. Auch wenn die Evaluation gezeigt hat, dass der Ansatz mit (festen) Saatpunkten gute Ergebnisse liefert, ist es (im Gegensatz zu einer interaktiven Segmentierung in 2D) recht schwierig, ein Objekt in 3D interaktiv zu segmentieren. Das liegt daran, dass der Saatpunkt im Raum verschoben wird und dabei die Seiten eines 3D-Objekts für eine zufriedenstellende Segmentierung überwacht werden müssen. Das Verfahren soll daher als nächstes zu einer Art iterativem Ansatz erweitert werden. Dabei segmentiert der Benutzer (interaktiv) zuerst mehrere Konturen in 2D. Anschließend wird ein 3D-Graph zur interaktiven Segmentierung aufgebaut, der allerdings in den drei vorher segmentierten 2D-Schichten bereits fixiert ist (Abb. 4). Diese 2D-Fixierungen schränken die Anzahl der möglichen s-t-Schnitte massiv ein [10] und unterstützen den Benutzer, auch in 3D einen geeigneten Saatpunkt interaktiv zu finden.

Danksagung. Ich danke den Neurochirurgen des UKGM in Marburg für ihr Mitwirken an der Studie, Robert Schwarzenberg für die Implementierung des Cube-Cut-Algorithmus, Fraunhofer MeVis in Bremen für die MeVisLab-Lizenz,

Abb. 4. Iterative Segmentierung: Zuerst werden mehrere Wirbelkonturen (obere Reihe, rot) mit einem interaktiven 2D-Ansatz wie aus Abb. 2 segmentiert. Danach wird ein 3D-Graph zur Segmentierung des Wirbelkörpers in 3D konstruiert, bei dem die drei schon segmentierten 2D-Konturen im 3D-Graphen fixiert sind. Diese Restriktionen des 3D-Graphen beeinflussen und unterstützen die Segmentierung der restlichen Konturen des Wirbelkörpers (grüne Konturen in der unteren Reihe). Die roten Konturen aus den Bildern der unteren Reihe korrespondieren mit den Konturen der Bilder der oberen Reihe. Rechts unten ist die voxelisierte Maske des Wirbelkörpers eingeblendet.

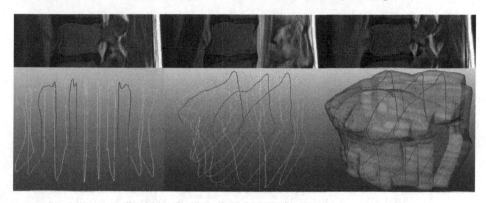

Edith Egger-Mertin für das Korrekturlesen und Fedorov et al. für die Prostata-datensätze: http://www.spl.harvard.edu/publications/item/view/2174

Literaturverzeichnis

1. Steger S, Sakas G. FIST: fast interactive segmentation of tumors. Abdom Imaging. 2011;7029:125–32.
2. Heckel F, Moltz JH, Tietjen J, et al. Sketch-based editing tools for tumor segmentation in 3D medical images. Comput Graph Forum. 2013.
3. Boykov Y, Kolmogorov V. An experimental comparison of min-cut/max-flow algorithms for energy minimization in vision. IEEE PAMI. 2004;26(9):1124–37.
4. Li K, Wu X, Chen DZ, et al. Optimal surface segmentation in volumetric images: a graphtheoretic approach. IEEE PAMI. 2006;28(1):119–34.
5. Egger J, Kapur T, Dukatz T, et al. Square-cut: a segmentation algorithm on the basis of a rectangle shape. PLoS One. 2012;7(2):e31064.
6. Egger J, Freisleben B, Nimsky C, et al. Template-cut: a pattern-based segmentation paradigm. Sci Rep. 2012;2(420).
7. Zou KH, Warfield SK, Bharatha A, et al. Statistical validation of image segmentation quality based on a spatial overlap index. Acad Radiol. 2004;2:178–89.
8. Boykov Y, Jolly MP. Interactive graph cuts for optimal boundary and region segmentation of objects in N-D images. Proc IEEE ICCV. 2001;1:105–22.
9. Vezhnevets V, Konouchine V. GrowCut-interactive multi-label N-D image segmentation. Proc Graphicon. 2005; p. 150–6.
10. Egger J, Bauer MHA, Kuhnt D, et al. A flexible semi-automatic approach for glioblastoma multiforme segmentation. Biosignal. 2010;60:1–4.

Volumen- und Oberflächenbestimmung vitaler Alveolar Makrophagen in vitro mit der Dunkelfeldmikroskopie

Dominic Swarat[1], Matrin Wiemann[2], Hans-Gerd Lipinski[1]

[1]Biomedical Imaging Group, Fachbereich Informatik, Fachhochschule Dortmund
[2]Institute for Lung Health (IBE R&D gGmbH), Münster
dominic.swarat@fh-dortmund.de

Kurzfassung. Das Volumen und die Oberfläche beweglicher Alveolarmakrophagen wurde mit Hilfe der Dunkelfeldmikroskopie unter in vitro-Bedingungen geschätzt. Dazu wurden aus 2D-Bildstapeln definierte Geometrieparameter selektiert und mit einem einfachen Geometriemodell abgeglichen. Die so bestimmten Oberflächen- und Volumenwerte zeigten nur geringfügige Unterschiede zu Daten einer Atomic-Force-Mikroskopie Untersuchung an einem Kontrollkollektiv sowie Daten aus der Literatur. Das Verfahren erscheint daher geeignet, um ungefärbte Makrophagen wiederholt dreidimensional abzubilden.

1 Einleitung

Alveolarmakrophagen sind als Teil der unspezifischen Immunabwehr unter anderem für die Erkennung und Phagozytose von Partikeln in der Lunge zuständig. Dabei verändern sie Zellvolumen und -oberfläche in typischer Weise. Die Aufnahmekapazität von Makrophagen für Partikel beeinflusst die Reinigungskapazität der Lunge („Clearance "), die zusammen mit anderen Expositionsgrößen Einfluss auf die Festlegung von Grenzwerten für die Partikelexposition besitzt [1].

Die Bestimmung des Zellvolumens ist nicht trivial. Für ein Zellkollektiv kann mit der so genannten Coulter Counter-Methode der Zelldurchmesser runder Zellen näherungsweise gemessen werden [2]. Die Beeinflussung von Größe und Oberfläche einzelner Zellen durch phagozytierte Partikel ist daher nur mit mikroskopischen Methoden messbar. Die Konfokale Laser Scanning Mikroskopie erscheint hier zunächst als Methode der Wahl, doch benötigt sie geeignete Fluoreszenzfarbstoffe, deren Auswirkung auf Zellfunktionen oft nicht gänzlich ausgeschlossen werden können. Dynamische Formveränderungen werden oft nur unzureichend erfasst, da das Signal-Rauschverhältniss bei wiederholten Messungen abnimmt, so dass kleine Details verloren gehen. Die Atomic Force Microscopy (AFM) zeichnet demgegenüber detailreiche Bilder adhärenter Zellen, arbeitet aber ebenfalls zu langsam, so dass nur einzelne fixierte Zustände beweglicher Zellen darstellbar werden.

In dieser Arbeit wird daher eine alternative Methode zur Volumenmessung vorgestellt, die auf der Auswertung von Bildstapeln beruht, die mittels Dunkelfeldmikroskopie gewonnen wurden. Diese Mikroskopietechnik wurden in den letzten Jahren durch verbesserte Beleuchtungssysteme weiterentwickelt und stellt sowohl Zellgrenzen als auch Partikel innerhalb und außerhalb der Zellen dar [3]. In Verbindung mit einer definierten Verschiebung der Beobachtungsebene können Bildstapel ganzer Zellen sehr schnell gewonnen werden, was die Beobachtung dynamischer Prozesse im Abstand weniger Sekunden erlauben könnte. Um die Leistungsfähigkeit des Verfahrens zu testen werden dazu die mittels Dunkelfeldmikroskopie gewonnenen Daten mit AFM Untersuchungen verglichen.

2   Material und Methoden

2.1   Zellen und Mikroskopieverfahren

Für die in vitro-Tests wurden Alveolar-Makrophagen (Zellinie: NR8383) aus der Lunge der Ratte verwendet. Diese wurden unter Zellkuluturbedingungen ($37°C$, $5\% CO_2$) auf Deckgläschen in F12-K Medium mit 15% fetalem Kälberserum kultiviert. Für die Dunkelfeldmikroskopie wurden die Deckgläschen in KRPG-Puffer überführt. Ausgewählte Zellen ($n = 27$) wurden mit einem CytoViva-Dunkelfeldsystem beleuchtet und bei 100-facher Vergrößerung mit einem Olympus BX40 Mikroskop mikroskopiert. Die Verschiebung der Fokusebene in z-Richtung erfolgte mit einem Piezo-Stepper in Verbindung mit einem analogen Steuergerät (30DC50,PiezoSystemJena). Digitale Bilder entstanden mit einer PCO Pixelfly VGA Kamera. Für die AFM Untersuchungen wurden Zellen mit 2,5% Glutaraldehyd in KRPG-Puffer fixiert. Lichtmikroskopisch ausgewählte Zellen wurden mit einem AFM (Veeco, Scanfeldgröße: $27 \times 27\,\mu m$, Auflösung: 128x128 px) in Flüssigkeit (KRPG-Puffer) gescannt und mit der Software Gwyddion in Bildstapelform räumlich rekonstruiert.

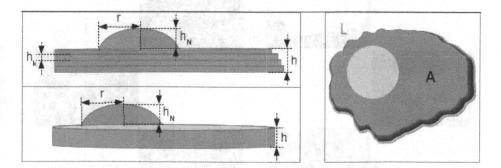

Abb. 1. Geometrisches Modell: Seitenansicht/geschichtet (oben links), Aufsicht (unten links), Seitenansicht/vereinfachtes Modell aus massiver planparalleler Platte (rechts).

2.2 Volumen- und Oberflächenbestimmung von Alveolarmakrophagen mit der Dunkelfeldmikroskopie

Die Abbildung 1 zeigt das verwendete geometrische Modell, das die flächige Ausdehnung des Zellrands sowie den kernhaltigen, näherungsweise halbkugeligen Zellkörper als geometrische Grundform aufweist. Im Bildteil (Abb. 1a) ist das Modell bestehend aus n äquidistanten Zellschichten gezeigt, der Bildteil (Abb. 1b) zeigt eine Aufsicht auf die oberste Schicht, mit der Lage des halbkugeligen Zellkörpers, im Bildteil (Abb. 1c) ist die basale Region der Zelle vereinfacht als gemittelte, planparallelen Platte gezeigt. Die analysierte Bildregion wurde auf jeweils eine Zelle begrenzt. Danach erfolgte die Einzelzellanalyse (jeweils 1600 × 1200 px Bildgröße; Programm: ImageJ). Für eine individuelle Kontrastanhebung sorgte eine automatische Grauwertspreizung, eine Rauschreduktion wurde mit Hilfe eines Gaußfilters erreicht ($\sigma = 1$). Bei der Bilderzeugung wurde die Dunkelfeld-Mikroskopebene mit Hilfe eines Piezo-z-Steppers zuerst auf den basalen Randbereichteil des Makrophagen fokussiert (Pseudopodium). Anschließend wurde der Fokus programmgesteuert zum apikalen Zellpol bewegt, um die Zellkörperhöhe im Bereich des Zellkerns h_N bestimmen zu können. Definierte, äquidistante Abstände der Fokusebenen wurden den Programmdaten der Piezosteuerung entnommen. Dabei wurden für n definierte, äquidistante Höhen (die untere Ebene, $n - 2$ Zwischenebenen und die Deckebene) die fokussierten Bildebenen ($50 \leq n \leq 70$) digitalisiert und gespeichert. Aus diesen Daten ließen sich für jeden analysierten Makrophagen auf der Grundlage eines einfachen geometrischen Modells sowohl das Zellvolumen als auch die Zelloberfläche schätzen. Neben der Höhenschätzung für den Zellkörper im Bereich des Nukleus und den

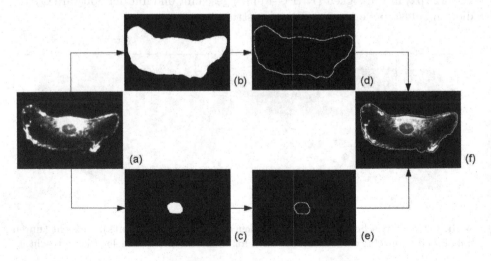

Abb. 2. Makrophage/Originalbild (a), Makrophagenfläche/binär (b), Zellkernbasisfläche/binär (c), Kontur des Makrophagenkörpers (d), Kontur des Zellkerns (e), Zusammenfassung der Konturen und Überlagerung mit dem Original (f).

Gesamtzellkörper können weitere Geometriefaktoren, wie Zellfläche und Kontur-
längen aus den 2D-Schichtbildern gewonnen werden (Abb. 2).

Für jede Höhe h_k wurde die korrespondierende Zellschicht als planparallele
Platte mit der Plattendicke $\Delta h_k = h_k - h_{k-1}$ angenommen. Ihre Fläche A_k ließ
sich mit Hilfe einer „Level Set Segmentation" aus den Bilddaten ermitteln, die das
Zellbild in ein Binärbild überführte, aus dem dann die Flächengröße bestimmt
werden konnte. Damit ergibt sich das Zellkörpervolumen als einfache Summe der
Produkte von Plattenhöhe Δh_k der zugehörigen Zwischenschichtplatte und deren
Fläche A_k. Ist die Dicke der Zwischenschichtplatten konstant ($\Delta h_k = \Delta h$ für alle
$k = 1, ..., n$) ergibt sich das Zellkörpervolumen V_B aus dem Produkt der mittleren
Fläche $\bar{A}$ der planparallelen Zwischenschichtplatten und der Gesamthöhe $h =
n \cdot \Delta h$ des Zellkörpers. Hinzugefügt werden muss jetzt nur noch das Volumen
des Zellkerns V_N, der nur zum Teil aus dem Zellkörper herausragt. Der Nukleus
kann durch ein Kugelsegment approximiert werden, dessen Volumen V_N mit Hilfe
der Zellkörperhöhe h_N und des Radius r des korrespondierenden Grundkreises
des Kerns aus den Bilddaten berechnet werden kann. Somit ergibt sich für das
Zellvolumen der Zusammenhang

$$V = V_B + V_N = \sum_{k=1}^{n} \Delta h \cdot A_k + V_N = h \cdot \bar{A} + \frac{\pi}{6} \cdot (3 \cdot r^2 + h_N^2) \cdot h_N \qquad (1)$$

Auf der Basis dieses geometrischen Modells lässt sich auch die Zelloberfläche
bestimmen. Dabei wird die Oberfläche durch insgesamt drei Teilflächen anhand
des Modells bestimmt: i) die Randfläche (sie ergibt sich aus dem Produkt der
mittleren Zellkörper-Konturlänge $\bar{L}$ und der Zellkörperhöhe h); ii) die zweifache
mittlere Zellkörperfläche abzüglich der Zellkernbasisfläche; iii) die Kugelsegment-
mantelfläche, also

$$A = \bar{L} \cdot h + 2 \cdot \bar{A} - \pi \cdot r^2 + \pi \cdot (r^2 + h_N^2) = \bar{L} \cdot h + 2 \cdot \bar{A} + \pi \cdot h_N^2 \qquad (2)$$

Um den Zellkernradius sowie die Zellkörperkonturlänge bestimmen zu können,
wurden aus den korrespondierenden Segmentbildern, welche den Zellkörper bzw.
den Zellkern zeigen, nach erfolgter Binärisierung die zugehörigen 1 px breiten
Konturen mit Hilfe eines Kantendetektors (Laplace) und der darauf folgenden Skeletierung erzeugt. Die Konturdaten liefern den Umfang des Zellkörpers
(„Konturlänge") L bzw. den Radius r des Zellkerns (Abb. 2). Die Höhe des Nukleus h_N lässt sich durch die Bestimmung der Grenzhöhe, an der die obere Spitze
des Zellkerns aus der Bildebene verschwindet, ermitteln.

3 Ergebnisse

Mit Hilfe der mit dem AFM und dem Dunkelfeldmikroskop erzeugten Bilddaten
wurden das Volumen V und die Oberfläche A der untersuchten Makrophagen
bestimmt. Die Abbildung 3 vergleicht typische 3D Volumendaten aus der AFM-
(Abb. 3a) und der Dunkelfeldmikroskopie (Abb. 3b). Die Visualisierung wurde
in beiden Fällen mit dem bekannten Marching-Cube-Verfahren durchgeführt.

Typische Volumen- und Oberflächenwerte betrugen 1050 μm^3 bzw. 1500 μm^2. Dabei zeigte sich, dass beide Methoden ähnliche Werte lieferten. Die relativen Differenzen zwischen den mit der AFM- bzw. der Dunkelfeldmikroskopie ermittelten Volumen- und Oberflächenwerten betrugen maximal 5%.

Interessanterweise lieferten für die Volumen- bzw. Oberflächenberechnung mit dem Dunkelfeldmikroskop bereits zwei Zwischenschichten sowie den beiden (oberen und unteren) Deckschichten hinreichend genaue Schätzungen, die dem aus allen Ebenen berechneten Werten zu mehr als 95% übereinstimmen. Daher konnten mit der Fläche aus vier gemittelten planparallelen Schichten und zwei Höhenbestimmungen Volumen- und Oberflächendaten der Makrophagen gewonnen werden, die denen der AFM-Messungen an einem Vergleiskollektiv entsprachen. Durch geeignete Anwendung der Bildverarbeitungsschritte konnten Volumen- und Oberflächenbestimmung eines vitalen Makrophagen innerhalb von 20 Sekunden durchgeführt werden. Hilfreich ist dabei, dass die Dunkelfeldmikroskopie in allen fokussierten Ebenen kontrastreiche Bilder liefert, die mit einfachen Bildverarbeitungsmethoden die erforderliche Flächen- und Höhenbestimmungen zulassen.

4 Diskussion

Die Volumen- und Oberflächenbestimmung (VOB) von Zellen wird üblicherweise mit Hilfe direkter 3D-Bildgebung (z.B. Laserscanning-Mikroskopie, LSM; Atomic-Force-Mikroskopie, AFM) durchgeführt. Allerdings haben diese Verfahren Nachteile. So können vitale Zellen im AFM nicht untersucht werden. Die LSM erfordert eine Anfärbung der Zellmembran, die während des gesamten Messzyklus ausreichend vorhanden sein muss („photobleeching"-Effekt). Zwar lassen

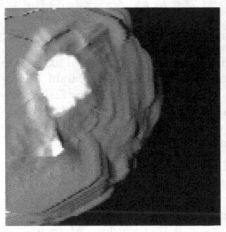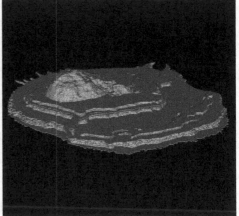

Abb. 3. 3D-Rekonstruktion und Visualisierung: AFM (links) und Dunkelfeldmikroskopie mit $n = 61$ (rechts).

sich auch VOB-Daten aus nur einem 2D-Bild durch Abgleich mit einem geeigneten geometrischen Zellmodell gewinnen [4], allerdings muss der Makrophage hier eine extrem flache Form annehmen, was nicht in allen in vitro Experimenten gegeben ist. Mit Hilfe der Dunkelfeldmikroskopie können Makrophagen oder andere Zellen dagegen mit sehr hohem Bildkontrast dargestellt werden. Durch die Höhenverschiebung des Präparates mit einem Piezo-z-Stepper lassen sich unterschiedliche Bildebenen problemlos fokussieren und als Bild in digitaler Form speichern.

Die gewonnenen Bilddaten lassen sich nahezu in Echtzeit so auswerten, dass durch den Abgleich mit einem einfachen geometrischen Zellmodell, welches die Zellmorphologie von in vitro-Makrophagen im wesentlichen widerspiegelt, sowohl die Zelloberfläche als auch das Zellvolumen reproduzierbar geschätzt werden kann. Da sich die VOB-Daten in sehr kurzer Zeit ermitteln lassen, sind Störeffekte, die durch Bewegungen der Makrophagen auftreten können, gering. Darüber hinaus werden auch dynamische Prozesse, die Volumen und Oberflächen verändern, darstellbar. Die im Rahmen der durchgeführten Experimente ermittelten Daten stimmten zudem mit solchen überein, die durch AFM-Parallelexperimente gewonnen wurden und auch in der Literatur [5] bekannt sind. Damit steht eine praktikable Methode zur VOB zur Verfügung, die im Rahmen von in vitro-Analysen vitaler Makrophagen in Kombination mit der Dunkelfeldmikroskopie erfolgreich eingesetzt werden kann.

Danksagung. Die Arbeit wurde mit Mitteln des Bundesministeriums für Bildung und Forschung (BMBF / FKZ 17PNT026) gefördert. Die Bilddaten zur AF-Mikroskopie stellte die Fa. Serend-IP GmbH, Münster zur Verfügung.

Literaturverzeichnis

1. Morrow PE. Contemporary issues in toxicology: dust overloading of the lungs: update and appraisal. Toxicol Appl Pharmacol. 1992;113(1):1–12.
2. Castranova V, Jones TA, Barger M, et al. Pulmonary responses of guinea pigs to consecutive exposures to cotton dust. Proc Cot Dust Res Conf. 1990;14:131–5.
3. Xiao L, Qiao Y, He Y, et al. Three dimensional orientational imaging of nanoparticles with darkfield microscopy. Anal Chem. 2010;82(12):5268–74.
4. Swarat D, Wiemann M, Lipinski HG. Volume and surface estimation of vital alveolar macrophages in vitro by 2D-Microscopy imaging. Biomed Tech. 2013;58(1):4289–90.
5. Krombach F, Münzing S, Allmeling AM, et al. Cell size of alveolar macrophages: an interspecies comparison. Environ Health Perspect. 1997;105(5):1261–3.

Interactive 3D Segmentation of Pleural Thickenings Simultaniously at Different Points of Time Using Graph Cut

Peter Faltin[1], Phan-Anh Nguyen[1], Kraisorn Chaisaowong[1,2], Thomas Kraus[3], Dorit Merhof[1]

[1]Institute of Imaging & Computer Vision, RWTH Aachen University
[2]King Mongkut's University of Technology North Bangkok, Thailand
[3]Institute and Out-Patient Clinic of Occupational Medicine, Uniklinik RWTH Aachen
peter.faltin@lfb.rwth-aachen.de

Abstract. A precise correction of segmentations within an acceptable amount of interaction time is a demanding task. In this paper, we present a method offering an intuitive way to correct the segmentation surface by user interaction, while including image information at the same time. An efficient segmentation of follow-up images is achieved by an automatic transfer of the segmentation results to a second point in time. Additionally, this leads to a more consistent follow-up assessment, since independent segmentations for both images might otherwise independently suffer from small deformations and image noise. We apply this method on pleural thickenings in follow-up CT scans. The thickenings are located at the pleura and typically have a relatively low resolution. The objective is a consistent segmentation and growth rate estimation of thickenings for the early diagnosis of malignant pleural mesothelioma.

1 Introduction

Pleural mesothelioma is a malignant form of cancer and is typically related to the previous exposure to asbestos fibers. Inhaled fibers can cause pleural thickenings. The thickenings are observable in thoracic CT data and act as an indicator for pleural mesothelioma. Their morphology can be complex. For a precise quantitative assessment automatic segmentation procedures [1] might need manual corrections by medical experts. With standard 2D segmentation methods this is a time consuming task and subject to strong inter- and intra-reader variability. To reduce the workload and to introduce more consistency for follow-up assessment, methods for comfortable and simultaneous segmentation of images at two points in time are desirable.

Existing interaction methods, to modify 3D surfaces, can be adapted for the segmentation correction of 3D volume data e.g. Proksch et al. [2]. Their methods allow a visual feedback from the image data during the correction process. The Live Wire tool [3] directly includes image information and allows the user to drag incorrectly positioned parts of the segmentation surface. The surface automatically snaps to edges, according to the displayed image slice. The range of influence for the interaction is limited by a spherical region of interest (ROI), placed around the mouse cursor. We suggest a new method based on Graph Cuts, which adopts the user interaction from the Live Wire tool, but operates in the voxel space.

2 Materials and methods

Fig. 1 visually compares our interaction approach to the well-known Graph Cuts based approach from Boykov et al. [4]. While dragging the surface, our approach offers a live preview, and allows a precise positioning before dropping the surface. In our method, a directed graph $\mathcal{G} = \langle \mathcal{V}, \mathcal{E} \rangle$, with a set of nodes $\mathcal{V}$ and a set of connecting edges $\mathcal{E}$ is constructed. Each node $v \in \mathcal{V}_v \subset \mathcal{V}$ corresponds to an image voxel at position $\mathbf{p}(v)$, with intensity value $\mathbf{I}(\mathbf{p}(v))$. Two special nodes, $\{s, t\} = \mathcal{V}_t = \mathcal{V} \setminus \mathcal{V}_v$, are introduced to represent the object and the background labels respectively. All nodes $v \in \mathcal{V}_v$ have incoming edges $(s, v)^T$ from the node s and outgoing edges $(v, t)^T$ to the node t, which form the set $\mathcal{E}_t \subset \mathcal{E}$ of so called t-links. Additionally, the set $\mathcal{E}_n \subset \mathcal{E}$ contains all edges $(q, r)^T$ and $(r, q)^T$ connecting a 26-neighborhood $r \in \mathbf{N}(q)$ of each voxel q. These links are called n-links. All edges $\mathbf{e} = (q, r) \in \mathcal{E}$ have a weight $w(\mathbf{e})$. The graph $\mathcal{G}$ is partitioned into two disjoint subsets $\mathcal{S}$ and $\mathcal{T}$ by a cut $\mathcal{C} \subset \mathcal{E}$, where $s \subset \mathcal{S}$ and $t \in \mathcal{T}$. Each edge $\mathbf{e} \in \mathcal{C}$ contributes its weight to the total cut cost. The cut with minimal costs, corresponding to the final segmentation, is found by applying the Min-Cut/Max-Flow algorithm suggested by Boykov et al. [4].

In this publication, only the front part of the thickening, facing the lung tissue, is segmented. For the backside, which could not be easily identified, a healthy lung model [1] is applied.

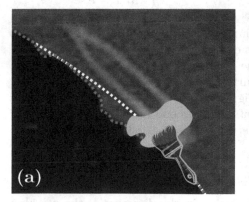 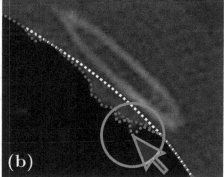

Fig. 1. Comparison between different interaction approaches to manipulate segmentation. Images show healthy lung contour (dotted, white) and initial segmentation (dotted, orange). (a) Typical approach: using a brush-like tool (gray). (b) Suggested approach: drag surface, which snaps in ROI (gray circle) to image data (dotted, green).

2.1 User interaction

The user interaction of dragging the surface is transferred into edge weights, by adding so-called hard constraints. These constraints are stored in an image H of same size as I. Each voxel $v \in \mathcal{V}_v$ has a corresponding hard constraint $H(p(v)) \in \{S, 0, T\}$. If the user drags the surface, in the first step, all hard constraints $H(p(v))$ of voxels $v \in \mathcal{V}_{v,\text{ROI}}$ inside the ROI are set to 0. In the next step, all hard constraints $H(p(v))$ of voxels $v \in \mathcal{V}_{v,\text{line}}$ on a line between the dragging start position p_{start} and the current mouse position p_{current} are set to S or T. This choice depends on if the users extends or reduces the segmentation and is determined by the surface normal n of the segmentation and the dragging direction, therefore

$$H(p(v)) = \begin{cases} S & \text{if } n^T \cdot (p_{\text{current}} - p_{\text{start}}) > 0 \\ T & \text{else} \end{cases}, \forall v \in \mathcal{V}_{v,\text{line}} \tag{1}$$

2.2 Edge weights

One of the most important criterions to separate the different image parts is their intensity. Intensity distributions for the two classes are used to calculate regional penalties based on the negative log-likelihoods [4]

$$R_s(v) = -\ln P(I(p(v))|v \in \mathcal{S}), R_t(v) = -\ln P(I(p(v))|v \in \mathcal{T}) \tag{2}$$

which are added to the edge weights. The conditional probabilities are extracted from training data. The t-link weights are given by

$$w((s,v)^T) = \begin{cases} 0 & H(p(v)) \equiv T \\ K & H(p(v)) \equiv S \\ \lambda R_s(v) & \text{else} \end{cases}, \quad w((v,t)^T) = \begin{cases} 0 & H(p(v)) \equiv S \\ K & H(p(v)) \equiv T \\ \lambda R_t(v) & \text{else} \end{cases} \tag{3}$$

where λ is a parameter to weight the influence of the intensity model and K is the maximum neighborhood weight, as defined in [4].

Another important criterion is the continuity of the segmenting surface, which is considered by penalizing the surface area of the segmentation boundary. A neighborhood system, as shown in Fig. 2(a), is utilized to calculate the weight terms $w_k(v)$, $v \in \mathcal{V}_v$ for all families k of neighborhood relations. The boundary terms are calculated in Riemannian metric D as suggested by Boykov et al. [4]

$$w_k^{\mathcal{R}}(v) = w_k^{\mathcal{E}} \frac{\det D(v)}{\left(u_k^T \cdot D(v) \cdot u_k\right)^2} \tag{4}$$

where u_k is a vector of unit length, pointing in the direction of the neighbor voxel, and $w_k^{\mathcal{E}}(p)$ is the corresponding boundary term in Euclidean metric. The anisotropic Riemannian metric depends on the image I

$$D(v) = g(|\nabla I(p(v))|) \cdot I_3 + (1 - g(|\nabla I(p(v))|)) \cdot u \cdot u^T \tag{5}$$

where $\boldsymbol{I_3}$ is the identity matrix and $g(x) = \exp(-\frac{x^2}{2\sigma^2})$. The Euclidean metric is

$$w_k^{\mathcal{E}} = \frac{\triangle\rho_k \cdot \triangle\varPhi_k}{\pi} \tag{6}$$

where $\triangle\rho_k$ is the closest distance between the lines within the family k, and $\triangle\varPhi_k$ is the angular differences between the nearest families of edge lines. Using a dense neighborhood this can be approximated using a spherical Voronoi diagram [5] and we chose $\triangle\varPhi_k = \frac{4\pi}{26}$. Typically, for CT data the voxel spacing $\delta_{x,y}$ in x- and y-direction is identical and the spacing in z-direction is $\delta_z > \delta_{x,y}$. For this special case the distances $\triangle\rho_k$ are reduced to 5 cases and given in Fig. 2(b). The n-link weights $w(e)$ are determined by the edge family k, with $\kappa : e \mapsto k$

$$w(e) = w_{\kappa(e)}^{\mathcal{R}}, \forall e \in \mathcal{E}_n \tag{7}$$

2.3 Simultaneous segmentation

For the transfer of the segmentation between different points in time, we assume that a non-rigid and volume preserving registration is available e.g. by applying the method suggested by Rohlfing et al. [6]. The labeling is transferred to the other point in time, and the signed distance function $\varPhi(\boldsymbol{p}(v))$, which is the closest distance for each point $\boldsymbol{p}(v)$ to the segmentation boundary, is extracted. The distance has a negative sign in the interior of the segmentation and a positive sign outside. Thickenings do not shrink over time but may grow. The volume-preservation is required during registration to effectively translate this knowledge into constraints: Shrinking is strongly penalized, while growing is only penalized if it is in an unreasonable range. In combination with the signed distance function

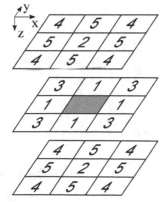

l	$\triangle\rho_l$
1	δ_z
2	$\delta_{x,y}(= \delta_{x,y})$
3	$\dfrac{\delta_z}{\sqrt{2}}$
4	$\dfrac{\delta_z \cdot \delta_{x,y}}{\sqrt{\delta_{x,y}^2 + \delta_z^2}}$
5	$\dfrac{\delta_{x,y} \cdot \sqrt{\delta_{x,y}^2 + \delta_z^2}}{\sqrt{2 \cdot \delta_{x,y}^2 + \delta_z^2}}$

(a) 26-neighborhood of the gray voxel. Each neighbor is labeled with number l of edge family.

(b) Corresponding closest distance within edge family.

Fig. 2. Relation between edge family and corresponding closest distance of edges.

$\Phi(\boldsymbol{p}(v))$, we chose the t-link weights at the second point in time

$$w'((s,v)^T) = \lambda \cdot R'_s(v) + \begin{cases} \frac{-\Phi(\boldsymbol{p}(v))}{1+|\Phi(\boldsymbol{p}(v))|} & \text{if } \Phi(\boldsymbol{p}(v)) < 0 \\ 0 & \text{else} \end{cases} \tag{8}$$

$$w'((v,t)^T) = \lambda \cdot R'_t(v) + \begin{cases} \alpha \left(\frac{\Phi(\boldsymbol{p}(v))}{\beta}\right)^\gamma & \text{if } \Phi(\boldsymbol{p}(v)) > 0 \\ 0 & \text{else} \end{cases} \tag{9}$$

where α, β, γ are parameters to influence the penalization. R'_s and R'_t are the intensity based penalties for the second point in time. The chosen penalties for the transfer in (8) and (9) are shown in Fig. 3(a).

In the graphical user interface both points in time are shown side-by-side and the user can see the live results of the interaction in both images.

3   Results

Our newly developed segmentation tool was tested in an initial evaluation by a group of 11 users and was compared to the Live Wire tool [3], which provides a similar user interface. Both tools were implemented using MITK [7] and tested in an identical scenario, where the users had 120 seconds to segment a given thickening. The tool presented in this paper was utilized for a simultaneous segmentation. Those results for the second point in time, where user interaction was only indirectly applied, were compared to results from the Live Wire tool, directly applied on the second point in time. The weight influence for the intensity model was chosen as $\lambda = 0.006$. The resulting segmentations were compared with a reference segmentation of the thickening. This reference was created by a voxel-wise majority decision of segmentations carefully carried out

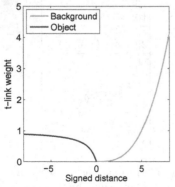

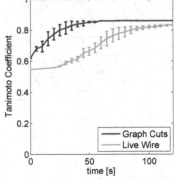

(a) Penalties to keep segmentation consistent, with $\alpha = 1, \beta = 5$ and $\gamma = 3$.

(b) Mean results off all users over time. Error bars show variance with factor of 10.

Fig. 3. Mean segmentation quality and applied penalties for segmentation transfer.

voxel-by-voxel by 3 experienced users. For performance analysis, the Tanimoto coefficient ($\frac{TP}{TP+FP+FN}$) was chosen as a quality criterion. User segmentation and reference segmentation were compared using the healthy lung model [1] as the backside. Resulting quality and variance for different users are plotted over time in Fig. 3(b). Both curves show similar improvement of quality over time, which converges to a Tanimoto coefficient of approximately 0.85. Different starting points were caused by the initial segmentation results of the Graph Cuts method without any user interaction. Both tools resulted in similar inter-user variances, visualized by error bars. Our proposed tool performed slightly better in case of variance and quality compared to the Live Wire tool; especially a faster convergence is achieved. Additionally, the users rated both tools according to their intuition, reaction time, precision, efficiency and usability. Our new tool was, averaged for all users, superior in all criteria except for the reaction time.

4 Discussion

The presented segmentation tool offers a convenient way to correct 3D segmentations, by combining image information and user interaction. Corrections from one point in time are successfully transferred to the other point in time. Initial tests indicate that it is superior to the similar Live Wire tool [3] in most criteria. The results achieved as a consequence of indirect user interaction at another point in time are even better than the results from the Live Wire tool directly applied on this image. A current limitation is the reaction time for a simultaneous segmentation, which is not comparable to the Live Wire tool applied on a single independent image. This will be addressed in future work by interleaving computation and interaction as well as GPU computing. One of the main tasks for the future will be to create a more comprehensive evaluation scenario to judge the tool's suitability for general segmentation correction.

References

1. Chaisaowong K, Bross B, Knepper A, et al. Detection and follow-up assessment of pleural thickenings from 3D CT data. Proc ECTI CON. 2008; p. 489–92.
2. Proksch D, Dornheim J, Preim B. Interaktionstechniken zur Korrektur medizinischer 3D-Segmentierungen. Proc BVM. 2010; p. 420–4.
3. Hachmann H, Faltin P, Kraus T, et al. 3D-Segmentierungskorrektur unter Berücksichtigung von Bildinformationen für die effiziente und objektive Erfassung pleuraler Verdickungen. Proc BVM. 2013; p. 296–301.
4. Boykov Y, Jolly MP. Interactive graph cuts for optimal boundary and region segmentation of objects in N-D images. Proc ICCV. 2001; p. 105–12.
5. Danvek O, Matula P. An improved riemannian metric approximation for graph cuts. Conf DGCI. 2011;6607:71–82.
6. Rohlfing T, Maurer Jr CR, Bluemke DA, et al. Volume-preserving nonrigid registration of MR breast images using free-form deformation with an incompressibility constraint. IEEE Trans Med Imaging. 2003;22:730–41.
7. Nolden M, Zelzer S, Seitel A, et al. The medical imaging interaction toolkit: challenges and advances. Int J Comput Ass Radiol Surg. 2013;8(3):1–14.

Regression Forest-Based Organ Detection in Normalized PET Images

Peter Fischer[1], Volker Daum[2], Dieter Hahn[2], Marcus Prümmer[2],
Joachim Hornegger[1]

[1] Pattern Recognition Lab and Erlangen Graduate School in Advanced Optical
Technologies (SAOT), FAU Erlangen-Nürnberg
[2] Chimaera GmbH
peter.fischer@fau.de

Abstract. The detection of organs from full-body PET images is a challenging task due to the high noise and the limited amount of anatomical information of PET imaging. The knowledge of organ locations can support many clinical applications like image registration or tumor detection. This paper is the first to propose an organ localization framework tailored on the challenges of PET. The algorithm involves intensity normalization, feature extraction and regression forests. Linear and nonlinear intensity normalization methods are compared theoretically and experimentally. From the normalized images, long-range spatial context visual features are extracted. A regression forest predicts the organ bounding boxes. Experiments show that percentile normalization is the best preprocessing method. The algorithm is evaluated on 25 clinical images with a spatial resolution of 5 mm. With 13.8 mm mean absolute bounding box error, it achieves state-of-the-art results.

1 Introduction

In order to correctly use positron emission tomography (PET) images for diagnosis, it is helpful for physicians to know the relation to the underlying anatomy. This information can be provided with the help of morphological images, for example computed tomography (CT) or magnetic resonance imaging (MRI). Nowadays, the standard scanners are hybrids of functional and morphological modalities, e.g. PET/CT or PET/MRI. Even in hybrid scanners, the images are not perfectly aligned due to motion artifacts and different acquisition times. This could be tackled by image registration. Image registration can be greatly enhanced by semantic information like known organ positions. Most of the publications on anatomy localization deal with CT images.

Seifert et al. segment organs and detect point landmarks automatically from full body CT images [1] using marginal space learning with probabilistic boosting trees and 3D Haar features. Detection of landmarks and organs is also performed in [2] with classification forests. The features used by Criminisi et al. are a generalization of 3D Haar features called visual features which emphasize long-range spatial context. This work was extended in [3] by using regression forests instead of classification forests. Pauly et al. transferred the approach using regression ferns and binary visual features to MRI [4]. In PET imaging literature, the focus of automatic localization methods is not on anatomy, but on tumors. Guan et al. include a rough body part localization by classifying feature curves from the PET volume using a hidden Markov model [5]. Montgomery et al. report a fully automated, unsupervised segmentation of PET volumes using Gaussian mixture models and a multiscale Markov random field [6].

This work localizes organs in the challenging environment of PET imaging using context-rich visual features, regression forests [3, 4], and intensity normalization. Multiple intensity normalization methods are analyzed and compared experimentally.

2   Materials and methods

2.1   Intensity normalization

Attenuation corrected PET images contain measurements of the count of positron emission decays in each voxel. The counts are a physical quantity, but they are not directly comparable for different acquisitions as Hounsfield units in CT. Reasons are the variability caused by the scanner, the injected dose, the tracer, the uptake time, and the human anatomy. Intensity normalization reduces the variability that the organ detection algorithm has to deal with.

The normalization of mean and variance of an image I makes subsequent features invariant to affine changes of intensity. An affine change of intensity is $I'(v) = a\,I(v) + b$ with the voxel $v \in \mathbb{R}^3$ and constants $a, b \in \mathbb{R}$. In normalization, the mean μ is set to 0, and the variance σ^2 to 1 using the transform $I_{\mathrm{MV}}(v) = \frac{I(v)-\mu}{\sigma}$. This nullifies the effects of affine intensity changes. Percentile normalization is in principle the same as the normalization of minimum and maximum values of the image. The difference is that outliers in the image are saturated before normalization. For the non-outlier intensities, this normalization removes affine transformations of the intensity. The percentile normalization works by $I_{\mathrm{PERC}}(v) = \frac{I(v)-I_{\mathrm{low}}}{I_{\mathrm{high}}-I_{\mathrm{low}}}$, with the low percentile I_{low} and the high percentile I_{high} set to intensities corresponding to an arbitrary percentage of the intensities of all voxels in the image. Standard uptake values (SUV) are used in radiology to diagnose the malignancy of tumors in PET imaging. SUV is the normalization $I_{\mathrm{SUV}}(v) = \frac{I(v)}{D/BW}$, with the patient body weight BW [g], the injected dose D [Bq], and the radioactivity concentration in a given voxel $I(v)$ [Bq/ml] [7]. The major difference between the above affine normalization schemes is the information source. Mean and variance normalization uses moments, whereas percentile normalization uses quantiles of the histogram. Both methods use only image information, as opposed to SUV which uses clinical and patient metainformation. The true transformation between images, especially of different patients, is not affine. Consequently, the normalizations presented so far cannot remove these variations. Nonlinear intensity variations also occur in magnetic resonance imaging. We transfer a sophisticated normalization scheme in MRI to PET, namely non-rigid registration of the image histogram to a reference histogram [8]. To avoid that the registration algorithm focuses on the background intensities, which constitute a dominant peak in the histogram, and to limit the number of histogram bins, extreme intensities are excluded from the registration [8]. This is achieved by masking values below the 80% percentile and above the 99% percentile.

2.2 Organ localization

Due to the human anatomy and the characteristics of imaging systems, the appearance and the relative position of anatomical structures is similar in medical images of the same modality. Consequently, the high amount of contextual information that is available should be exploited by the features. A successful feature framework in medical object localization are the visual features from Criminisi et al., which capture anatomical structures and their relative positions [2, 3, 4]. The features consist of the relationship of cuboid regions with a random offset to the voxel under consideration and with random size. One benefit of visual features is that context can be captured well over a long range. Visual features are especially suited for PET imaging because the involved averaging makes them robust to the high noise of PET and the context information allows them to cope with the low discriminability of small voxel neighborhoods. Instead of intensity normalization, it is possible to make the features themselves invariant to intensity changes by replacing the difference in [2] with a binary comparison [4]. However, information about the relative magnitude of the features is lost because of the binarization. Another issue is that some feature regions necessarily lie outside of the image for some voxels due to the random offsets. For full-body PET images, the feature value for these boxes can set to zero, assuming no tracer concentration outside of the image. This assumption is only violated in the area of the legs, but as the field of view is similar for all images, the violation has only a small influence.

In this work, organs in PET images are detected using the nonlinear, multidimensional regression algorithm of regression forests. The output of the regression is a vector containing the bounding boxes of several organs [3]. The cost function for tree training is based on class affiliation [9], which in this case are the organs. The affiliation to an organ is modeled by a Laplacian density with the empirically set parameter $\lambda = 100 \, \text{mm}$. The number of features that are examined during training in each node is called randomness ρ. In each leaf of the tree, a Gaussian density is stored as a probabilistic approximation of the training samples. During testing, the trees of the forest are combined by weighted averaging. For an image, all the samples are combined by adding the mean value of the Gaussian of the leaf in which the samples end up in, weighted by the inverse of the trace of the covariance matrix of the respective leaf. In addition, only the 10% of samples with highest weight are retained, the others are discarded. Regression forests are well suited because they incorporate multidimensional outputs, are fast, and easy to parallelize. Regression is superior to voxel-wise classification in PET imaging, because the involved averaging makes the estimates robust to the high noise level.

2.3   Experiments

Comparison of intensity normalization methods The intensity normalization methods are compared using organ localization and histogram errors. The organ localization error is the absolute difference of the estimated and the true bounding boxes. Measures to compare the PET image histograms are the Sum of Squared Differences (SSD) and the symmetric Kullback-Leibler Divergence (SKLD). The histograms are computed with 256 equally sized bins, except for percentile normalization, where the number of bins is reduced to reflect the compression of the intensity range. The histogram error reflects the similarity of the intensity distributions of different PET images.

The random forest in this experiment consists of 8 trees with a maximal depth of 10. $\rho = 100$ visual features are searched in each node during forest training with a maximum size of 200 mm and offset of 500 mm. Training is performed on 16 images and testing on 4 images not in the training set. In percentile normalization, 0% and 99.5% percentiles are used.

Organ localization In the PET images, brain, liver, left and right kidney, and bladder are located. The regression forest has 14 trees of depth up to 9. The randomness is $\rho = 500$. Percentile normalization is performed with 0% and 99.5%. The visual features are thresholded to a maximum size and offset of 200 mm. There are 25 PET images with a spatial resolution of 5 mm in each direction. All are acquired with the tracer fluorodeoxyglucose (FDG). From each image, 1% of the voxels are drawn for training to reduce training time. The results are computed using 5-fold cross validation.

3   Results

3.1   Comparison of intensity normalization methods

The results are summarized in Tab. 1. The lowest histogram errors are achieved by SUV normalization. This shows that SUV is a good choice in clinical evaluation of PET images. Percentile normalization reduces the SKLD error, but shows no improvement in SSD. Non-rigid histogram registration is most flexible and thus expected to give the lowest errors. Instead, it increases both errors, because PET histograms show little structure that can be aligned [5]. As histogram registration is worsening the total histogram alignment, its organ localization error is not investigated. The organ localization test errors agree only partially with the histogram errors. Without preprocessing, the algorithm achieves a test error of 15.6 mm. Mean-variance normalization and binary comparison increase the test and train error, which can be explained by the change of the background intensity and by the missing magnitude information, respectively. With 11.7 mm

Table 1. This table compares mean absolute bounding box errors over all organs and the histogram errors for different preprocessing methods.

Preprocessing Method	Train Error [mm]	Test Error [mm]	Histogram Error [SKLD]	Histogram Error [SSD]
None	8.1	15.6	0.055	3.1e12
Mean-Variance	28.5	26.9	0.034	6.3e12
Percentile	6.5	11.7	0.013	3.5e12
SUV	6.7	13.9	0.0004	1.6e10
Histogram Registration	–	–	0.061	3.4e12
Binary Comparison	9.7	18.1	–	–

test error, percentile normalization is the best in our experiments. The left and middle of Fig. 1 show an unprocessed and a percentile normalized PET image.

3.2 Organ localization

The mean organ localization error is 13.8 ± 7.5 mm. This is higher than the corresponding experiment in Tab. 1 due to the cross-validation. Separated into single organs, we achieve an error of 15.4 ± 11.3 mm for the brain, 13.0 ± 4.9 mm for the liver, 13.4 ± 6.5 mm for the left and 11.1 ± 5.5 mm for the right kidney, and 15.9 ± 6.4 mm for the bladder. The errors compare favorably with the ones from the literature, e.g. 15.0 mm for organ localization in MRI [4] and 16.7 mm for organ localization in CT [3]. The average runtime of training is 5 h for 20

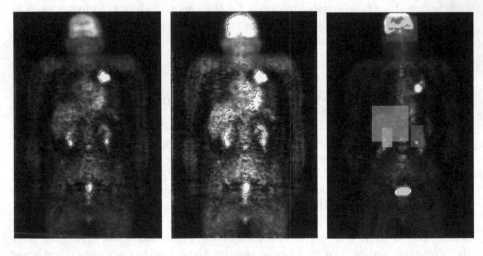

Fig. 1. Left is a slice of an attenuation-corrected PET image. In the middle is the same slice with normalized percentiles. On the right, a typical organ localization result is shown.

images and the runtime of testing is 10 min for 5 images. In Fig. 1, a typical organ localization result is shown overlaid onto the PET image.

4 Discussion

This paper presents an algorithm for automatic detection of organs in PET images. This is achieved with nonlinear regression of organ bounding boxes using a regression forest. Visual features with long-range spatial context are the input of the regression algorithm. Different intensity normalization methods are proposed to cope with the unstandardized intensities of PET. Experimental evaluation shows that percentile normalization works best because it removes outliers and affine transformations between the image intensities. The final organ localization error, computed using 5-fold cross-validation, is 13.8 mm on average over all images and organs. In the future, the inclusion of organs and landmarks into image registration could be analyzed. It should be determined whether any improvement over traditional PET/CT and PET/MRI is achievable.

Acknowledgement. We thank the nuclear medicine department of the Universitätsklinikum Erlangen for providing the images and medical advice. The authors gratefully acknowledge funding of the Erlangen Graduate School in Advanced Optical Technologies (SAOT) by the German Research Foundation (DFG) in the framework of the German excellence initiative.

References

1. Seifert S, Barbu A, Zhou SK, et al. Hierarchical parsing and semantic navigation of full body CT data. Proc SPIE. 2009;7259:725902-1-8.
2. Criminisi A, Shotton J, Bucciare S. Decision forests with long-range spatial context for organ localization in CT volumes. Proc MICCAI PMMIA. 2009; p. 69-80.
3. Criminisi A, Shotton J, Robertson DP, et al. Regression forests for efficient anatomy detection and localization in CT studies. Proc MICCAI MCV. 2010; p. 106-17.
4. Pauly O, Glocker B, Criminisi A, et al. Fast multiple organ detection and localization in whole-body MR Dixon sequences. Proc MICCAI. 2011; p. 239-47.
5. Guan H, Kubota T, Huang X, et al. Automatic hot spot detection and segmentation in whole body FDG-PET images. Proc ICIP. 2006; p. 85-8.
6. Montgomery DWG, Amira A, Zaidi H. Fully automated segmentation of oncological PET volumes using a combined multiscale and statistical model. Med Phys. 2007;34:722-36.
7. Kelly M. SUV: Advancing Comparability and Accuracy. Siemens; 2009.
8. Jäger F, Hornegger J. Nonrigid registration of joint histograms for intensity standardization in magnetic resonance imaging. IEEE Trans Med Imaging. 2009;28(1):137-50.
9. Dantone M, Gall J, Fanelli G, et al. Real-time facial feature detection using conditional regression forests. Proc CVPR. 2012; p. 2578-85.

Polar-Based Aortic Segmentation in 3D CTA Dissection Data Using a Piecewise Constant Curvature Model

Cosmin Adrian Morariu[1], Daniel Sebastian Dohle[2], Tobias Terheiden[1], Konstantinos Tsagakis[2], Josef Pauli[1]

[1]Intelligent Systems Group, Faculty of Engineering, University of Duisburg-Essen
[2]Department of Thoracic and Cardiovascular Surgery, Universitätsklinikum Essen
adrian.morariu@uni-due.de

Abstract. Immediate open surgery represents nowadays the only possibility to treat acute aortic Type A dissections, involving the ascending aorta. However, this procedure is correlated with high perioperative mortality rates. Due to the complex vascular anatomy of the ascending aorta and aortic arch, a minimally invasive therapy would only prove feasible by manufacturing custom-designed stent-grafts for each patient according to morphological characteristics obtained from CT data. In order to overcome the inherent difficulties linked to the segmentation of severe aortic dissections, this contribution introduces a novel polar-based segmentation approach implying a piecewise constant curvature model for the outer aortic cross-sectional boundary. Subsequently, the resulting aortic mesh is refined by an efficient narrow-band 3D level-set method.

1 Introduction

The proximity to the aortic valve, coronary arteries and supraaortic branches outlines the necessity of patient-specific stent-grafts for the endovascular treatment of aortic Type A dissections. This type of dissections involve the ascending aorta and are currently treated by conventional open surgery. Unfortunately, elderly patients with multiple comorbidities are deemed unamenable for open repair, where mortality rates reach up to 30% [1].

Aortic segmentation has gained special attention in recent years as it represents a crucial task for various clinical applications including surgical planning and stent-graft deployment. There has been done extensive research in the area of vessel segmentation in general, but only few approaches are suited for the localization of the dissected aorta, which possesses a much larger width than other vessels and which often exhibits a non-circular cross-sectional shape due to the dissection. Blood entering through an initial tear in the intima layer of the aortic wall leads to the formation of a false lumen, separated from the true channel by a membrane, which may be split or highly tortuous as shown in Fig. 1(b). The presence of the dissection membrane represents another factor cumbering the feasibility of generic vessel segmentation algorithms applied to aortic dissections, as we aim at the simultaneous detection of both lumina.

Previous research with focus on aortic segmentation can be categorized into deformable models approaches [2], iterative graph-based algorithms [3], parametric analytical models [4] and joint approaches including segmentation and registration [5]. The method described by [3] is applied to datasets without pathologies for detection of thoracic aorta calcifications. Therefore, the authors consider an entropy-based cost term around an initial circular boundary.

2   Materials and methods

The premises of this approach concern the ideal aortic shape and appearance are not given in our CT datasets, as the acute dissection bears the existence of more than one lumen and discloses irregular shapes in axial slices, especially at aortic arch level. A segmentation scheme with focus on aortic dissections is discussed in [2]. By performing the Hough transformation, circles are being extracted in several cross-sectional slices around the center of the aortic arch. They serve as an initial mesh for an elastically deformable model. The analytic intensity model highlighted in [4] incrementally fits a 3D cylinder segment to the image intensities within a 3D ROI in order to estimate the vessel radius and centerline. This model is extended in [5] by combining it with an intensity-based elastic image registration functional.

This contribution proposes a novel polar-based segmentation approach operating on extracted cross-sectional slices, orthogonal to the vessel centerline. The clinician is required to select a subvolume of choice within the input CT dataset by manually placing 3 points in order to trigger the automated segmentation process. At the same time, these points serve for a cubic spline interpolation with lagrangian end conditions as a coarse approximation of the aortic centerline. The spline is sampled at a constant interval of twice the slice spacing, wherein each sampled 3D point becomes the center of a plane orthogonal to the spline. In a first step, only both multiplanar reformatted (MPR) planes passing through the ending points of the spline are being constructed and preprocessed in order to obtain a suitable Canny-edge image for a subsequent Hough transformation (HT) for circles. The preprocessing comprises a contrast-limited adaptive histogram equalization and a nonlinear, inhomogeneous anisotropic diffusion filtering. The anisotropic filter is employed iteratively, as proposed in [6] for filtering of MRI data. Advantages of anisotropy consist in preserving or even sharpening object boundaries while removing noise in homogeneous areas.

After performing the HT on both planes orthogonal to the aortic centerline passing through the ending points of the spline, the circle centers having the lowest euclidian distances to the corresponding spline ending points are being chosen. The radii R_{Start} and R_{End}, associated to the selected circle centers, represent rough estimates for the aortic boundary at the proximal end of the ascending aorta, respectively at the distal end of the descending aorta. Based on R_{Start} and R_{End}, we calculate the half-width pixel-sized length N of the quadratic ROI for extracting all planes along the equidistantly sampled aortic spline by $N = \max(50, \max(R_{Start}, R_{End}))$. Each extracted MPR-ROI with the corresponding spline point as center is being split into M circular sectors of equal degrees and transformed into polar coordinates around its center. For $\Phi = 360$ degrees and $M = 10$ circular sectors we obtain a block length of $L = \frac{\Phi}{M} = 36$ degrees per circular sector, which allows an aortic boundary model of constant curvature for each sector in cartesian space (Fig. 1(b)) and therefore a constant radius $R(\varphi)$ per block in polar space (Fig. 1(a)), with $1 \leq \varphi \leq \Phi$. This piecewise constant curvature boundary model should incorporate both lumina of the dissected aorta, being robust to the often highly folded and discontinuous dissection membrane. We overcome this hindrance by not allowing $R(\varphi)$ to fall below a certain R_{min}^{i} for the i-th MPR-ROI. Oversegmentation caused by boundary gaps, where the delimitation between aortic lumina and surrounding tissue is non-existent, is avoided by setting an upper barrier R_{max}^{i}. Based on the aforementioned R_{Start} and R_{End} we compute a linear increment $r_{step} = \frac{R_{End} - R_{Start}}{n_{Spline} - 1}$ for the "expected" aortic radius in each MPR-ROI, wherein n_{Spline} denotes the number of sampled points along the aortic centerline. Depending on the pathological severity of each aortic dissection case, we have to tackle the problem of sudden significant changes of the vessel diameter within adjacent slices. For this reason we allow 40% deviance in each direction from the "expected" radius ($r_{dev} = 0.4$), so that $R_{max/min}^{i} = (R_{Start} + (i - 1) \cdot r_{step}) \cdot (1 \pm r_{dev})$ for the i-th MPR-ROI. The average intensity

$$\bar{I}_{R(\varphi)} = \left[\sum_{\varphi=1}^{\Phi} R(\varphi)\right]^{-1} \cdot \sum_{\varphi=1}^{\Phi} \sum_{r=1}^{R(\varphi)} I(\varphi, r) \qquad (1)$$

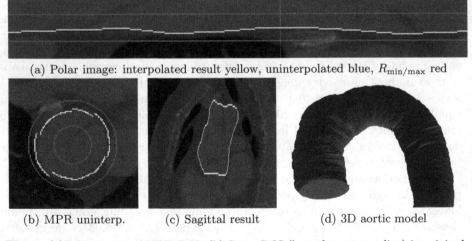

(a) Polar image: interpolated result yellow, uninterpolated blue, $R_{min/max}$ red

(b) MPR uninterp.   (c) Sagittal result   (d) 3D aortic model

Fig. 1. (a)Polar image of MPR-ROI. (b) Same ROI (but of greater radius) in original cartesian coordinates with uninterpolated result in yellow and $R_{min/max}$ in red. (c) Result in one of the sagittal slices. (d) 3D volume revealing enlarged ascending aorta.

of the already segmented region described by $R(\varphi)$ is compared to the average value of the 1-pixel width arc belonging to the k-th circular sector ($0 \leq k < M$)

$$\bar{I}_{k,R(\varphi)} = L^{-1} \cdot \sum_{\varphi=1}^{L} I(k \cdot L + \varphi, R(k \cdot L + \varphi) + 1)) \qquad (2)$$

in order to check whether this arc should be added to the aortic cross-section. We iteratively consider the region delimited by $R(\varphi)$ at different time steps starting with t_0, for which $R_{t_0}(\varphi) = R_{\min}$, $1 \leq \varphi \leq \Phi$. A homogeneity function

$$h_k(R_t(\varphi)) = \begin{cases} 0 & \text{if } |\bar{I}_{R_t(\varphi)} - \bar{I}_{k,R_t(\varphi)}| > \lambda_t \\ 1 & \text{if } |\bar{I}_{R_t(\varphi)} - \bar{I}_{k,R_t(\varphi)}| \leq \lambda_t \\ -6 & \text{if } R_t(\varphi) > R_{\max} \text{ for } k \cdot L < \varphi \leq (k+1) \cdot L \end{cases} \qquad (3)$$

is evaluated within each iteration for an arc of the k-th circular sector. Using this homogeneity function the update-equation of all k circular sectors during an iteration step is being formulated as

$$R_{t+\Delta t}(\varphi) = R_t(\varphi) + \sum_{k=0}^{M-1} h_k(R_t(\varphi)) \cdot \delta_k(\varphi) \qquad (4)$$

$\delta_k(\varphi)$ denotes the unit mass concentrated at $\forall \varphi$ within the arc of the k-th circular sector, with $\delta_k(\varphi) = 1$ if $k \cdot L < \varphi < (k+1) \cdot L$ and 0 otherwise. In case that $R_{t+\Delta t}(\varphi) = R_t(\varphi)$ for all M circular sectors, then the convergence criterion of our algorithm has been fulfilled. Equations (3) and (4) show that if the radius of the aortic region contained within one sector exceeds $R_{\max}$, then it is being decreased by 6 pixels. Simultaneously, the adaptive homogeneity threshold

$$\lambda_{t+\Delta t} = \begin{cases} \lambda_t & \text{if } R_t(\varphi) \leq R_{\max} \text{ for } 1 \leq \varphi \leq \Phi \\ \lambda_t \cdot 3/4 & \text{otherwise} \end{cases} \qquad (5)$$

is diminished by a factor of 3/4. This implies the preservation of the initial threshold $\lambda_{t_0} = 0.03$ until $R_t(\varphi)$ exceeds $R_{\max}$ within any of the circular sectors.

Finally, in order to obtain a continuous $R(\varphi)$ over $1 \leq \varphi \leq \Phi$ we interpolate the segmentation result over all circular sectors after algorithm convergence. The resulting aortic cross-sections from all MPR slices are connected in 3D to a volume (Fig. 1(d)), which is subsequently refined by a sparse-field level set method [7]. The volume's 3D closed aortic surface is defined as the initial zero level set. Due to the tremendous 3D voxel data we consider only the 3x3x3 vicinity of the zero level set, resulting in 5 layers w.r.t. to the maximal city-block distance of 2 around the zero-level-set. The energy functional to be minimized within this narrow-band relies on the well-known Chan-Vese region-based energy.

The presented approach has been evaluated on 11, respectively parameter-optimized on further 8 CTA datasets from patients with aortic Type A dissection. The evaluation datasets from different Siemens CT scanners (Sensation 16, Emotion 6, Definition, Sensation 4) contain 87 to 1034 axial slices with a slice spacing ranging from 0.7 to 6 mm. The in-plane resolution of the axial slices (each of 512x512 voxels) varies between 0.445 and 0.863 mm.

Table 1. Mean and standard deviation for 11 CTA datasets of aortic dissection.

Refinement	3D Level Set	Without
DSC	0.9232 ± 0.0219	0.8955 ± 0.0329
Precision	0.8920 ± 0.0444	0.8258 ± 0.0596
Recall	0.9589 ± 0.0329	0.9815 ± 0.0255

3   Results

In order to achieve a quantitative assessment of our algorithm's capabilities we compare the result of the automatic 3D segmentation with manual annotations performed by a vascular surgeon on the original axial slices of the 11 CTA datasets. The voxelwise comparison of the volumes resulting from automatic segmentation, respectively from ground truth, leads to the four possible combinations: true negatives (TN), true positives (TP), false negatives (FN) and false positives (FP). The latter three do not depend on axial data size and serve to evaluate the accuracy of our segmentation in terms of the Dice Similarity Coefficient $DSC = 2TP/(FN+2TP+FP)$, Precision $P = TP/(TP+FP)$ and Recall $R = TP/(TP+FN)$. For the 11 datasets we obtain a mean DSC value (also known as F1 score) of 92.3%, which is the harmonic mean of $P = 89.2\%$ and $R = 95.9\%$. Without refinement by 3D narrow-band level-sets, the DSC decreases by 2.77% (Tab. 1).

Fig. 1(b) shows the segmentation result (yellow) obtained in one of the MPR slices. The corresponding polar image is depicted in Fig. 1(a). All aortic boundaries delineated in MPR-ROIs are interpolated in 3D to a volume (Fig. 1(d)), which is compared to the ground truth volume. The slice spacing in 5 out of 11 CT datasets is much coarser (3 – 6 mm) than the average within-slice resolution (0.6 mm). Minor inaccuracies occur when performing segmentation on

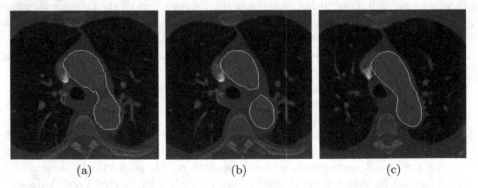

(a)   (b)   (c)

Fig. 2. Intersection of segmented 3D volumes with an axial slice just below the aortic arch (a),(b) and within the arch (c). Minor inaccuracies of the segmentation in MPR-ROIs lead to not delineating the ascending and descending aorta separately in (a). Improved result is due to 3D level-set refinement in (b).

some MPR-ROIs extracted from these datasets. An example is illustrated in Fig. 2(a), where the ascending and descending aortic cross-sections are not located separately after interpolating the results of MPR planes to a volume and intersecting this volume with an original axial slice (just below the aortic arch). The sparse-field 3D level-sets prove to be appropriate to remedy the oversegmentation (Fig. 2(b)). Another successful segmentation result is shown in Fig. 1(c) after intersecting the aortic volume with a sagittal slice. The overlap of the volume with an axial slice within the aortic arch also exhibits a good segmentation outcome (Fig. 2(c)). The computation time for segmenting the aortic arch within a CTA dataset is 36.5 ± 28.7 s (2.66 GHz Intel Core i5, 8 GB RAM and Matlab).

4 Discussion

We introduced a novel adaptive polar-based model of piecewise constant curvature for segmenting the aortic cross-sectional boundary. An inherent advantage of this approach resides in its reliable applicability to datasets with severe pathologies (e.g. acute aortic Type A dissections). Higher R compared to P indicate a slight oversegmentation, which occasionally occurs in some of 5 CTA datasets comprising coarse slice spacing of 3 – 6 mm. Despite the partial volume effect and the aorta rapidly changing appearance and shape from slice to slice within the aforementioned datasets, the proposed approach yields accurate segmentation results. Further work will focus on the automated quantification of morphological specifics of the ascending aorta in order to enable minimally invasive endovascular techniques, which are presently confined to the descending aorta and, partly, to the aortic arch.

References

1. Moon MC, Greenberg RK, Morales JP, et al. Computed tomography-based anatomic characterization of proximal aortic dissection with consideration for endovascular candidacy. J Vasc Surg. 2011;53(4):942–9.
2. Kovács T, Cattin P, Alkadhi H, et al. Automatic segmentation of the vessel lumen from 3D CTA images of aortic dissection. Proc BVM. 2006; p. 161–5.
3. Avila-Montes OC, Kukure U, Kakadiaris IA. Aorta segmentation in non-contrast cardiac CT images using an entropy-based cost function. Proc SPIE. 2010; p. 76233J–1–8.
4. Wörz S, von Tengg-Kobligk H, Henninger V, et al. 3-D quantification of the aortic arch morphology in 3D CTA data for endovascular aortic repair. IEEE Trans Biomed Eng. 2010;57(10):2359–68.
5. Biesdorf A, Rohr K, Feng D, et al. Segmentation and quantification of the aortic arch using joint 3D model-based segmentation and elastic image registration. Med Image Anal. 2012;16(6):1187–201.
6. Gerig G, Kubler O, Kikinis R, et al. Nonlinear anisotropic filtering of MRI data. IEEE Trans Med Imaging. 1992;11(2):221–32.
7. Whitaker RT. A level-set approach to 3D reconstruction from range data. Int J Comput Vis. 1998;29(3):203–31.

Automatic Classification of Salient Boundaries in Object-Based Image Segmentation

Carmela Acevedo[1,2], Teodora Chitiboi[1,2], Lars Linsen[2], Horst Karl Hahn[1,2]

[1]Fraunhofer MEVIS, Bremen
[2]Jacobs University Bremen
c.acevedo@jacobs-university.de

Abstract. We present a supervised classification approach for image segmentation that operates in an object-based image representation and combines object features with boundary features. While classical algorithms focus on either regions (i.e. objects) or edges (i.e. boundaries), we offer a hybrid solution that takes both aspects into consideration. To illustrate the capacity of this approach, we apply the proposed classification to CT bone segmentation.

1 Introduction

Object-based image analysis (OBIA) alleviates many of the problems of pixel-based segmentation. Since it offers the possibility of encoding context information in its representation. Compared to individual pixels which face the scale problem of not covering the extent of an image feature, the objects represent pixel regions of certain properties such as shape, orientation, intensity statistics, and relations to other regions.

First formally defined Hay and Castilla [1], OBIA made its way to medical image analysis in applications such as the ones presented by Schwier et al. [2] based on the framework proposed by Homeyer et al. [3]. Aplin and Smith [4] present recent advances of object-based image classification. They mention that using edge detectors to initially identify image regions could improve the result. However, the current OBIA frameworks do not offer the possibility to combine region features with the border properties of a particular object and perform automatic classification.

We propose a supervised classification approach that operates on an object level and employs, besides region properties, features describing the strength and continuity of object boundaries. Our algorithm can identify salient boundaries which would otherwise be missed because of small discontinuities or leaks.

2 Classification based on boundary and object features

Given an image, we obtain an initial over-segmentation (Fig. 1(a)) using the watershed implementation by Hahn et al. [5] on the image gradient. Our goal is to merge regions that belong to the same structure while preserving salient borders.

For this we consider as boundary features the border strength (correspondence to a high gradient) and continuity (with respect to adjacent borders), as described in [6]. These allow us to distinguish between real and over-segmentation caused borders. We also define the border straightness as the ratio between the straight-line distance between its endpoints and its actual pixel length.

In our supervised classification approach, a user manually selects samples of borders that are to be merged and kept (Fig. 1(a)). These border samples and their features are used to train a Random Forest classifier. By applying this classifier to the rest of the borders (Fig. 1(b)), we merge the pairs of objects whose borders are not classified as actual object boundaries (Fig. 1(c)). Afterwards, we introduce intrinsic object features complement border features in a second Random Forest classification iteration. These describe the differences and ratios between size and intensity of neighboring objects. We obtain the classification and segmentation results (Fig. 1(d) and 1(e)).

3 Results

We obtained the boat object while conserving the boundaries for its internal structure (Fig. 2). In order to distinguish between foreground and background interactive watershed [5] requires numerous manually placed markers to reproduce a similar result (Fig. 1(f)).

Next, we applied our approach to medical images to axial CT scans showing the hip. We train our classifier on one slice in order to classify the entire stack of images. Fig. 2 shows the two iterations of our process on one slice and the result for a second slice, both showing meaningful results.

One limitation is that, our approach is sensitive to the choice of training samples. Choosing inappropriate samples leads to misclassification. However,

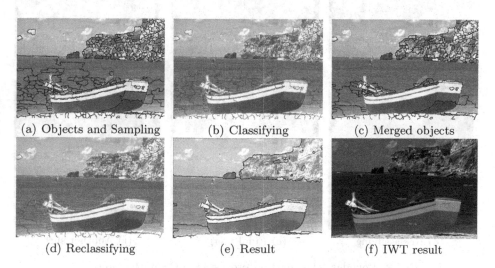

(a) Objects and Sampling   (b) Classifying   (c) Merged objects

(d) Reclassifying   (e) Result   (f) IWT result

Fig. 1. Boundary classification process on sample image.

we assume that the user has knowledge about the image content and makes suitable choices. Nevertheless, in the future, we plan to eliminate samples that represent outliers before classification. We also aim to provide the user with a visual connection between the boundaries and their feature space.

4   Conclusion

We have presented a supervised classification approach for image segmentation that combines region and boundary features. In an object-based image representation, one can use this approach to define merging criteria for pairs of neighboring objects to reconstruct larger, significant image structures, while preserving salient borders. We have tested this idea on regular shapes (artificial and anatomical) with promising results.

References

1. Hay G, Castilla G. Object-based image analysis: strengths, weaknesses, opportunities and threats (SWOT). Proc OBIA. 2006;36:4–5.
2. Schwier M, Chitiboi T, Hülnhagen T, et al. Automated spine and vertebrae detection in CT images using OBIA. Int J Numer Method Biomed Eng. 2013;29(9).

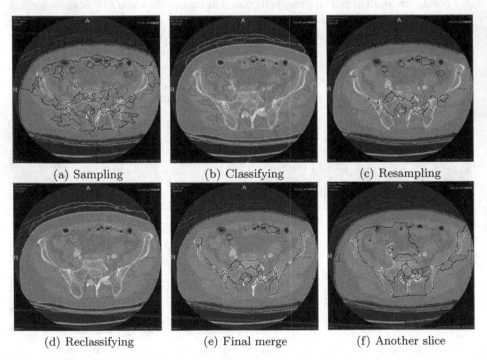

(a) Sampling   (b) Classifying   (c) Resampling

(d) Reclassifying   (e) Final merge   (f) Another slice

Fig. 2. Boundary classification process on a CT of the hip bones.

3. Homeyer A, Schwier M, Hahn H. A generic concept for OBIA. Proc VISAPP. 2010;2:530–3.
4. Aplin P, Smith G. Advances in object-based image classification. Proc ISPRS. 2008.
5. Hahn HK, Peitgen HO. IWT-interactive watershed transform. Proc SPIE. 2003;5032:643–53.
6. Chitiboi T, Homeyer A, Linsen L, et al. Object-based boundary properties. Proc BVM. 2013; p. 199–204.

Entwicklung und Vergleich von Selektionsstrategien zur atlasbasierten Segmentierung

Jonas Beuke[1], Andre Mastmeyer[1], Dirk Fortmeier[1,2], Heinz Handels[1]

[1]Institut für Medizinische Informatik, Universität zu Lübeck
[2]Graduate School for Computing in Medicine and Life Sciences, Universität zu Lübeck

beukej@miw.uni-luebeck.de

Kurzfassung. Um die Multi-Atlas-Segmentierung der Leber zu beschleunigen, wurde ein Ansatz zur Vorauswahl der ähnlichsten Bilder nach affiner Registrierung untersucht. Die Auswahl der Datensätze wurden mit den Metriken Mean Squares Mutual Information und Normalized Correlation vorgenommen. Die Qualität der Selektion wurde nach der nicht-linearen Registrierung und anschließender Label-Fusion mit dem Dice-Koeffizienten bewertet. Es ergab sich eine Reduktionsmöglichkeit der Anzahl der aufwändigen nicht-linearen Registrierung von 50% bis 70% bei gleichzeitiger Verbesserung der Segmentierungsqualität.

1 Einleitung

Diese Arbeit beschäftigt sich mit der effizienten Multi-Atlas-Segmentierung von Lebern für ein patientenindividuelles Virtual-Reality-Training der perkutanen transhepatisches Cholangiodrainage (PTCD). Die Segmentierung der Leber stellt ein wichtiges Objekt im benötigten Patientenmodell dar. Um die Segmentierungen weitestgehend automatisiert zu erstellen, wurde daher in dieser Arbeit die multi-atlas-basierte Segmentierung untersucht. Zur Beschleunigung des Verfahrens wurden drei Metriken zur Auswahl der am besten passenden Bilder nach der affinen Registrierung getestet, wodurch die Anzahl der zeitaufwändigen nicht-linearen Registrierungen reduziert werden soll. Ein ähnlicher Ansatz wurde von Wu et al. [1] bereits für MRT-Daten des Gehirns getestet. Es wird allerdings auch darauf hingewiesen, dass die verwendeten neun bzw. dreizehn Atlanten u.U. zu wenig sind und eine höhere Anzahl von Atlanten bessere Ergebnisse liefern könnte. Diese Lücke schließen Aljabar et al. [2] mit der Verwendung von 275 Datensätzen.

2 Material und Methoden

Als Atlanten, also bereits bekannte Segmentierungen anderer Bilder, wurden 59 CT-Bilder aus der radiologischen Abteilung des Universitätsklinikums Lübeck verwendet, welche von Radiologen manuell segmentiert wurden. Die Bilder enthalten den Bereich von knapp unterhalb des Herzens bis zum Beckenkamm. Die Patientenliege und eventuelle Kabel wurden entfernt [3]. Diese Atlanten werden bei der Multi-Atlas-Segmentierung genutzt, um aus bekannten Segmentierungen anderer Patienten die Segmentierung eines neuen, unsegmentierten Datensatzes zu schätzen. Dazu werden die Atlanten durch ein Registrierungsverfahren so verformt, dass sie dem neuen Bild ähnlich werden und dann durch ein Fusionsverfahren zusammengefasst. Die Registrierungen wurden mittels Methoden aus der institutseigenen Programmbibliothek durchgeführt [4]. Um die hier vorgestellte Methode der besten Atlanten zu evaluieren, wurde in einer Leave-One-Out-Kreuzvalidierung jeweils ein Atlas als Referenz ausgewählt und die restlichen 58 auf diesen registriert. Anschließend wurden die im ITK [1] implementierten Metriken Mean Squares, Mutual Information und Normalized Correlation zwischen den Bildern berechnet, um Rangordnungen der besten Bilder in der jeweiligen Metrik zu erstellen. Um die Ergebnisse zu verbessern, wurden vor der Metrikberechnung zunächst die Grauwertbilder maskiert, sodass nur noch die Leber Grauwerte verschieden von Null aufweist und die Metriken organspezifisch sind. In die Label-Fusion unter Anwendung der Vote Rule [5] gehen pro

---

[1] http://www.itk.org/

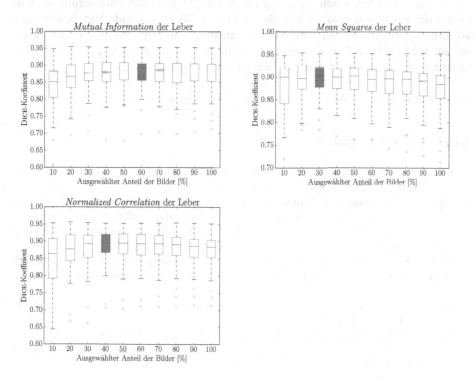

Abb. 1. DICE-Koeffizienten nach der Label-Fusion für die verschiedenen Metriken.

Experiment nur die besten 10% bis 100% in 10%-Schritten ein. Die Vote Rule ist ein einfaches Verfahren, bei dem per Mehrheitsentscheid die Segmentierungen voxelweise zusammengefasst werden. Sie wurde den komplexeren Verfahren wie bspw. dem SIMPLE-Algorithmus [6] vorgezogen, da nur der Effekt der Vorauswahl untersucht werden soll. Um zu überprüfen, inwieweit niedrige Prozentanteile ähnlich gute Endsegmentierungen liefern wie hohe Anteile, wurden die DICE-Koeffizienten zwischen den als Goldstandard angenommenen manuellen Segmentierungen und den fusionierten Segmentierungen berechnet.

3   Ergebnisse

Abb. 1 zeigt die DICE-Koeffizienten der Segmentierungen nach der Label-Fusion für die drei Metriken. Es konnte festgestellt werden, dass je nach Metrik die Auswahl von 30% bis 50% optimal ist, wobei Mean Squares die höchste Reduktionsmöglichkeit liefert.

4   Diskussion

Es reicht aus, wenige ausgewählte Atlanten zu verwenden und damit Rechenzeit zu sparen. Außerdem ergibt sich eine gleichzeitige Qualitätsverbesserung im Vergleich zur Verwendung von 100% der Atlanten. Weitergehende Untersuchungen könnten beispielsweise eine verbesserte automatische Extraktion der Körperbox in den Bildern betreffen, da externe Geräte u.ä. einen starken Einfluss auf die Qualität der nicht-linearen Registrierung haben.

Danksagung. Diese Arbeit wird von der DFG gefördert (DFG-HA 2355/10-1).

Literaturverzeichnis

1. Wu M, Rosano C, Lopez-Garcia P, et al. Optimum template selection for atlas-based segmentation. NeuroImage. 2007;34(4):1612–8.
2. Aljabar P, Heckemann R, Hammers A, et al. Classifier selection strategies for label fusion using large atlas databases. Proc MICCAI. 2007; p. 523–31.
3. Mastmeyer A, Fortmeier D, Maghsoudi E, et al. Patch-based label fusion using local confidence-measures and weak segmentations. Proc SPIE. 2013.
4. Murphy K, van Ginneken B, Reinhardt JM, et al. Evaluation of registration methods on thoracic CT: the EMPIRE10 challenge. IEEE Trans Med Imaging. 2011;30:1901–20.
5. Kittler J, Hatef M, Duin RPW, et al. On combining classifiers. IEEE Trans Pattern Anal Mach Intell. 1998;20(3):226–39.
6. Langerak TR, Van der Heide UA, Kotte ANTJ, et al. Label fusion in atlas-based segmentation using a selective and iterative method for performance level estimation (SIMPLE). IEEE Trans Med Imaging. 2010;29(12):2000–8.

Lokalisierung von Knochenmarkzellen für die automatisierte morphologische Analyse von Knochenmarkpräparaten

Sebastian Krappe[1], Katja Macijewski[2], Elisabeth Eismann[1], Tobias Ziegler[1],
Thomas Wittenberg[1], Torsten Haferlach[2], Christian Münzenmayer[1]

[1]Fraunhofer-Institut für Integrierte Schaltungen IIS, Erlangen
[2]MLL Münchner Leukämie Labor GmbH, München
sebastian.krappe@iis.fraunhofer.de

Kurzfassung. Die morphologische Analyse von Knochenmarkpräparaten ist bedeutend für die Leukämiediagnose. Bisher wird dabei das Auszählen und Klassifizieren der unterschiedlichen Knochenmarkzellen manuell unter dem Mikroskop durchgeführt und ist zeitaufwändig, z.T. subjektiv und mühsam. Aus diesem Grund wird eine Automatisierung der Analyse von Knochenmarkpräparaten angestrebt. Die automatische Lokalisierung der Zellen stellt dabei die Basis für die nachfolgenden Verarbeitungsschritte, d.h. für die Segmentierung und automatische Klassifikation, dar. Das entwickelte Verfahren löst diese Aufgabe durch zwei unterschiedliche Ansätze für Bilder mit einem niedrigen und einem hohen Zellanteil. Das vorgestellte Verfahren wird mit 400 Knochenmarkbildern aus 200 unterschiedlichen Präparaten evaluiert. Für diese Bilder ergibt sich für die Detektion eine durchschnittliche Sensitivität von 97% bei einer mittleren Falschdetektionsrate von 8%.

1 Einleitung

Zur Abklärung von Abweichungen im Differentialblutbild wird eine manuelle, zytologische Untersuchung des Knochenmarks unter dem Mikroskop benötigt. Die morphologische Auswertung wird des Weiteren zur Ursachenabklärung bei Blutarmut, zum Ausschluss eines Knochenmarkbefalls bei Lymphknotenvergrößerungen und bei Verdacht auf Leukämie durchgeführt. Diese mikroskopische Beurteilung bildet die Basis für die Erstellung einer Diagnose und ist Entscheidungshilfe für die weiterführende Diagnostik.

Durch steigende Kosten im Gesundheitswesen und den demographischen Wandel wird eine Zentralisierung und Automatisierung der zytologischen Knochenmarkuntersuchungen benötigt. Zur Unterstützung dieses Prozesses werden Verfahren und Systeme für die Analyse von Knochenmarkspräparaten entwickelt [1]. Diese Präparate werden mit einem automatisierten Mikroskopiesystem digitalisiert und auf einem Rechner analysiert. In den aufgenommenen Bilddaten werden Auswerteregionen bestimmt, in denen die die dort vorliegenden Zellen automatisch lokalisiert werden sollen.

Eine der großen Herausforderungen bei der automatischen Analyse von Knochenmarkpräparaten ist die enorme Probenvielfalt. Zum Einen existieren unterschiedliche Präparationstechniken, zum Anderen ist die Probenqualität abhängig von der Qualität des manuellen Ausstrichs. So können Zellen entweder vereinzelt oder in Zellclustern vorliegen. Ein automatisches Lokalisierungsverfahren soll zusätzlich auch mit der Vielzahl von mehr als einem Dutzend Klassen umgehen können, die für eine Analyse benötigt wird. Es lässt sich eine große Varianz der Zellbilder zwischen Zellen einer Klasse und eine hohe Ähnlichkeit der Zellbilder unterschiedlicher Klassen feststellen.

Bekannte Segmentierungsverfahren für Knochenmark [2, 3, 4] tendieren dazu, einzelne Zelle in mehrere Segmente zu zerlegen, was für eine automatische weitere Analyse nicht geeignet ist. Aus diesem Grund ist ein Verfahren zur automatischen, eindeutigen Bestimmung des Zellzentrums gewünscht, sodass sich solche Segmentierungsverfahren über die Position des Zellzentrums optimieren lassen. Somit können gefundene Segmente einer einzelnen Zelle zusammengefasst werden.

Für die anschließende weitere Aufteilung einer Zelle in Plasma- und Kernbestandteile, sowie für die automatische Klassifikation sollte eine Zelle nicht mehrfach detektiert bzw. in mehrere Segmente zerfallen, da die Charakterisierung über Eigenschaften der ganzen Zelle erfolgt. Jede Zelle soll nur einmal gezählt und automatisch klassifiziert werden, da ansonsten die prozentuale Verteilung der Zellen bei der automatischen Klassifikation nicht mit der Realität übereinstimmt und somit falsche Schlüsse gezogen werden könnten.

2   Material und Methoden

Für die Entwicklung und Evaluation des Lokalisierungsalgorithmus werden 400 Knochenmarkbilder verwendet, die aus 200 unterschiedlichen Knochenmarkpräparaten stammen. Die Bilder decken dabei ausschließlich von Experten ausgewählte Bereichen ab, die zur morphologischen Analyse geeignet sind. Durch diese Vielzahl an Präparaten sollen möglichst viele Zelltypen und Variationen in Bezug auf die Ausstrichqualität, auf den Hintergrund, auf Artefakte oder auf Verschmutzungen abgedeckt werden. Diese Aufnahmen wurden mit einer CCD-Kamera erfasst, die an einem Mikroskop der Firma Zeiss (Axio Imager Z2) angebracht ist. Die Auflösung der Bilder ist 2452×2056 Pixel und die Pixelgröße der Kamera beträgt $3{,}45\,\mu m \times 3.45\,\mu m$. Bei der Bildakquisition wurde ein $40\times$-Ölobjektiv (Zeiss Plan-Apochromat) mit einer numerischen Apertur von 1,4 benutzt. Zur Evaluation wurden auf den 400 Bildern 21393 Zellzentren manuell markiert, d.h. durchschnittlich etwa 53 Zellzentren pro Bild.

Für die Lokalisierung von Knochenmarkzellen in Mikroskopbildern wird zunächst der Anteil der Zellfläche pro Bild bestimmt. Je nach Vordergrundanteil wird ein Verfahren für wenig oder eine Methode für viel Vordergrund ausgewählt (Abb. 1). Hierfür wird das Farbbild – wie in [2] beschrieben – mit Hilfe eines gewichteten Quotienten der Farbkanäle Grün und Blau zunächst in ein Grauwertbild überführt. Über das Otsu-Verfahren [5] wird ein Binärbild erzeugt, aus dem der Vordergrundanteil über das Auszählen weißer und schwarzer Pixel berechnet wird (Abb. 1(d)). Der Schwellwert für die Auswahl der Methode wurde mit Hilfe der 400 Bilder empirisch bestimmt und liegt bei 0.09. Für die Lokalisierung von Zellen in Bildern mit geringem Zellinhalt genügen einfache, weniger rechenaufwändige Verfahren. Liegen Zellen in Bildern mit hohem Zellinhalt in Clustern vor, lassen sich einzelne Zellen durch fortgeschrittenere Methoden gut trennen.

2.1 Wenig Vordergrund

Bei einem geringem Anteil des Vordergrundes werden im erzeugten Binärbild (Abb. 1(d)) zunächst Löcher innerhalb weißer Zellbereiche durch morphologische Operationen aufgefüllt und durch binäres Öffnen und Schließen bearbeitet, wobei der Radius des Strukturelements 20 Pixel beträgt [6]. Einzelne weiße Regionen werden extrahiert, die dann als Masken für die nachfolgende Wasserscheidentransformation [7] dienen. Ausgangspunkt der Wasserscheidentransformation ist ein Gauß-gefiltertes Grauwertbild, das zuvor zur Schätzung des Vordergrundanteils berechnet wurde. Als potentielle Zellzentren werden geometrische Schwerpunkte der gefundenen Regionen benutzt, die eine Mindestgröße von 2500 Pixel überschreiten. Im folgenden Schritt werden diese möglichen Zellzentren wie folgt in eine Graphendarstellung umgewandelt. Zellzentren werden in Knoten überführt und zwischen zwei Knoten werden Kanten hinzugefügt, falls der Abstand eine maximale euklidische Distanz von 70 Pixel nicht überschreitet. In diesem Graph werden stark zusammenhängende Komponenten mit Hilfe des Algorithmus von Tarjan berechnet, der auf der Tiefensuche beruht [8]. Für Komponenten, die mehr als einen Knoten enthalten, werden vollständige Graphen bestimmt. Anschließend wird eine Überdeckung der Komponente mit einer möglichst kleinen Anzahl von ermittelten, vollständigen Graphen berechnet [8]. Jeder so bestimmte vollständige Graph kann als eine Zusammenfassung von mehreren benachbarten, potentiellen Zellzentren interpretiert werden (Abb. 2(a)). Bei der Schwellwertbildung zur Bestimmung des Vordergrundanteils ergeben sich bei in Clustern vorliegenden Zellen größere zusammenhängende Vordergrundbereiche, die nicht einzelnen Zellen entsprechen und somit durch nachfolgende Verarbei-

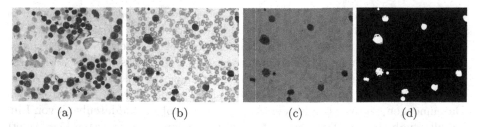

(a)   (b)   (c)   (d)

Abb. 1. Bestimmung des Vordergrundanteils: (a) Aufnahme mit viel Vordergrund (b) Aufnahme mit wenig Vordergrund (c) skalierter, gewichteter Quotient der Farbkanäle Grün und Blau (d) binarisiertes Bild nach Anwendung des Schwellwertverfahrens.

tungsschritte weiter aufgetrennt werden müssen. Bei hohem Vordergrundanteil wird wie in [2] zunächst eine Hintergrundkorrektur durch eine Approximation des Hintergrundes mit Hilfe eines 2D-Polynoms dritten Grades durchgeführt. Der Vordergrund wird über einen Mittelwertfilter variabler Größe geschätzt. Anschließend wird die Bestimmung des Vordergrunds über einen „Fast Marching"–Algorithmus [9] realisiert. Die dazugehörige Geschwindigkeitsfunktion verwendet die Distanz im Farbraum zwischen dem aktuell betrachteten und dem Pixel in der Vordergrundschätzung, sowie die Kantenstärke an der entsprechenden Stelle. Im nächsten Schritt wird zur Glättung ein Gauß-Filter auf das Ergebnisbild angewendet. Durch den sogenannten „Color Structure Code" [10] können homogene Regionen extrahiert werden, die zur Erzeugung eines geordneten Graphen benutzt werden. In diesem Graph lassen sich die Blätter als potentielle Zellzentren (Abb. 2(b)) identifizieren [2]. Ähnlich wie bei dem o.g. Fall mit wenig Vordergrund werden hier die potentiellen Zellzentren in einen Graphen überführt. Die Knoten von stark zusammenhängenden Komponenten werden dabei durch deren Schwerpunkt ersetzt.

2.2 Bewertungsmaße

Die Sensitivität pro Bild wird mit den beschriebenen Kennzahlen wie folgt berechnet: Sensitivität $= \mathrm{TP}/(\mathrm{TP} + \mathrm{FN})$. Für die Falschdetektionsrate pro Bild gilt: Falschdetektionsrate $= \mathrm{FP}/(\mathrm{FP} + \mathrm{TP})$.

3 Ergebnisse

Bei den 400 evaluierten Bildern ergibt sich eine durchschnittliche Sensitivität von 97% bei einer mittleren Falschdetektionsrate von 8%. Abb. 2(c) und Abb. 2(d) zeigen jeweils ein Beispiel für das Ergebnis bei wenig und bei viel Vordergrund. Die von Hand annotierten Zellzentren sind mit grünen Kreisen, die automatisch berechneten Zellzentren mit grünen Kreuzen visualisiert. In beiden Bildern wurden alle Zellen korrekt lokalisiert.

4 Diskussion

Das beschriebene Verfahren zur automatischen Bestimmung der Zellzentren in Knochenmarkbildern liefert sehr überzeugende Ergebnisse, sodass mehrere Einsatzzwecke möglich sind. Zum Einen lassen sich beispielsweise Segmentierungsverfahren für Knochenmarkzellen, wie sie etwa in [2, 3, 4] beschrieben sind, durch die gewonnene Information über die Lage des Zellkerns optimieren. Zum Anderen lassen sich durch die automatisierte Lokalisierung einzelne Zellen in großen Datenmengen, wie sie etwa für den Aufbau einer großen Bilddatenbank von Einzelzellaufnahmen von Nöten ist, extrahieren, die dann von Experten klassifiziert werden können. Des Weiteren kann ein solches Verfahren das Training und die Qualitätssicherung für die morphologische Analyse von Knochenmarkpräparaten unterstützen [11].

Die automatische Lokalisierung von Knochenmarkzellen liefert im Zuge der Entwicklung eines automatischen Analysesystems für Knochenmarkpräparate die Basis für die Segmentierung und die nachgeschalteten Verarbeitungsschritte zur Merkmalsextraktion und Klassifikation. Sie ist somit von großer Bedeutung und wird weiterentwickelt, um die Performanz der automatischen Analyse zu erhöhen. Das Ziel ist es, möglichst alle Zellen zu detektieren, wobei dabei eventuell auftretende, falsch-positive Zellzentren in der nachfolgenden Segmentierung und Klassifikation aussortiert werden könnten. Eine detaillierte Auswertung der Lokalisierungsleistung nach unterschiedlichen Kriterien (z.B. Zellklassenspezifische Sensitivität, Einfluss des Ausstrichtyps und der Probenqualität) ist geplant.

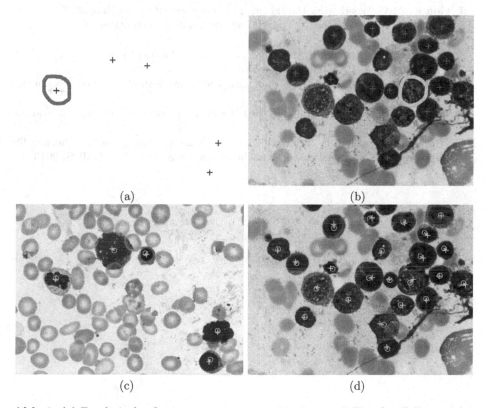

Abb. 2. (a) Ergebnis der Optimierung bei wenig Vordergrund. Einzelne Zellen werden durch ein blaues Kreuz dargestellt. Zellzentren, die durch die Optimierung zusammengefasst werden, sind türkis markiert. Die neue, optimierte Lage des Zellzentrums dieser Zellzentren ist in schwarz visualisiert. (b) Potentielle Saatpunkte bei viel Vordergrund vor der Optimierung. Grün markierte Zelle wird doppelt detektiert. (c) Evaluationsbild bei wenig Vordergrund: manuelle Annotation (grüne Kreise) und automatische Lokalisierung (grüne Kreuze). Die in (a) doppelt detektierte Zelle wird nun nur noch einmal detektiert. (d) Evaluationsbild bei viel Vordergrund: manuelle Annotation (grüne Kreise) und automatische Lokalisierung (grüne Kreuze). Die in (b) doppelt detektierte Zelle wird nun nur noch einmal detektiert.

Literaturverzeichnis

1. Krappe S, Haferlach T, Macijewski K, et al. Automated morphological analysis of bone marrow samples for leukemia diagnosis. Proc Forum Life Science. 2013.
2. Zerfass T, Haßlmeyer E, Schlarb T, et al. Segmentation of leukocyte cells in bone marrow smears. Comp Based Med Syst. 2010; p. 267–72.
3. Nilsson B, Heyden A. Model-based segmentation of leukocytes clusters. Proc Pattern Recognit. 2002;1:727–30.
4. Nilsson B, Heyden A. Segmentation of complex cell clusters in microscopic images: application to bone marrow samples. Cytometry A. 2005;66A(1):24–31.
5. Otsu N. A threshold selection method from gray-level histograms. IEEE Trans Syst Man Cybern. 1979;9(1):62–6.
6. Gonzalez RC, Woods RE. Digital Image Processing. Prentice Hall; 2007.
7. Roerdink JBTM, Meijster A. The watershed transform: definitions, algorithms and parallelization Strategies; 2000.
8. Cormen TH, Leiserson CE, Rivest RL, et al. Introduction to Algorithms. 2nd ed. Cambridge, MA, USA: MIT Press; 2001.
9. Sethian JA. Level Set Methods and Fast Marching Methods. 2nd ed. Cambridge University Press; 1999.
10. Priese L, Sturm P. Introduction to the color structure code and its implementation; 2003.
11. Krappe S, Efstathiou E, Haferlach T, et al. Training und Qualitätssicherung für die morphologische Analyse von Knochenmarkpräparaten. Proc GMDS. 2013.

Cell Segmentation and Cell Splitting Based on Gradient Flow Tracking in Microscopic Images

Julian Hennies, Jan-Philip Bergeest, Simon Eck, Karl Rohr, Stefan Wörz

Dept. Bioinformatics and Functional Genomics, Biomedical Computer Vision Group
University of Heidelberg, BIOQUANT, IPMB, and DKFZ Heidelberg
j.hennies@stud.uni-heidelberg.de

Abstract. We introduce a new approach for segmentation and splitting of cells in different types of microscopy images. Our approach is based on gradient flow tracking followed by local adaptive thresholding to extract nuclei and cells from the background. In comparison to previous flow tracking-based approaches, we introduce a new criterion for the detection of sinks, a new scheme for their combination, and filtering steps for more robust and accurate results. Experiments using different types of image data show that the approach yields good results for single and touching cells of different sizes, shapes, and textures. Based on quantitative results we found that that our approach outperforms previous approaches.

1 Introduction

Segmentation of cells in microscopy images is needed for interpretation of biological experiments. The gained information is important, for counting cells, for cell type analysis, or for cell tracking over time. Since high-throughput techniques generate a large amount of image data, automated image analysis methods are required to evaluate image data in a time-efficient and reproducible manner. However, image characteristics differ significantly depending on the applied microscopy technique and the cell type. In this work, we propose a new approach for accurate cell segmentation in different types of microscopy images. The approach needs to cope with touching cells and cells of different shape, intensity, and texture features as well as with high levels of image noise.

In previous work on cell segmentation, often methods based on thresholding Otsu's method [1] and the watershed transform [2] were used. However, disadvantages are a usually high rate of over- or undersegmentation, especially when cells are touching or overlapping. In addition, approaches using gradient-based flow tracking techniques have been proposed [3, 4, 5], which cope well with touching or overlapping cell nuclei. However, these methods are often only used and validated for cell nuclei segmentation [3, 4]. Additionally, when nuclei strongly differ in shape or show elongated elliptical shape, the risk of oversegmentation significantly increases [4], or a pre-segmentation step is needed, which increases the computational cost [5].

In this contribution, we introduce a new approach for segmentation and splitting of different cell types in microscopy images obtained by different techniques such as fluorescence or bright field microscopy. The approach is based on gradient flow tracking in conjunction with a local adaptive thresholding step. In contrast to [3], where the sinks of a gradient vector field are determined using a heuristic criterion, our approach introduces a new criterion which is based on a mathematically well founded definition of sinks. In addition to the distance between sinks, we use further criteria for the combination of sinks to avoid oversegmentation and to be able to segment cells that differ strongly in shape. Furthermore, in contrast to previous work [3], our approach enables to segment large cells with strong texture characteristics by including different measures and filtering steps for more robust and accurate results. We have successfully applied our approach to different types of image data, including synthetic images with different noise levels, Hoechst stained DNA images, images of fluorescence labeled Drosophila melanogaster cell nuclei, and Escherichia coli brightfield microscopy images. A quantitative experimental comparison showed that our new approach yields better results than approaches based on thresholding, the watershed transform, and a previous gradient flow tracking approach [3].

2   Materials and methods

In the following, we first describe the general segmentation scheme based on gradient flow tracking. Then, we present our new approaches for the determination and combination of sinks as well as for the elimination of undesired attraction basins which are caused by image artifacts. Finally, we describe the used filtering steps which include filters for noise reduction and morphological operations.

2.1   Segmentation based on gradient flow tracking

The idea of gradient flow tracking is based on the fact that the image gradient at the border of cells generally points towards the corresponding centers. By using gradient diffusion for smoothing the vector field, this directional information can be extended to the interior and exterior of the cells, which also reduces deviations of the gradient direction caused by image noise. Following the gradient direction for each pixel until a sink is reached yields a separation of an image into attraction basins, which contain in the ideal case a single cell and some background.

Our approach for segmentation and splitting of cells is based on four main steps [3]: i) gradient vector diffusion, ii) gradient flow tracking, iii) combination of sinks and attraction basins, and iv) extraction of the cell by local adaptive thresholding for each attraction basin. The used gradient vector diffusion is based on the Navier-Stokes equation, which describes the motion in fluids, and can be understood as a (feature-preserving) smoothing process of the gradient field [6]. The diffused gradient field $\mathbf{v}(x, y) = (u(x, y), v(x, y))$ is used for the gradient flow tracking step. For every pixel $\mathbf{x} = (x, y)$, trajectories are determined by following the gradient direction until a sink is reached, which is the case when the angle of two subsequent vectors is larger than $\frac{\pi}{2}$. All pixels which lead to the same sink are grouped as one attraction basin. If the Euclidean distance between two sinks is below a certain threshold T_{dis} (below two pixels), the sinks and their corresponding attraction basins are combined to form larger attraction basins. This prevents splitting of cells into several adjacent attraction basins, which would subsequently lead to oversegmentation. The local adaptive thresholding step is performed for each attraction basin individually to extract the cell from background. The threshold is determined by Otsu's method [1].

2.2 Determination and combination of sinks

In contrast to [3], where sinks are determined by the angle of subsequent positions in a trajectory, we determine sinks using the divergence $div(\mathbf{v})$ of the gradient field, which is computed as follows

$$div(\mathbf{v}(u,v)) = \frac{\partial u(x,y)}{\partial x} + \frac{\partial v(x,y)}{\partial y} \tag{1}$$

If the divergence is below a threshold T_{div} the according position is a sink.

In our case, the sinks are determined and combined before the flow tracking step, which is performed as backtracking by starting at the sinks. This avoids time consuming combination of attraction basins. To increase the rate of correctly combined sinks (to avoid over- and undersegmentation), an additional criterion based on the difference of intensity values is introduced to combine sinks: The connecting line $l(\mathbf{s}_1, \mathbf{s}_2)$ between two sinks $\mathbf{s}_1$ and $\mathbf{s}_2$ is determined and the intensity profile along this line is used to calculate a relative difference d_{rel} between the maximum and minimum intensity value

$$d_{rel} = \frac{\max(g(x,y) \,|\, (x,y) \in l(\mathbf{s}_1, \mathbf{s}_2)) - \min(g(x,y) \,|\, (x,y) \in l(\mathbf{s}_1, \mathbf{s}_2))}{\max(g(x,y) \,|\, (x,y) \in l(\mathbf{s}_1, \mathbf{s}_2))} \tag{2}$$

where $g(x,y)$ denotes the intensity value of the original image at the position (x,y). If d_{rel} is below a threshold T_{int} then the sinks are combined ($T_{int} = 0.25$). Note that the new criterion is only applied to sinks with a distance below T_{dis}. By using (2), we can use a much larger value of T_{dis} compared to [3] without increasing undersegmentation, while at the same time over segmentation caused by small values of T_{dis} is significantly reduced. Moreover, to eliminate attraction basins which do not contain a cell and which may be found during the previous steps, it has been proven effective to determine the variance of intensity values in each attraction basin and to eliminate those with low variance.

2.3 Filtering steps

To improve the results in the presence of image noise and image artifacts, we apply different image filters to the original image depending on the type of image data. To reduce texture features of cells without altering edge information we use a median or a tophat filter. In addition, we apply a Gaussian filter to reduce image noise. To improve the segmentation results, different morphological operations are applied to the labeled image. To correct pixels of background label within cells, morphological closing and hole filling is performed. Finally, we apply morphological opening to eliminate pixels which are not connected to the cell of the same label (found, close to cell borders in images with high noise level).

3 Results

We have applied our new approach to synthetic images as well as to different types of microscopy images. The results of our approach have been validated based on ground truth data and we have performed an experimental comparison to a previous approach based on gradient flow tracking [3] and to Otsu-based segmentation with subsequent cell splitting using a watershed algorithm.

3.1 Synthetic images

To evaluate the robustness of our approach with respect to image noise we used synthetic images. These images showed occasionally touching rod-shaped objects with different levels σ_n of additive Gaussian noise ($\sigma_n = 1, 2, 3, 5, 10, 20, 30, 50$). In total 100 objects were generated for each noise level. Our approach successfully segmented and split all objects for most noise levels ($\sigma_n \leq 20$). Only few cases of over- and undersegmentation were found in images with the highest noise levels ($\sigma_n = 30, 50$). For $\sigma_n = 30$, 98 % of the objects were segmented correctly (Fig. 3.1a and b) and for $\sigma_n = 50$ still 91 % of the objects could be segmented without over- and undersegmentations.

3.2 Drosophila melanogaster cell nuclei images

We have used D. melanogaster Kc167 fluorescence labeled cell nuclei images where ground truth data is available [7]. Note that these images are similar to the type of images which were used to validate the method in [3]. Using our approach, we achieved quite good segmentation results with over- and undersegmentation rates of 2.0 % and 1.8 %, respectively, and a mean Dice coefficient of

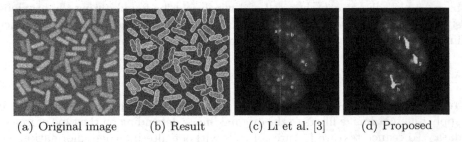

(a) Original image   (b) Result   (c) Li et al. [3]   (d) Proposed

Fig. 1. a) Synthetic image with additive Gaussian noise ($\sigma_n = 30$) and segmentation result by our approach (b). Determined sinks for NIH3T3 cells using the previous (c) and our approach (d).

Table 1. Segmentation results of a watershed-based approach, the previous approach [3], and our new approach on Drosophila and NIH3T3 cell nuclei images.

Experiment		Watershed	Li et al. [3]	Proposed method
Drosophila	Oversegmentation	2.9 %	2.9 %	2.0 %
$n = 400$ nuclei	Undersegmentation	3.1 %	2.4 %	1.8 %
	Dice coefficient	85 %	86 %	87 %
NIH3T3	Oversegmentation	(14.9 %)	—	2.7 % (1.4 %)
$n = 1667$ nuclei	Undersegmentation	(3.2 %)	—	2.6 % (0.4 %)
($n = 225$ nuclei)	Dice coefficient	(85 %)	—	93 % (94 %)

87 % (based on 400 nuclei, Tab. 1). In contrast, using the previous approach [3] over- and undersegmentation rates were 2.9 % and 2.4 %, respectively, the Dice coefficient was 86 %. The watershed-based approach led to over- and undersegmentation rates of 2.9 % and 3.1 %, respectively, with a Dice coefficient of 85 %.

3.3   Hoechst stained NIH3T3 cell nuclei images

We also used Hoechst stained NIH3T3 cell nuclei images (49 images with a total of 1667 cell nuclei [8]) which showed relatively large cell nuclei (average size of about 8000 pixels) which could not be segmented using the previous method [3]. The reason is that due to the size and the inhomogeneous texture of the cell nuclei, the sinks were distributed randomly and far apart from each other within each nucleus (Fig. 3.1c), leading to false splitting events of almost every nucleus. In contrast, our new approach determined groups of sinks which are more closely located to the center of a cell (Fig. 3.1d) and thus yielded good segmentation results for all 1667 nuclei with low rates of over- and undersegmentation (2.7 % and 2.6 %, respectively) as well as a high accuracy (Dice coefficient of 93 %; Tab. 1). For the watershed-based approach, due to inhomogeneous background in most images, only 225 nuclei in 8 of the 49 images could be segmented. For these 225 nuclei, the watershed-based approach yielded over- and undersegmentation rates of 14.9 % and 3.2 %, respectively, which is much worse compared to our approach (1.4% and 0.4 %).

3.4   Escherichia coli cell images

Moreover, we used E. coli brightfield microscopy images to demonstrate the capability of our approach to segment rod-shaped objects (Fig. 2). The watershed-based approach tended to over segment rod-shaped cells (Fig. 2b, red arrow) or showed inaccurate cell borders between touching cells (Fig. 2b, blue and green arrow). When using the previous approach [3], sinks are irregularly distributed along the cell. The distances between sinks of touching cells and the distances between sinks of a single cell often did not differ enough to sufficiently determine whether the sinks are to be combined or not, which often resulted in over-

Fig. 2. Segmentation results for E. coli brightfield microscopy image using watershed-based segmentation (b), the previous approach (c), and our new approach (d).

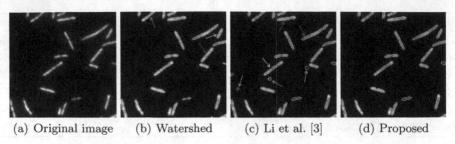

(a) Original image   (b) Watershed   (c) Li et al. [3]   (d) Proposed

(Fig. 2c, red arrows) or undersegmentation (Fig. 2c, yellow arrow). Artifacts were sometimes found in background regions (Fig. 2c, green arrows). Our proposed approach improved the segmentation result especially due to the additional criterion (2) to combine sinks (Fig. 2d). Additionally, all artifacts were eliminated by excluding attraction basins with small variance.

4   Discussion

We introduced a new approach for cell segmentation and splitting in various types of microscopy image data. Our approach is based on gradient flow tracking followed by local adaptive thresholding to extract nuclei and cells from the background. Experiments using, fluorescence microscopy images or Hoechst stained DNA images showed that the approach yields good results for single and touching cells of different sizes, shapes, and textures. Based on quantitative results we found that our approach outperforms previous approaches. In future, an extension of our approach to 3D image data is planned.

References

1. Otsu N. A threshold selection method from grey level histograms. Proc IEEE. 1979;9:62–6.
2. Vincent L, Soille P. Watersheds in digital spaces: an efficient algorithm based on immersion simulations. Proc IEEE. 1991;13:583–98.
3. Li G, Liu T, Tarokh A, et al. Segmentation of touching cell nuclei using gradient flow tracking. J Microsc. 2008;231:47–58.
4. De Vylder J, Philips W. Computational efficient segmentation of cell nuclei in 2D and 3D fluorescent micrographs. Proc SPIE. 2011;7902.
5. Surut Y, Phukpattaranont P. Overlapping nuclei segmentation using direction-based flow tracking. IEEJ Trans Elec Electron Eng. 2013; p. 387–94.
6. Davatzikos C, Prince JL, Bryan RN. Image registration based on boundary mapping. Proc IEEE. 1996;15:112–5.
7. Ljosa V, Sokolnicki KL, Carpenter AE. Annotated high-throughput microscopy image sets for validation. Nat Methods. 2012;9:637.
8. Coelho L, Shariff A, Murphy R. Nuclear segmentation in microscope cell images: a hand-segmented dataset and comparison of algorithms. Proc IEEE. 2009; p. 518–21.

An ImageJ Plugin for Whole Slide Imaging

Daniel Haak[1], Yusuf Z. Filmwala[1], Eric Heder[1], Stephan Jonas[1], Peter Boor[2],
Thomas M. Deserno[1]

[1]Department of Medical Informatics, Uniklinik RWTH Aachen
[2]Institute of Pathology, Uniklinik RWTH Aachen
dhaak@mi.rwth-aachen.de

Abstract. Whole slide imaging (WSI) has become important in medicine
and pathology, and challenges processing and management of high-resolution images with up to 10 GB of data. Open source tools such as ImageJ
do not sufficiently support high volume data and require manual interaction in otherwise automatic workflows. We present an open source
ImageJ plugin for automatic processing of Nanozoomer Digital Pathology Images (NDPI). In a batch-orientated workflow, the plugin provides
an image processing pipeline including data conversion, segmentation,
tiling, region of interest detection, thresholding, and quantification. The
plugin is exemplarily applied to quantitative analysis of renal histology
images. However, the general design supports other WSI file formats and
analysis tasks.

1 Introduction

Whole slide imaging (WSI) plays an increasingly important role in medical diagnostics, educations and research [1]. Particularly in pathology, WSI is used in
routine diagnostics and telemedicine. WSI yields high-resolution images of up
to 10 GB uncompressed data, scanning the entire glass slide. Since this volume
is exceeding common memory size of computers, specialized requirements have
to be met by WSI tools and formats. Hence, WSI is separately specified in standards such as Digital Imaging and Communications in Medicine (DICOM) [2],
which, however, are not sufficiently supported yet by the vendors.

Particularly for image processing in research, open sources tools such as the
Insight Segmentation and Registration Toolkit (ITK), the Visualization Toolkit
(VTK), the Medical Imaging Interaction Toolkit (MITK) [3], and ImageJ [4]
have been established. ITK and VTK provide methods for image processing and
visualization, respectively, and MITK combines their functionality for image-
based medical interaction. However, all f these tools do not aim at WSI-analysis
and corresponding WSI-formats stay unsupported. Although – in particular for
digital pathology – various macros and plugins are provided [5], ImageJ still
lacks in seamless handling of WSI. Researchers and physicians have to manually
crop snapshots, iteratively perform analysis on each part separately, and then
join the results, which is time-consuming and error-prone.

In this work, we present an open source plugin for ImageJ providing an
automatic analysis pipeline for WSI. Our workflow follows the basic idea of

indeed performing analysis on large images but outsourcing processing steps to lower-resoluted images, if possible.

2   Material and methods

We demonstrate our plugin by quantifying Nanozoomer Digital Pathology Images (NDPI) to quantitatively assess the scarring tissue (fibrosis) of mice kidneys.

2.1   Application domain

Assessment of fibrosis in mice kidneys requires the quantification of immuno-histochemical stained WSI. This is done by pixel counting of stained areas in renal tissue (Fig. 1). Here, the slide is stained for collagen type 3, a typical extracellular matrix protein deposited in exaggerated manner in kidney fibrosis. The extent of this deposition correlates with the extent of fibrosis and thereby with the extent of kidney injury and loss of kidney function. For automatization of this method, an WSI processing pipeline consisting of conversion, tissue segmentation, tiling, region of interest (ROI) and threshold setting, analysis and joining of results is provided.

2.2   NDPI format

WSI are acquired with specialized scanners for high-resolution recordings. The vendors provide proprietary file formats. For example, the NanoZoomer 2.0-HT (Hamamatsu Corporation, Japan)[1] acquires data in the pyramidal NDPI format. Specifications are unknown to the public, but an excerpted view has been published by the OpenSlide project[2]. An NDPI file consists of a single Tagged Image File Format (TIFF) files with customized tags, including a pyramid of Joint Picture Expert Group (JPEG)-compressed TIFF-files. The various magnification levels are stored as a multi-plane image stack forming a so-called pyramid. A viewer is provided, which is limited for data processing or analysis only supporting navigation and zooming through the image.

---

[1] http://www.hamamatsu.com/
[2] http://openslide.org/

Fig. 1. Histological WSI of renal tissue after coloration of starring tissue area.

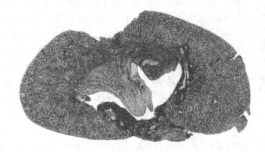

Table 1. Resolutions and data volume sizes and of a typical NDPI file.

Magnification	Resolution (in pixels)	Compressed (in MB)	Uncompressed (in MB)
×40	77.824 × 44.032	676,10	9.574,22
×10	19.456 × 11.008	44,30	627,45
×2.5	4.864 × 2.752	2,50	39,21
×0.625	1.216 × 688	0,17	2,45
×0.15625	304 × 172	0,01	0,15

In our application, the dimension of the highest resolution in the pyramid is 77.824 × 44.032 pixels, resulting in a data volume of approximately 670 MB and 9.5 GB in compressed JPEG and TIFF formats, respectively (Tab. 1).

2.3 Conversion

A couple of tools for handling of WSI file formats, such as NDPI, are offered by the open source community [6]. Bio-Formats[3] of the Open Microscopy Environment consortium is a Java library, which supports up to 127 scientific image formats and their conversion to common formats, such as TIFF or JPG. Using Bio-Formats, the NDPI file is converted into multiple TIFF files, each file containing the data of one NDPI magnification level.

2.4 Tissue segmentation

Usually, tissue regions are relevant for analysis. Hence, the highest-resoluted image is segmented into tissue and background areas. Several tissue segments can be processed consecutively. Nevertheless, the segmentation boundaries are calculated on a lower-resoluted image and upscaled, since the highest resolution may exceed the free memory. This is done with ImageJ segmentation and masking functionality. The desired tissue boundary is extracted using likelihood features, which have been trained on a series of WSI. Then, the upscaled ROI boundaries of tissue areas (t-ROIs) are stored.

2.5 Tiling

Due to their large volume, tissue segmentation and further processing steps cannot be performed directly on the highest-resolution images. Hence, the images have to be tiled, which means building a physical tessellation of the original image on the hard disk, which allows reading it in parts instead of entirely. For this, the free memory space of the Java Virtual Machine (JVM) is determined and a maximum image size calculated. Using this information, valuable tiles are created and stored on the file system. Meanwhile, a Java object is created, which holds references of the tiled parts, tile sizes and (x, y)-coordinates

---

[3] http://www.openmicroscopy.org/site/support/bio-formats4/

of tile placements. This information allows interpretation of tiles as one whole image. Among others, the Java Advanced Imaging (JAI) application programming interface (API)[4] contains methods for tiling of images and processing of tiles. During tiling, the t-ROIs are considered and irrelevant background area is directly removed.

2.6 Input parameters

Usually, specific tissue ROIs need analysis rather than the entire area. Hence, tools for ROI selection are provided. The ImageJ ROI Manager[5] provides extensive methods for user-interactive ROI drawing. Considering that according to tissue segmentation ROIs have to be defined on lower-resolution images and upscaled, the ImageJ ROI Manager has been modified with the user-selected ROI referred to as s-ROI.

Beside a ROI, a threshold is required for each image. Based on the gray scale, the threshold defines the pixels which have to be counted during analysis. The optimal threshold depends on specific image characteristics, which is visualized to the user by colorizing pixels in a lower resolution using ImageJ Threshold[6] (Fig. 1).

2.7 Quantitative analysis and batch processing

For analysis, the entire image information is needed. Thus, analysis is performed on the highest resolution. Due to limited memory capacity, this image may have been tiled and tiles are processed sequentially. Recorded tile size and the (x, y)-coordinates support whole image assessment, representing the complete ROI. If the s-ROI has been set, a final ROI of each tile is computed, which is then processed with ImageJ standard methods.

Automated batch processing is provided by an image queue. Since batch processing in ImageJ is only supported by macro scripting, and in addition a fixed workflow with user-interaction is needed here at all, an graphical user interface (GUI) has been developed, which visualizes progress information and analysis results. For each tile or each tile-specific ROI, the ratio between the number of pixels with a gray value above the threshold and all ROI pixels is calculated, and the average ratio of all tiles is determined.

3   Results

The resulting workflow is composed of interactive and automatic modules (Fig. 2). The user adds multiple NDPI files to the batch. Conversion, tissue segmentation, and – depending on the free memory – tiling is performed. The tissue segments

---

[4] http://tinyurl.com/nevbveo

[5] http://tinyurl.com/ldveabw

[6] http://tinyurl.com/kwhof2m

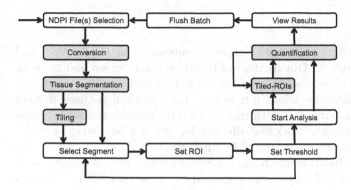

Fig. 2. Workflow of the proposed ImageJ plugin. White and gray boxes denote user interaction and automatic modules, respectively.

and associated NDPI file names are listed to the user, who can select individual segments and sets ROIs and thresholds repeatedly for any number of images in the batch. As soon as one image of the batch is ready for processing, the user starts automatic analysis of all images in the queue. The required parameters are provided automatically. Considering tiling, quantification is done on each tile and the ratio of stained area for all tiles is visualized. At any time, the user is allowed to flush the batch and to remove images and results.

Figure 3 shows the NDPI pyramid including the highest and second-highest magnifications levels, which are – after conversion – used by our ImageJ plugin for user-interaction and quantitatively analysis, respectively. The microscopy slide contains two tissue segments (t-ROIs), each including one s-ROI, which has been set by the user. For analysis, the s-ROIs are upscaled and projected on the highest-resolution image, resulting in a final ROI for all affected tiles.

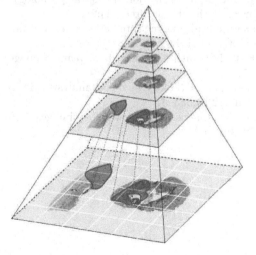

Fig. 3. NDPI pyramid with five magnification levels and user-selected s-ROIs on two tissue segments.

4 Discussion

In this paper, we presented an ImageJ plugin for automatic analysis of WSI and applied it to renal histology. Our method is based on a conversion and tiling of WSI in NDPI format and processing in ImageJ standard components. Compared to the physician's manual workflow, our automatized method is time-effective and less error-prone, in particular with respect to inter-individual observer variability. The batch-orientated workflow allows selection of input parameters for multiple tissue segments before starting the analysis.

Since the included Bio-Formats library supports conversion of various WSI file formats, also formats of other scanners, such as Leica LAS AF LIF, should be processable. However, tissue segmentation is currently optimized for renal histology data, but should be applicable on other tissue types, such as liver, by training of specific likelihood features. Furthermore, various analysis algorithm can be integrated. However, analysis is performed on each tile individually, which limits analyzing methods.

In future, our plugin should be extended by further integration of analysis algorithms for automatic cell and point counting on histological WSI. Support of DICOM's WSI standard will be integrated, too. The pyramidal structure (Fig. 3) is similar that of the DICOM Supplement 145, which will simplify DICOM compliance.

References

1. Daniel C, Rojo MG, Klossa J, et al. Standardizing the use of whole slide images in digital pathology. Comput Med Imaging Graph. 2011;35(7):496–505.
2. Singh R, Chubb L, Pantanowitz L, et al. Standardization in digital pathology: supplement 145 of the DICOM standards. Pathol Inf J. 2011;2(1):23.
3. Nolden M, Zelzer S, Seitel A, et al. The medical imaging interaction toolkit: challenges and advances. Int J Comput Assist Radiol Surg. 2013;8(4):607–20.
4. Schneider CA, Rasband WS, Eliceiri KW. NIH image to ImageJ: 25 years of image analysis. Nat Methods. 2012;9(7):671–5.
5. Rangan GK, Tesch GH. Quantification of renal pathology by image analysis (Methods in Renal Research). Nephrology. 2007;12(6):553–8.
6. Deroulers C, Ameisen D, Badoual M, et al. Analyzing huge pathology images with open source software. Diagn Pathol. 2013;8(1):92.

Kategorisierung der Beiträge

Bildverbesserung und -darstellung, 13, 36, 42, 54, 78, 84, 90, 96, 102, 126, 174, 204, 210, 240, 276, 318

Merkmalsextraktion und Segmentierung, 7, 13, 19, 30, 60, 66, 108, 114, 132, 138, 144, 150, 156, 162, 192, 198, 204, 210, 216, 228, 234, 258, 264, 288, 336, 354, 366, 372, 378, 384, 390, 396, 400, 409

Objekterkennung und Szenenanalyse, 13, 19, 24, 66, 108, 120, 132, 138, 162, 186, 288, 306, 312, 324, 330, 336, 348, 384, 403

Quantifizierung von Bildinhalten, 13, 19, 30, 42, 108, 180, 192, 204, 234, 246, 264, 415

Multimodale Aufbereitung, 54, 90, 180, 294, 306, 360

Art des Projektes

Grundlagenforschung, 24, 60, 168, 234, 246, 270, 312, 348, 354, 396

Methodenentwicklung, 13, 24, 30, 36, 42, 48, 54, 60, 66, 84, 90, 96, 102, 108, 114, 120, 126, 138, 144, 150, 156, 162, 168, 186, 192, 204, 210, 216, 222, 234, 240, 246, 252, 258, 264, 282, 300, 324, 330, 336, 342, 348, 354, 366, 378, 384, 390, 400, 403, 409, 415

Anwendungsentwicklung, 42, 66, 72, 78, 108, 114, 120, 132, 162, 168, 180, 186, 204, 246, 270, 276, 318, 342, 360, 372, 384, 400, 409

Klinische Diagnostik, 13, 19, 48, 114, 174, 204, 210, 234, 246, 252, 276, 306, 318

Autorenverzeichnis

Stichwortverzeichnis